Percutaneous Venous Blood Sampling in Endocrine Diseases

Renan Uflacker   Reingard Sörensen
Editors

Percutaneous Venous Blood Sampling in Endocrine Diseases

With 122 Illustrations

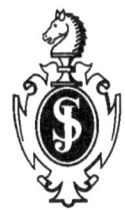

Springer Science+Business Media, LLC

Renan Uflacker
Vascular and Interventional Radiology
Med-Imagem
Hospital Beneficiencia Portuguesa
Rua Maestro Cardim 769
Sao Paulo, SP 01323, Brazil

Reingard Sörensen
Cardiovascular and Interventional Radiology
Klinikum Steglitz
Freie Universität Berlin
Abteilung Röntgendiagnostik
Hindenburgdamn 30
D-1000 Berlin 45, Germany

Library of Congress Cataloging-in-Publication Data
Percutaneous venous blood sampling in endocrine diseases / editors,
    Renan Uflacker and Reingard Sörensen.
        p. cm.
    Includes bibliographical references and index.
    ISBN 978-1-4612-7688-3   ISBN 978-1-4612-2830-1 (eBook)
    DOI 10.1007/978-1-4612-2830-1

    1. Endocrine glands—Diseases—Diagnosis. 2. Hormones—Analysis.
3. Hormones—Sampling. 4. Veins—Puncture. I. Uflacker, Renan.
II. Sörensen, Reingard.
    [DNLM: 1. Endocrine Diseases—blood. WK 100 P429]
    RC648.P43 1992
    616.4—dc20
    DNLM/DLC
    for Library of Congress   91-5156

Printed on acid-free paper.

Production managed by Karen Phillips; Manufacturing supervised by Jacqui Ashri.
Typeset by Asco Trade Typesetting Ltd., Hong Kong.

9 8 7 6 5 4 3 2 1

Preface

This book discusses contemporary features of diagnosis of endocrine diseases using the radiologic technique of percutaneous venous blood sampling for hormone assay. A comprehensive survey of the field is provided by the contributing authors, who have considerable expertise in the subject. Some have published several articles in the literature; others have extensive clinical experience.

The approach to many of the endocrine diseases has been markedly improved during the last two decades because of selective venous blood sampling, not only in the diagnosis of the condition but especially in the precise localization of the hormone-producing lesion and its clinical significance.

Scattered information on venous blood sampling is available in the literature, but there is no comprehensive text dealing with the subject, creating, therefore, a lacuna the could be filled by this project.

This book is intended to be a practical guide for vascular and interventional radiologists, internists, surgeons, endocrinologists, and other physicians who care for patients with endocrine diseases. The intention is to provide a practical text covering anatomical data, clinical problems related to the diagnosis of the endocrine diseases, patient preparation for the sampling, blood sampling techniques, sample manipulation and storage, laboratory data, and clinical significance of the hormone sampling and assay.

Renan Uflacker
Reingard Sörensen

Contents

Contributors

Claudio E. Kater, M.D.
Associate Professor of Medicine
Director, The Adrenal and
    Hypertension Unit
Division of Endocrinology
Department of Medicine
Escola Paulista de Medicina
P.O. Box 20.266
04034, São Paulo, SP, Brazil

Lothar Moltz, M.D
Professor of Obstetrics and Gynecology
Institute of Gynecological Endocrinology,
    Fertility, and Family Planning
Knesebeckstr 35
1000 Berlin 12, Germany

Hans H. Schild, M.D.
Professor of Radiology
Department of Radiology
Johannes-Gutenberg-University
    Medical School
Langenbeckstrasse 1
6500 Mainz 1 Germany

Reingard Sörensen, M.D.
Cardiovascular and Interventional Radiology
Klinikum Steglitz, Freie Universität Berlin
Hindenburgdamn 30
D-1000 Berlin 45 Germany

Thomas A. Sos, M.D.
Professor of Radiology
Cornell Medical School–New York Hospital
Division of Cardiovascular Radiology
525 East 68th Street
New York, NY 10021
U.S.A.

T.R. Strack, M.D.
Department of Endocrinology
Johannes-Gutenberg-University
    Medical School
Langenbeckstrasse 1
6500 Mainz 1 Germany

Renan Uflacker, M.D.
Head of Vascular and
    Interventional Radiology
Med-Imagem
Hospital Beneficencia Portuguesa
Rua Maestro Cardim 769
São Paulo, SP, 01323
Brazil

Jose Gilberto H. Vieira, M.D
Associate Professor of Medicine
Chief, Laboratory of Hormones
Division of Endocrinology
Department of Medicine
Escola Paulista de Medicina
P.O. Box 20.266
04034 São Paulo, SP, Brazil

Selective Venous Sampling for the Differential Diagnosis of Female Hyperandrogenemia

—— *Lothar Moltz and Reingard Sörensen* ——

Introduction

Hyperandrogenism is one of the most common female endocrinopathies. It may be due to (a) glandular causes (ovarian and/or adrenal hypersecretion of androgenic steroids), (b) extraglandular causes (increased peripheral conversion of preandrogens, decreased specific plasma androgen binding, target organ hypersensitivity, or administration of androgenic drugs; or (c) a combination of these factors. Extremely high elevated peripheral androgen levels are suggestive of an androgen-producing tumor of the ovaries or the adrenals.

Numerous methods have been used to determine the origin of the excess androgen production, because none of the circulating androgens has an exclusive gonadal or adrenal source. Plasma concentrations reflect the sum of entry into the circulation from glandular secretions and extraglandular tissue production, as well as their hepatic and extrahepatic clearance. The estimation of secretion rates is complicated by the complexities of ovarian and adrenal steroidogenesis (episodic, diurnal, cyclic, and age-related variations; 1). Dynamic function tests also cannot reliably discriminate between steroids of ovarian and adrenal origin due to nonspecific pharmacodynamic effects (2). In contrast to common belief, estrogen-suppressible ovarian and glucocorticoid-suppressible adrenal neoplasms as well as adrenocorticotropic hormone (ACTH)-responsive ovarian and human chorionic gonadotropin (HCG)-responsive adrenal tumors, have been described (3). Even with the improved resolution of computed tomography and ultrasound, the detection of ovarian and adrenal tumors remains difficult if their sizes are smaller than the sizes of the organs (4,5). In adults, real-time ultrasound equipment and specific high-frequency transducers are able to demonstrate the right adrenal gland in 95% of patients; however, the left side can only be seen in 71% (6,7).

Other radiographic procedures such as retrograde venography fail to demonstrate ovarian tumors and cause a stress-induced uncontrolled output of adrenal steroids. Moreover, gross morphology and functional pathology do not necessarily correlate (3,8). Therefore, negative results on ultrasound and computed tomography do not exclude the presence of tumorous hyperandrogenism. Selective catherization techniques are known to be reliable methods to study direct glandular secretion (9,10). This combined radiologic-endocrinological procedure involves retrograde transfemoral sampling of both ovarian and adrenal veins to determine their androgen content. Demonstration of the gradients between glandular effluent levels and peripheral concentrations establishes the amount of secretion.

Steroid gradients serve as semiquantitative

estimates; they reflect hormone output more closely when compared with the absolute effluent levels (8,11). Yet this approach is also associated with difficulties and potentially significant errors: the inability to calculate secretion rates without determination of actual glandular blood flow during the procedure; the lack of knowledge of intraglandular androgen metabolism; the influence of premedication, stress, and application of contrast media on the secretion of hormones, and the uncertainty of problems related to correct identification of catheter placement during sampling procedures. This could result in an admixture of peripheral blood with the effluent of the secreting organ (12). Nevertheless, the method of catheterization and venous sampling provides useful information on ovarian and adrenal nontumorous or tumorous androgen secretion.

Diagnostic Procedures

Clinical Features

The clinical history should provide information on

1. the beginning, duration, and progress of sign of hyperandrogenism;
2. race, family history, growth, and weight;
3. thelarche, pubarche, menarche, and menopause;
4. partus, abortion, basal temperature measurements, and previous surgery;
5. methods and frequency of hair removal, and amount of daily hair loss;
6. irregularities of the menstrual cycle, amenorrhea, sterility, medication, and therapeutic trials;
7. accompanying diseases of thyroid, liver, kidneys, neurological disorders, and anorexia.

The most important clinical data are summarized in Table 1.1. Nontumorous (NTM) patients (group II) are divided into three subgroups—IIa: NTM patients without clinical signs of polycystic ovaries (PCO), $n = 17$, IIb: NTM patients with laparoscopically confirmed PCO ($n = 33, 37$), and IIc: NTM patients with histologically proven hyperthecosis (HYP, $n = 10, 40$). All patients have either elevated

testosterone (T) and/or dehydroepiandrosterone sulfate (DHEA-S) levels. Except for the normal volunteers (N, $n = 8$, group I), all patients underwent laparoscopy prior to catheterization to rule out macroscopically visible ovarian neoplasm. These studies include also patients with histologically proven ovarian A_{mors} (TM, $n = 7$, group III). Hormonal drugs had not been taken by any of the women during the 6 months preceding catheterization.

Physical Examination

The physical examination provides information on the type, localization, distribution, and the grade of hyperandrogenism; the symptoms of virilism; and various other stigmata, such as habitus, weight, height, striae, struma, preliminary pubes, and distribution of fat.

The gynecological examination evaluates the external and internal genital parts (clitoris, ovaries), the quality of the cervical mucus, and the cytology of the vagina.

Laboratory Tests

Hormone Status

Plasma testosterone (T) and dehydroepiandrosterone sulfate (DHEA-S) are the most important hormones in the workup of patients with hyperandrogenemia: T is the indicator of ovarian and adrenal androgen secretion; DHEA-S is almost exclusively the product of the zona reticularis of the adrenal gland. No androgen-producing tumors without elevation of plasma T and DHEA-S have been described so far (7). The laboratory tests for determination of the plasma hormone content should be done according to a standardized protocol in order to reduce the influence of cyclic, circadian, and episodic variations of steroid secretion (Table 1.2).

Long-Term Dexamethasone Suppression Test

Dexamethasone (DXM) should be given in relation to body weight 1 to 2.5 mg for 2 weeks. DXM is known to suppress adrenal androgen secretion and is used to differentiate adrenal

Table 1.1. Clinical findings and peripheral androgen levels in 75 women who underwent selective catheterization for progredient hirsutism.

	I N = 8	IIa NTM = 17	IIb NTM + PCO = 33	IIc NTM + HYP = 10	III TM = 7
Age (years)	21–40	16–33	18–52	14–67	26–65
Height (cm)	157–168	134–174	148–173	153–173	157–168
Weight (kg)	47–62	44–79	43–90	45–104	57–85
Menstrual status[a]	regular, biphasic	4 × A/3 × O/10 × E	11 × A/9 × O/13 × E	1 × PM/4 × A/2 × O/2 × E	4 × PM/3 × A
Hirsutism	no	12	30	10	7
Alopecia	no	5	16	5	7
Virilism[b]	no	1	0	4	7
Pelvic examinations (enlarged ovaries)	normal	0	7	3	1
Laparoscopic findings (evidence for PCO)	–	0	33	7	3
Precatheterization peripheral T (ng/ml)	0.20–0.47	0.24–1.78	0.38–1.88	1.2–2.51	1.51–8.67
Precatheterization peripheral DHEA-S (ng/ml)	1,100–2,630	1,810–15,660[c]	1,100–8,650	400–5,300	600–2,640

N, healthy volunteers; NTM, nontumorous; TM, tumorous; PCO, polycystic ovaries; HYP, hyperthecosis.
[a] PM, postmenopausal; A, amenorrheic; O, oligomenorrheic; E, eumenorrheic.
[b] Including deepening of voice, male body habitus, clitoromegaly, baldness.

Table 1.2. Standardized protocol for ovarian and adrenal vein sampling.

Discontinuation of hormone therapy 6 weeks before catheterization
No premedication
Within the early follicular phase (days 3–7) except oligoamenorrheic patients
Between 8 and 10 A.M.
Three serial blood samples at 5 to 10 minutes intervals of all four vessels in a randomized fashion

and ovarian hyperandrogenemia. If androgen levels are examined before and after DXM suppression the origin of androgen excess can be localized. Adrenals are adequately suppressed if cortisol (compound F) is less than 40 ng/ml and DHEA-S is less than 400 ng/ml. The problem is that the DXM long-term suppression test is not reliable, according to the results of studies in the literature. DXM not only suppresses adrenal androgens but ovarian androgen biosythesis as well (see Clinical Result, below).

Noninvasive Imaging

Ultrasound, computed tomography (CT), scintigraphy, and venography are able to visualize adrenal tumors up to 1 cm and ovarian tumors up to 3 cm in diameter. These methods (except ultrasonography) have the disadvantage of radiation exposure to the gonads. This is expected to be especially high in adrenal scintigraphy (Table 1.3). Magnetic resonance imaging (MRI) still has limited significance compared with CT due to the problem of respiratory motion and the difficulties in obtaining

Table 1.3. Diagnostic methods for localization of androgen-producing tumors.

Method	Spacial resolution (diameter in cm)		Radiation exposure (rem)	
	Ovaries	Adrenals	Ovaries	Adrenals
Laparoscopy	>1.0	–	–	–
Ultrasound	>3.0	>1.0	–	–
CT	>3.0	>1.0	2.5	0.5
Scintigraphy	–	>1.0	65	34
Venography	<1.0	<1.0	0.8	0.8

From ref. 7.

appropriate pulse sequences (13). Randomized studies comparing CT and MRI in the region of adrenal or ovarian tumors are not yet available. There is evidence that MRI is able to distinguish metastatic/malignant disease and nonmalignant tumors of the adrenal glands; however, there has been no mention of the limit of the size of the lesions detectable.

Indications

For medical management of the patients, it is necessary to differentiate between normal, nontumorous, and tumorous hyperandrogenism. Hyperandrogenemia without tumor is usually due to increased hormone production by the ovaries and/or the adrenal glands. Only in rare instances is it caused by androgen-producing tumors. Multiple methods have been tried to locate the source of excess androgen production, however, most of these techniques proved not to be reliable. Selective catheterization is at the present time the most sensitive method for preoperative identification of an androgen-secreting neoplasm. Catheterization procedures should be performed if the patient's peripheral plasma T levels are greater than 1.5 ng/ml, plasma DHEA-S levels are greater than 7,000 ng/ml, and if other imaging modalities have failed to locate the lesion (these values apply only if normal plasma levels of T-assay method are less than 0.5 ng/ml).

Anatomy and Anatomical Variations

Knowledge of the anatomy of the ovarian and adrenal veins and their variations is essential for the correct placement of the catheter (Fig. 1.1). Anatomical studies on complete venographic examinations demonstrate the vascular collaterals and anastomoses (12,14).

Left Adrenal Vein

Usually the left adrenal vein drains into the left renal vein (Fig. 1.2). The purity of the effluent hormone is expected to be influenced by multi-

Figure 1.1. Anatomical variations and anomalies of adrenal and ovarian veins in women.

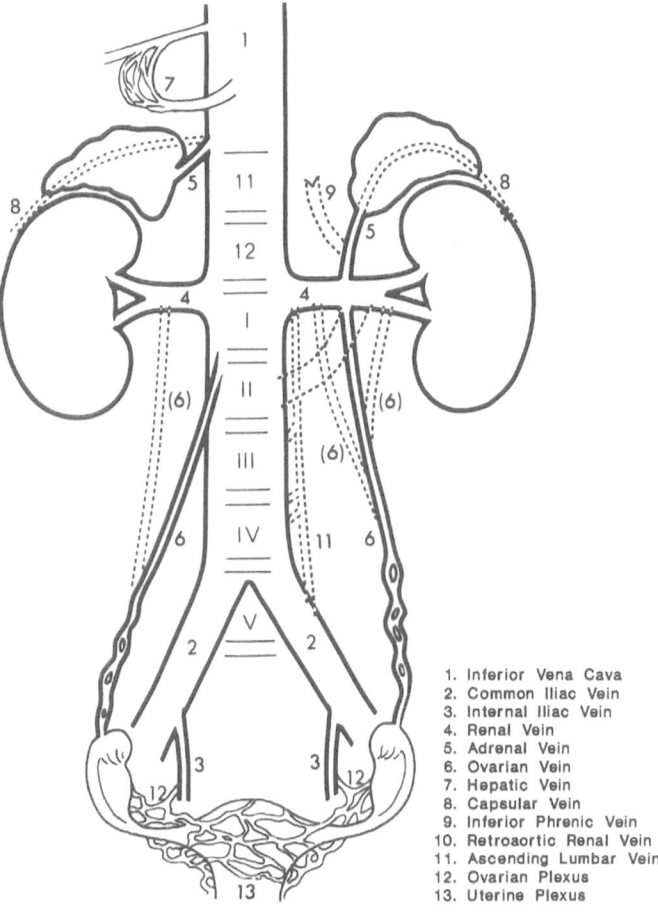

1. Inferior Vena Cava
2. Common Iliac Vein
3. Internal Iliac Vein
4. Renal Vein
5. Adrenal Vein
6. Ovarian Vein
7. Hepatic Vein
8. Capsular Vein
9. Inferior Phrenic Vein
10. Retroaortic Renal Vein
11. Ascending Lumbar Vein
12. Ovarian Plexus
13. Uterine Plexus

ple inflowing veins: the inferior phrenic vein (74%), renal capsular veins (60%), small communicating veins of the renal vein (35%), ureteral veins (19%), veins of the epidural and paravertebral plexus (17%), and anastomoses of the ovarian vein (2%; Fig. 1.3). Duplication of the left adrenal vein is rare.

The inferior phrenic vein joins the left adrenal vein. Selective sampling of only the inferior phrenic vein, however, leads to erroneous hormone concentration measurements (Fig. 1.4).

Right Adrenal Vein

The right adrenal vein is smaller and thinner than the left. The vein drains into the inferior vena cava approximately 2 to 3 cm above and posterolateral to the right *renal* vein (Fig. 1.5). Its direct drainage into the inferior vena cava

creates more difficulties in finding the orifice during catheterization procedures, due to its proximity to the right hepatic vein. Small hepatic veins are often very difficult to differentiate from right adrenal veins. Lecky et al. (15) has published a table that characterizes signs that differentiate the right adrenal and small hepatic veins (Table 1.4; Fig. 1.6). Anastomoses are found to originate from capsular veins of the kidney (45%), from the epidural and intervertebral plexus (26%), from connections with the renal vein (23%), from hepatic veins (8%), from the inferior phrenic veins (6%), and from ureteral veins (2.1%; 12,14; Fig. 1.7).

Left Ovarian Vein

Just opposite the left adrenal vein, the left ovarian vein empties into the left renal vein (Fig. 1.8). Opacification of the vein can be difficult

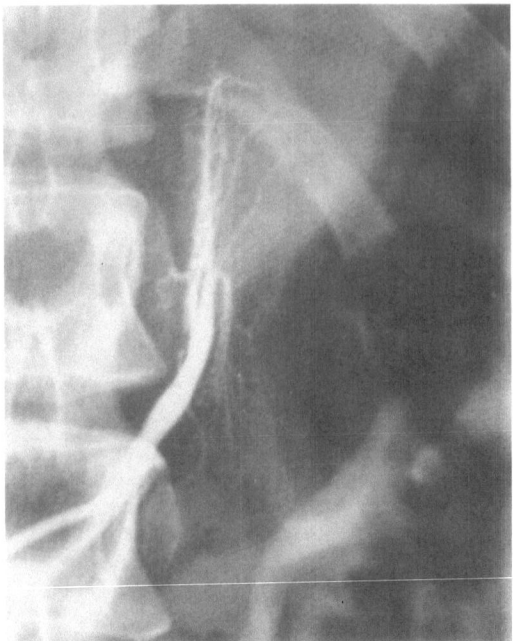

Figure 1.2. Normal left adrenal vein.

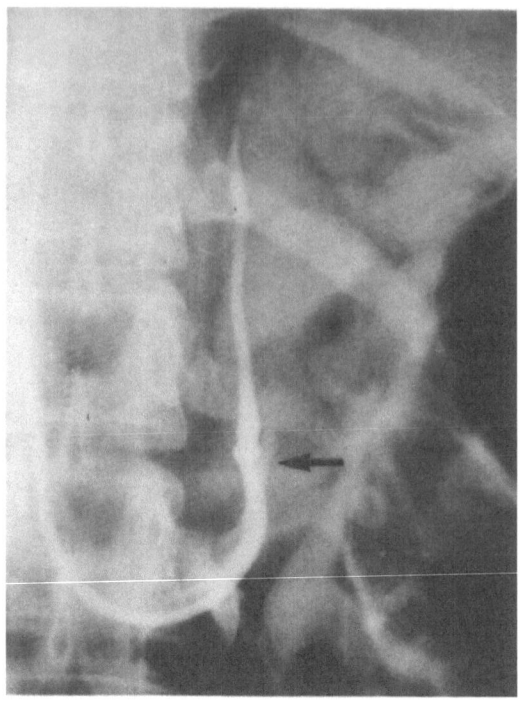

Figure 1.4. Selective catheterization of the inferior phrenic vein. The arrow demonstrates the origin of the left adrenal vein.

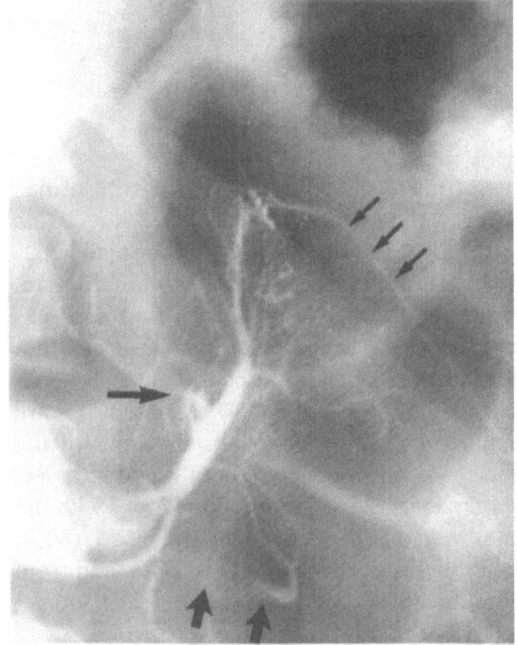

Figure 1.3. Veins that drain into the left adrenal vein. Inferior phrenic vein (arrow) with venous valve, renal vein (two arrows), capsular veins (three arrows).

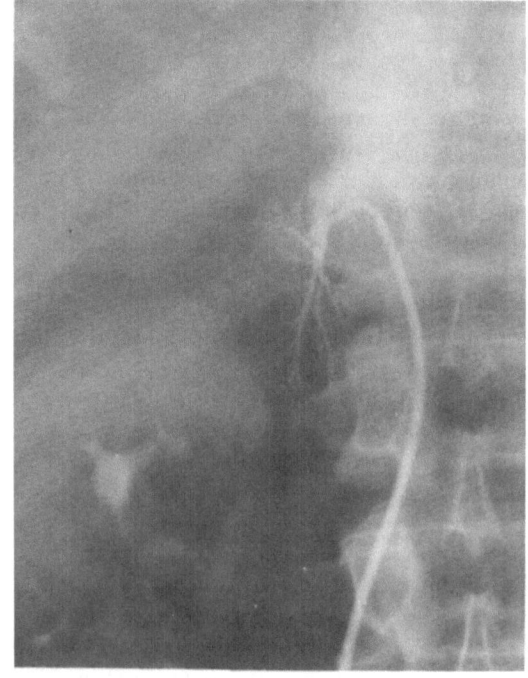

Figure 1.5. Normal right adrenal vein.

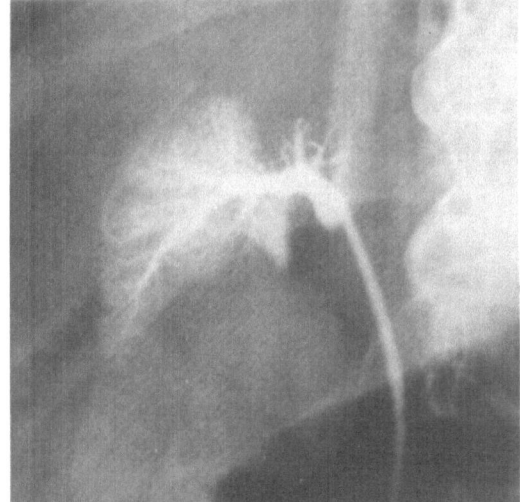

A

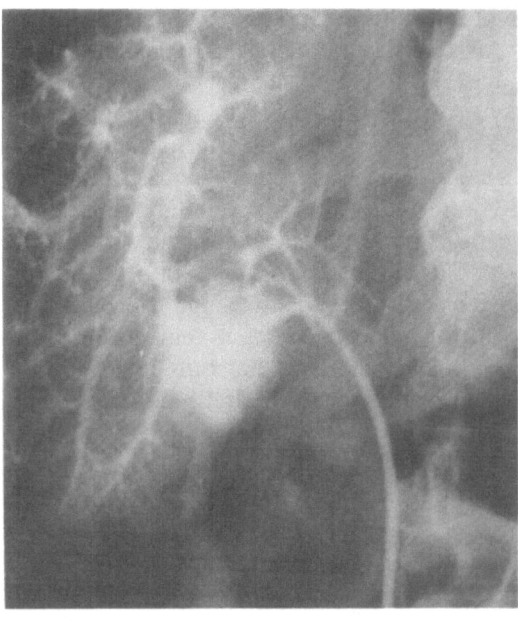

B

Figure 1.6. **A,B,C:** Right hepatic veins mimicking right adrenal veins.

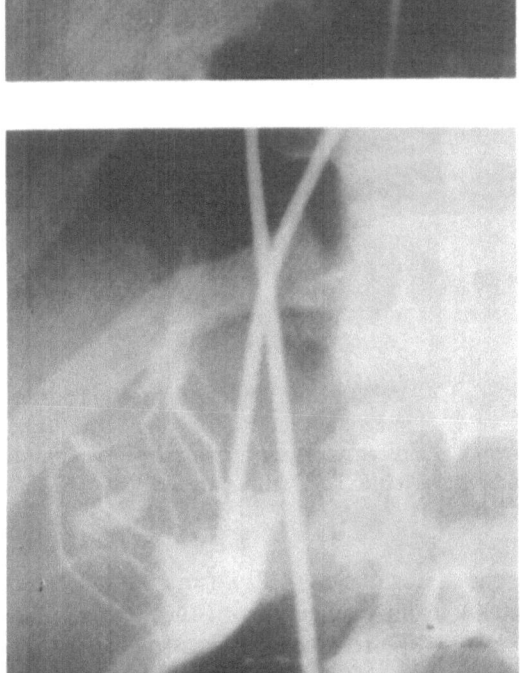

C

due to competent venous valves of the proximal ovarian vein. With the new catheter techniques these valves can be surpassed and samples can be collected. One can expect approximately 12 different connecting veins to contribute to the ovarian venous blood (12; Fig. 1.9). Contributions of veins of the epidural and paravertebral plexus (36%), the internal iliac vein (28%), multiple ovarian veins (28%), veins of the parietal abdominal wall (25%), the ascending lumbar veins (22%), small renal veins (18%), veins of the sacral plexus with connections to the opposite side (17%), ureteral veins (11%), renal capsular veins (8%), veins from the inferior mesenteric vein (3%), and the gluteal vein (3%) could be found giving admixture of blood samplings.

The ascending lumbar vein is described as

having a connecting branch to the renal vein in 9% of patients and could lead to incorrect samplings (Fig. 1.10A). The ascending lumbar vein may also empty into the distal portion of a double renal vein (Fig. 1.10B). Retroaortic venous rings should be identified by the injection of contrast media. This anomaly shows the preaortic portion wider than the retroaortic part. The adrenal vein drains into the upper portion and the ovarian vein into the preaortic or into the undivided renal vein prior to the hilus. If the renal vein has only a retroaortic portion, the adrenal vein drains either prehilar or directly into the inferior vena cava (Fig. 1.11). The most difficult variation to catheterize is a horseshoe kidney.

Right Ovarian Vein

The right ovarian vein drains directly into the inferior vena cava either at the entrance of the right renal vein or up to 5 cm below the renal vein (Fig. 1.12). Anastomoses and veins with contributory flow to the ovarian vein could be expected to originate from the uterine plexus

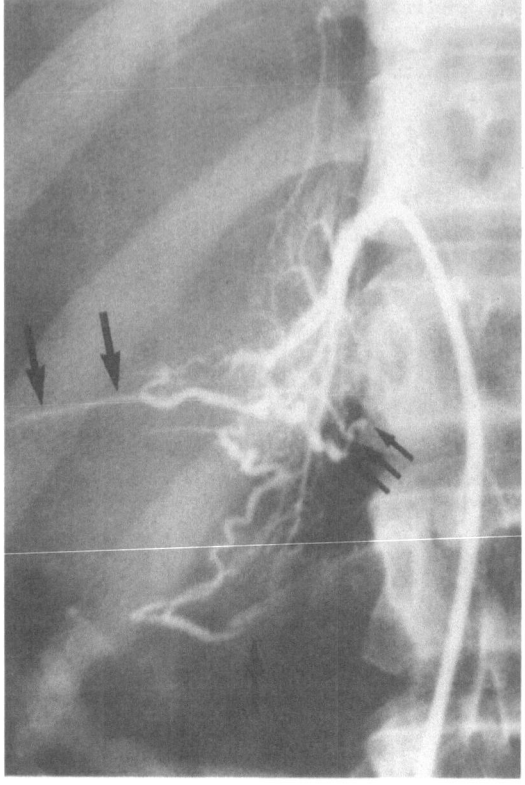

Figure 1.7. Venous contributions to the right adrenal vein: connecting vein to the renal vein (one arrow), renal capsular veins (two arrows), epidural and paravertebral veins (three arrows).

Table 1.4. Differentiation between right adrenal vein and hepatic veins.

	Right adrenal vein	Hepatic vein
Vena caval location of vein orifice	Posterior lateral or posterior	Lateral or anterior lateral
Angle of vein from inferior vena cava	Acute; sharply angulated	Less sharp, or straight
Contrast reflux into other hepatic veins	Rare	Common
Contour ends at visible liver edge	Never	Common
Suprarenal "capping" of kidney	Frequent	Rare
Persistent tissue "blush"	Rare, except extravasation	Common
Patient discomfort and pressure	Common	Very rare or never
Aspiration of blood	Difficult	Usually easy
Cortisol content related to IVC sample	Higher	Lower

Modified from ref. 15

of the opposite side (43%), from parietal veins (40%), from connections to the internal iliac vein (37%), from the peridural veins (34%), from the renal vein (29%), from the ascending lumbar vein (23%), from the ureteral veins (14%), and from renal capsular veins (6%). The ovarian vein drains into the renal vein in about 3 to 11% (Fig. 1.13).

Catheterization

Catheterization techniques should be performed following a standarized protocol (Table 1.2). The procedure can either be carried out on an outpatient basis or the patient could be admitted for 24 hours to guarantee closed post-catheterization monitoring. The patient should receive no premedication to avoid iatrogenic

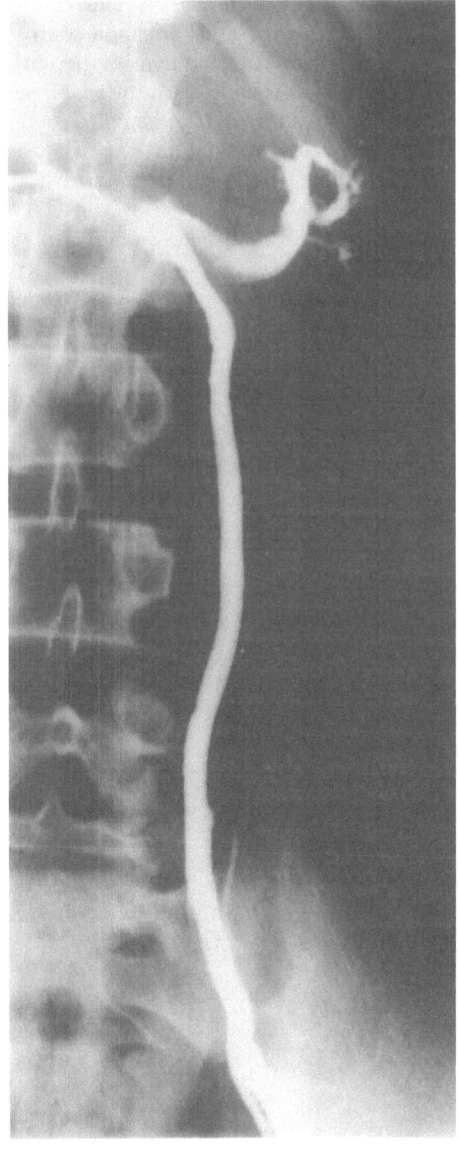

A

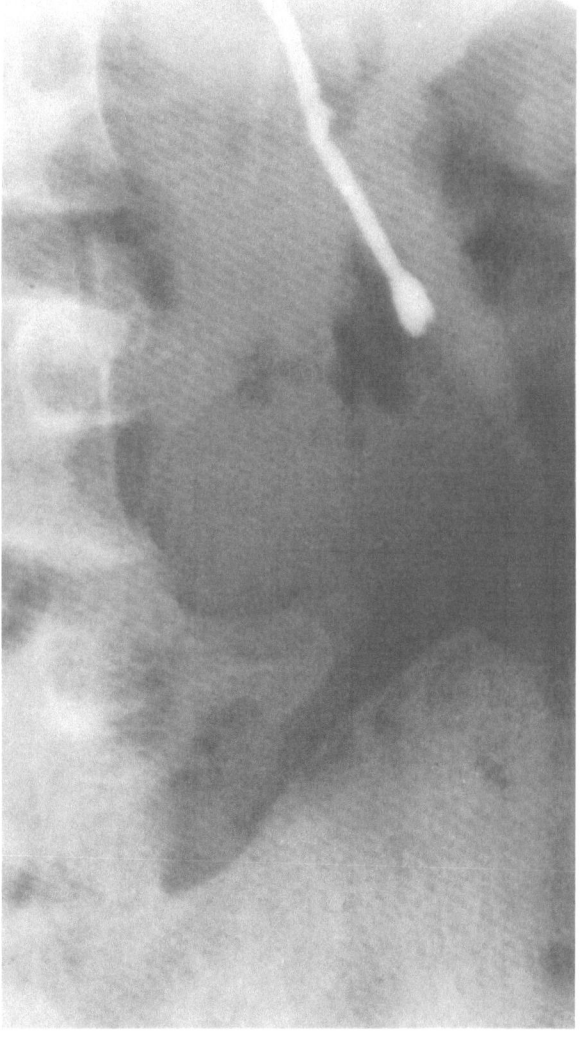

B

Figure 1.8. Left ovarian vein. **A**: Single left ovarian vein emptying into the left renal vein. **B**: Left ovarian vein with competent venous valve in the midportion. The valve prevents distal flow of contrast media; sampling, however, is possible.

secretion of adrenal steroids. The procedure takes place during the early follicular phase (days 3 to 7)—except in postmenopausal or amenorrheic individuals—between 8 and 10 A.M. to reduce interference from cyclic and circadian variations of androgen secretion.

A femorovisceral catheter (cobra-shaped, Sidewinder I and II, internal diameter 1.17 mm; one or two side holes 1 mm apart from the catheter tip, Fig. 1.14) is introduced percu-taneously under local anesthesia via the femoral approach (Seldinger). This catheter can be turned inside the inferior vena cava into six different shapes (Fig. 1.15; 12,14,15,16) to fit the different angled origins of both adrenal and ovarian veins. The high flow thin wall catheters are used now; we have found, however, that they have poorer torque control than the larger size catheters, especially if they are shaped within the venous system.

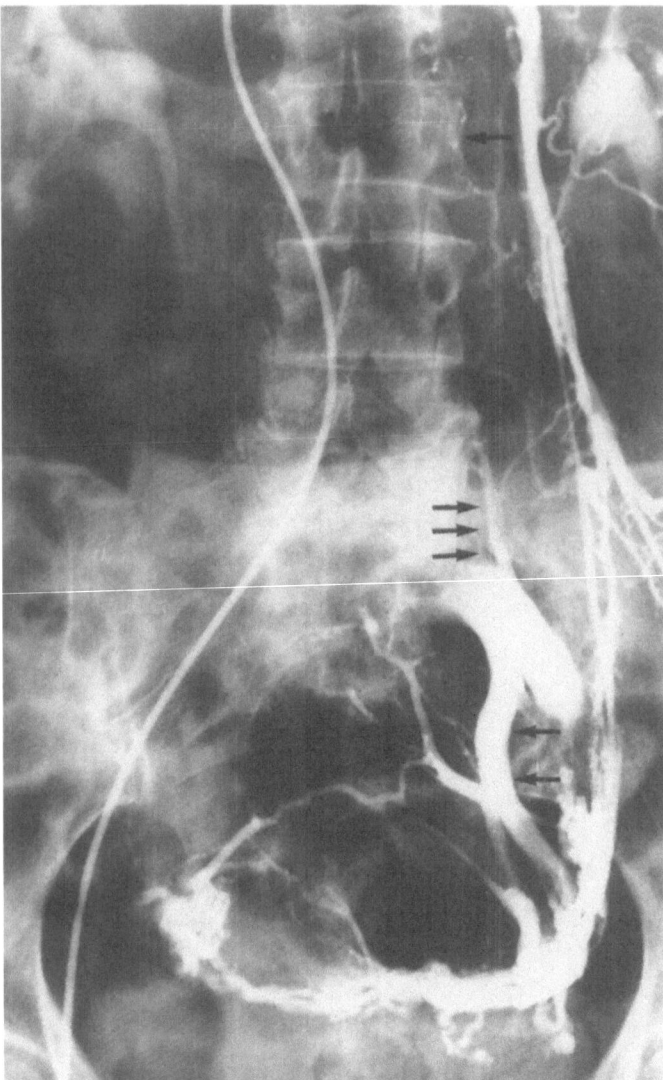

Figure 1.9. Left ovarian vein. Venography of the most common contributory and connecting veins: peridural plexus (one arrow), internal iliac vein (two arrows), and multiple ovarian veins (concomitant veins); ascending lumbar vein (three arrows).

The catheter tip is guided into the orifices of both adrenal and ovarian veins in random sequence. Three serial samples (8 to 10 ml) are obtained at 5- to 15-minute intervals for all four vessels to compensate for episodic variations in steroid secretions. After each sampling, fluoroscopic control during the injection of up to 0.5 ml of a nonionic contrast media is used to confirm the correct position of the catheter tip. This is routinely followed by flushing with saline solution after withdrawal of the catheter tip. Steroid levels determined in samples considered subselective by radiographic criteria should be disregarded. In androgenized patients, samples are drawn both before and 20 to 30 minutes after intravenous injection of 8 to 12 mg of dexamethasone. In addition, three peripheral blood samples are drawn either from an antecubital vein or from the iliac vein. Retrograde venography is not carried out because of complications accompanying this technique. Retrograde venography with the injection of 3 to 6 ml of contrast media has a definite effect on adrenal steroid release; 0.5 ml is well tolerated and does not affect hormone effluence (Fig. 1.16).

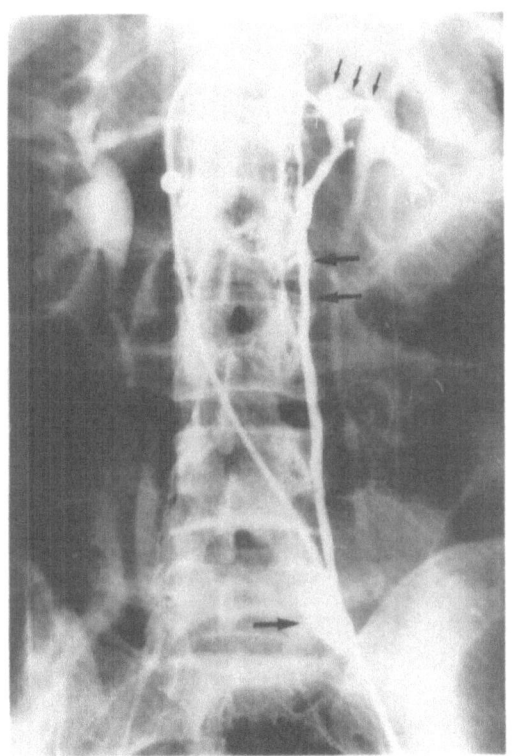 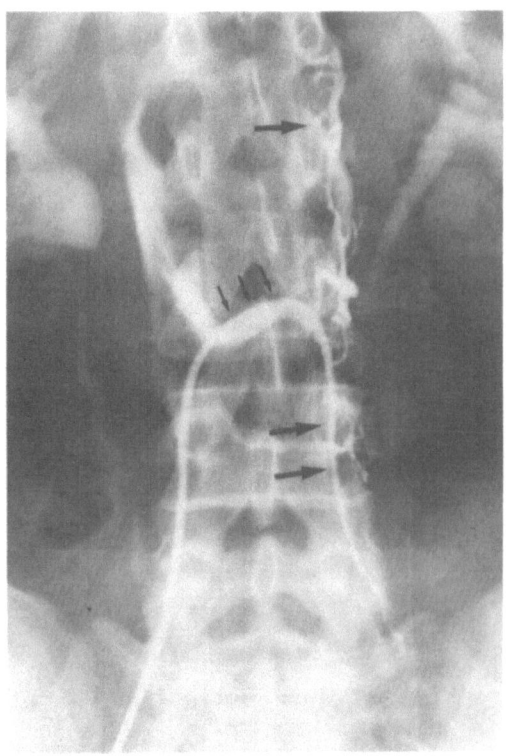

A   B

Figure 1.10. Ascending lumbar vein (two arrows). **A:** Connecting vein between the renal vein (three arrows) and the internal iliac vein (one arrow). This is not an ovarian vein! **B:** Inflowing ascending lumbar vein (two arrows) which empties into a small renal vein (three arrows). Paravertebral veins (one arrow).

Accuracy of Catheterization Technique and Blood Sampling

The following method-related data reflect our experience with a total of 75 catheterizations. Accurate placement of the catheter (selectivity) at the orifices of the adrenal and ovarian effluents was directly assessed by "fluoroscopy" ($n = 75$) and additional venography ($n = 67$). The left adrenal vein was most reliably entered (97.3%); the left ovarian vein was the vessel most difficult to catheterize (66.7%). Correct positioning in the right adrenal and ovarian vein was verified in 82.7% and 79.7%, respectively. One patient had had a right ovariectomy prior to the examination. Accurate placement of all four glandular effluents was achieved in 45% ($n = 34$); three of four and two of four veins were positively identified in 81% ($n = 61$) and 100% ($n = 75$) of our cases, respectively.

Steroid levels determined in subselective samples were disregarded in calculation of the three groups for accuracy of the catheterization techniques. They were, however, efficient enough to localize the tumor (Table 1.5).

Table 1.5. Accuracy of catheterization.

	NL ($n = 8$)	NTM ($n = 60$)	TM ($n = 7$)	Total ($n = 75$)
LOV	8	36	6	50 (66.7%)
ROV	7	47	5[a]	59 (78.7%)
LAV	8	58	7	73 (97.3%)
RAV	6	49	7	62 (82.7%)

NL, normal volunteers; NTM, nontumorous patients; TM, patients with tumors; LOV, left ovarian vein; ROV, right ovarian vein; LAV, left adrenal vein; RAV, right adrenal vein.
[a] Ovarectomy.

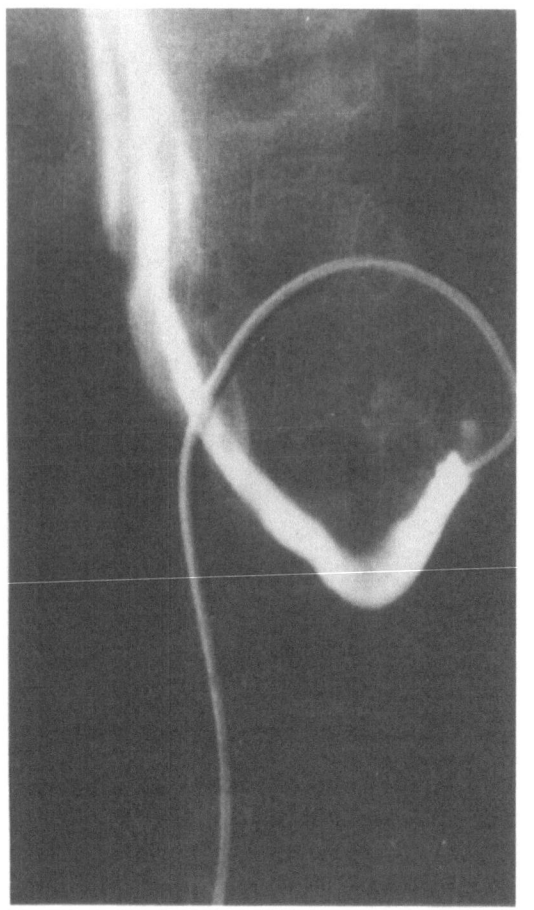 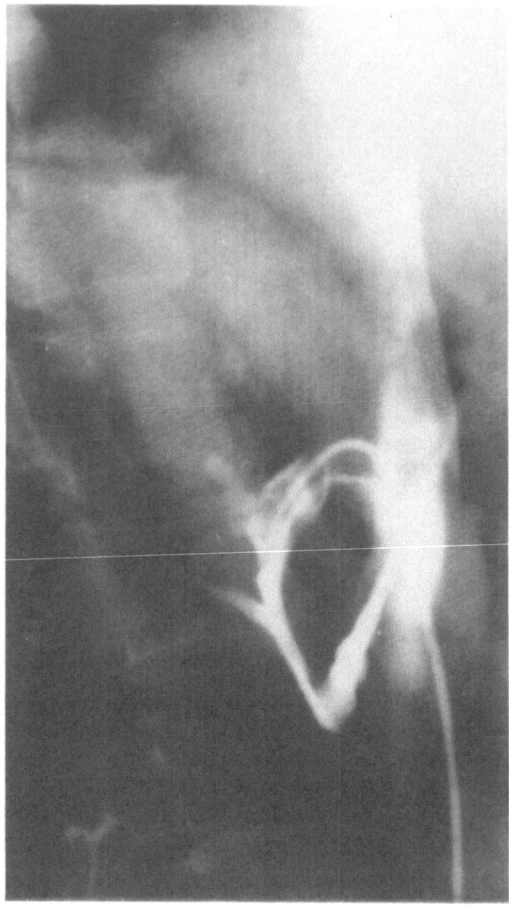

A   **B**

Figure 1.11. Circumaortic venous ring. **A**: Anterior-posterior projection. **B**: Lateral projection.

Influence of Contrast Media on Hormone Release

Retrograde injection of contrast media into adrenal veins induces changes of the adrenal secretory activity. This depends on the amount being injected (Fig. 1.16). While venography (3 to 6 ml) causes extremely high elevation of adrenal vein cortisol (compound F; 420 ± 194 ng/ml before and 2.310 ± 1.409 ng/ml after venography), less elevation is observed for testosterone (T; 0.95 ± 0.53 ng/ml before and 1.65 ± 0.55 ng/ml after venography) and dehydroepiandrosterone sulfate (DHEA-S; 1.850 ± 1.440 ng/ml before and 2.920 ± 1.810 ng/ml after venography). Injections of minute volumes of contrast material (less than 0.5 ml: "fluroscopic control") has no significant effect on adrenal androgen release (F = 380 ± 136 ng/ml before and 798 ± 349 ng/ml after fluoroscopy; T = 1.42 ± 1.21 ng/ml before and 1.37 ± 1.04 ng/ml after; DHEA-S = 2.140 ± 1.610 ng/ml before and 2.270 ± 1.530 ng/ml after fluoroscopy).

Side Effects and Complications of Catheterization

The nature and incidence of side effects are usually related to the contrast media injected into the glands. They are minor according to the literature (12,14,16,17). They include extravasation of contrast media into the adrenal parenchyma (Fig. 1.17), small hematomas at

Figure 1.12. Right ovarian vein and its contributions: uterine plexus with veins to the contralateral side (three arrows), parietal veins (two arrows), internal iliac vein (one arrow).

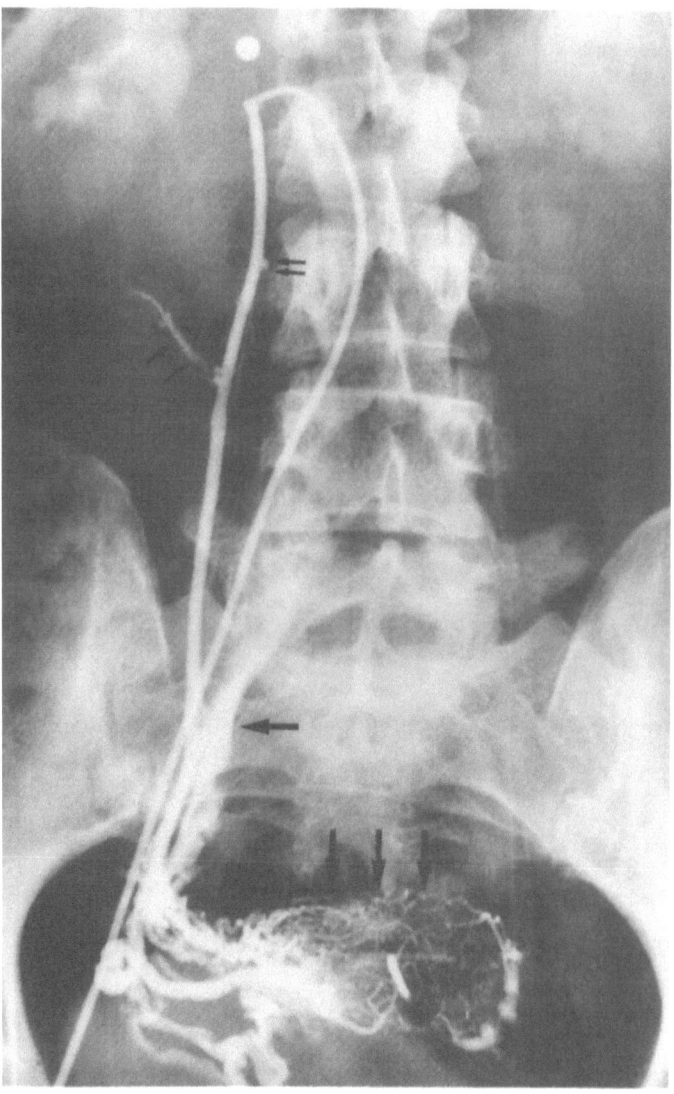

the puncture site, and allergic reactions. Serious complications are described (15,17); however, they appear to be rare. There were no major complications in our series. The length of the procedure in skilled hands is approximately 45 minutes on the average. The procedure usually causes minor discomfort.

Radiation exposure to the gonads has been measured employing an Alderson phantom (12). Twenty minutes of fluoroscopy resulted in a total radiation dose of 800 mrem at the level of the gonads; seven radiographic exposures were calculated to give an additional 1.5 mrem.

Endocrinologic Results

Stress Factor and Hormone Release During Sampling

Catheterization itself causes relatively little stress. Peripheral compound F during the procedure prior to venography (212 ± 111 ng/ml) is described to be not significantly different ($p > 0.05$) from a normal outpatient control group (140 ± 60 ng/ml). Likewise, peripheral F does not differ significantly according to the literature (12,18, (Fig. 1.18). This study was performed with an ionic contrast media (meg-

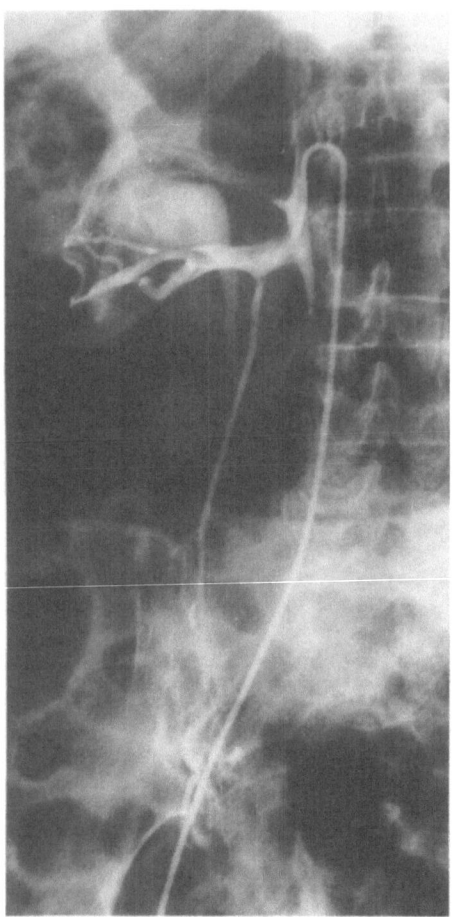

Figure 1.13. Right ovarian vein draining into the right renal vein.

lumine diatrizoate). At present, there has been no study performed after the introduction of the nonionic substances.

Hormone Analysis

The following serum steroids have been determined by direct radioimmunoassay (19): dehydroepiandrosterone sulfate (DHEA-S), 17-hydroxyprogesterone (17-OHP; commercial kit, Sorin Biomedica, Saluggia, Italy), and cortisol (F). Testosterone (T) and dihydro-T (DHT), androstenedione ($\triangle_4$-A), and dehydroepiandrosterone (DHEA) have been estimated by radioimmunoassay after celite chromatography. The reliability of T and F results was monitored by external quality control (WHO Matched Reagent Program).

Statistical Analysis

Steroid gradients, i.e., the difference between ovarian and adrenal and peripheral vein levels (OPG, APG), serve as semiquantitative estimates of the momentary secretory activity (11). Steroid concentration and gradients are given as means ± standard deviations (m ± SD). Wilcoxon's test for paired variants is used for statistical analysis of data obtained in a special group of patient (e.g. group I–III). The Mann-Whitney test for unpaired variants is applied for statistical comparison of results gathered between the different (sub)groups.

Clinical Results

Normal Women

In the past, interpretation of catheterization findings in hirsute patients was often speculative due to the absence of information regarding androgen gradients in healthy women with proven normal ovulatory cycles. The wide range of individual T and DHEA-S concentrations evaluated in peripheral veins as well as in the four glandular effluents is depicted in Fig.

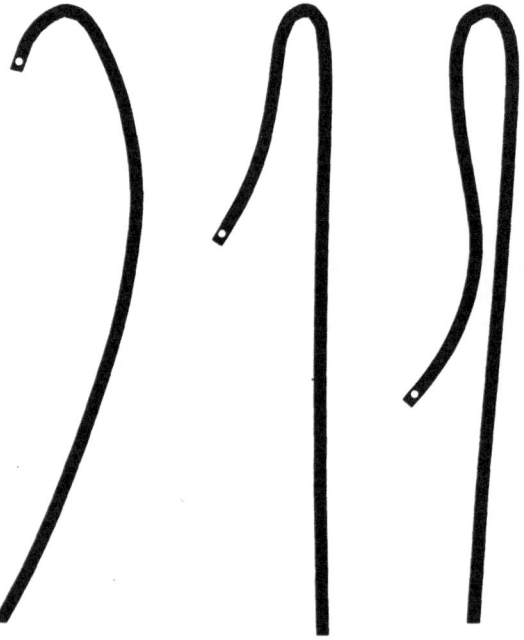

Figure 1.14. Angiographic catheters for sampling of adrenal and ovarian veins.

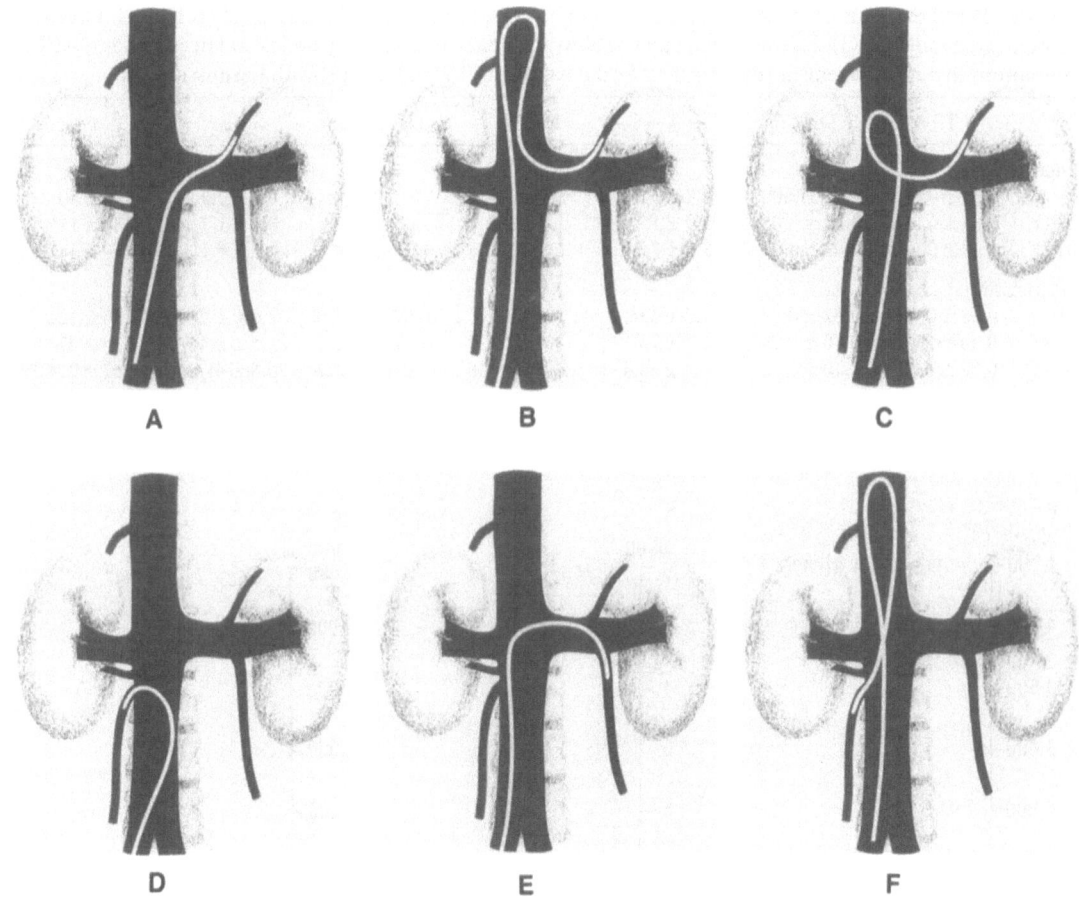

Figure 1.15. Four-vessel blood sampling technique. The six shapes of the cobra catheter employed for adrenal and ovarian vein catheterization. **A**: Catheter straight forward. **B**: Catheter with large loop. **C**: Catheter with short twisted loop. **D**: Catheter with short bend. **E**: Catheter with long bend. **F**: Catheter with large twisted loop.

1.19 (18). Large interindividual variations of DHT, A, DHEA, S, 17-OHP, and F levels can be observed in each vessel as well. These studies (18; Table 1.6) reveal that the gonads do not secrete significant amounts of T during the early follicular phase. There were similar findings in five women who were catheterized intraoperatively (20). Although in vitro studies have demonstrated the capacity of the human follicle to synthesize androgens (21), the in vivo data demonstrate that this potential is not utilized at the beginning of the cycle.

Our observations also contradict the reported ovarian contribution of 33 to 66% to the circulating T pool assumed for this stage on the basis of peripheral T changes after dexamethasone administration (22,23). The discrepancy is understandable in view of the nonspecificity of glucocorticoid suppression tests (7). In contrast to the absence of gonadal T, DHT, and F secretion, the ovaries did generate significant quantities of $\triangle_4$-A, DHEA-S, and 17-OHP between day 3 and 7 of the cycle. To our knowledge, the observations of significant OPGs (i.e., 2,100 and 570 ng/ml, respectively) for DHEA-S in two individuals is the first direct evidence for its partially gonadal origin. It explains the cyclic changes of DHEA-S reported in an adrenalectomized woman (24). However, it cannot be ruled out definitely that this finding is due to ovarian secretions of unknown steroids other than DHEA-S that cross-react with the antiserum used in our laboratory, e.g., androsterone or etiocholanolone conjugates.

Table 1.6. Peripheral vein steroid concentrations (PV), ovarian peripheral gradients (OPG), and adrenal peripheral gradients (APG) determined in eight healthy women with ovulatory cycles and in 60 patients with nontumorous hyperandrogenism (mean ± standard deviation). (From Ref. 18, with permission.)

	T	DHT	A	DHEA	DHEA-S	17-P	F
Normal							
PV	0.36 ± 0.16	0.25 ± 0.09	0.9 ± 0.3	5.1 ± 2.0	1,860 ± 850	0.6 ± 0.2	170 ± 50
OPG	0.03 ± 0.09	0.05 ± 0.05	1.0 ± 1.1	1.7 ± 1.8	191 ± 72	0.9 ± 1.7	−38 ± 11
APG	0.48 ± 0.57	0.69 ± 0.60	8.3 ± 7.9	141.8 ± 261.6	706 ± 824	6.3 ± 6.1	610 ± 1,329
Nonneoplastic							
PV	0.68 ± 0.43	0.32 ± 0.13	2.2 ± 2.0	8.8 ± 8.9	3,137 ± 1,774	2.0 ± 3.0	216 ± 121
OPG	0.40 ± 1.10	0.10 ± 0.20	3.4 ± 7.0	14.6 ± 100.0	−288 ± 523	4.5 ± 8.4	−35 ± 47
APG	0.88 ± 1.30	1.10 ± 0.90	14.4 ± 38.4	327.0 ± 367.0	854 ± 1,223	20.8 ± 41.3	1,252 ± 2,023

From ref. 18, with permission.

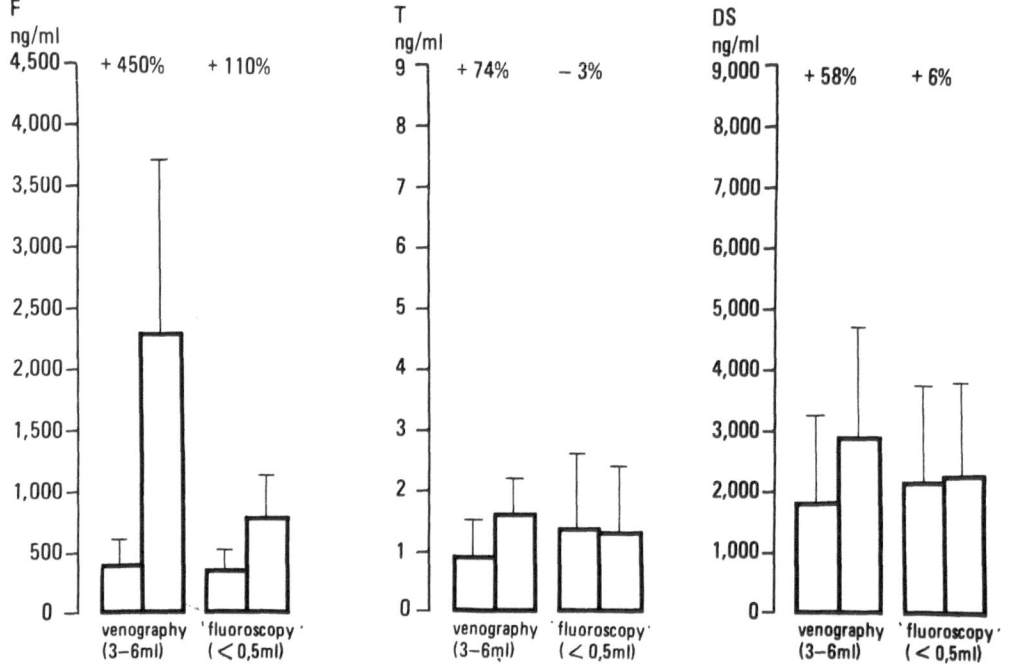

Figure 1.16. Effects of contrast media on adrenal steroid release in nine patients with hyperandrogenemia. F, cortisol; T, testosterone; DHEA-S, dehydroepiandrosterone sulfate. The percentage values denote the mean changes of adrenal vein steroid levels induced.

The adrenals are considerably more active than the gonads during the early follicular phase; this is apparent for all seven steroids measured. Previously it had been thought the DHT arises exclusively from peripheral conversion of $\triangle_4$-A and T (23,25). Our study indicates that DHT is directly secreted by normal adrenals, thus supporting in vitro findings (26).

The adrenal DHEA-S gradients are relatively small despite a high production rate; they reflect the low metabolic clearance rate characteristic of this steroid (23). Random, nonsimultaneous catheterization of the four glandular veins revealed no significant differences between the respective effluent concentrations on the left and right sides. It appears that the

Figure 1.17. Extravasation into the parenchyma of the right adrenal gland after retrograde venography.

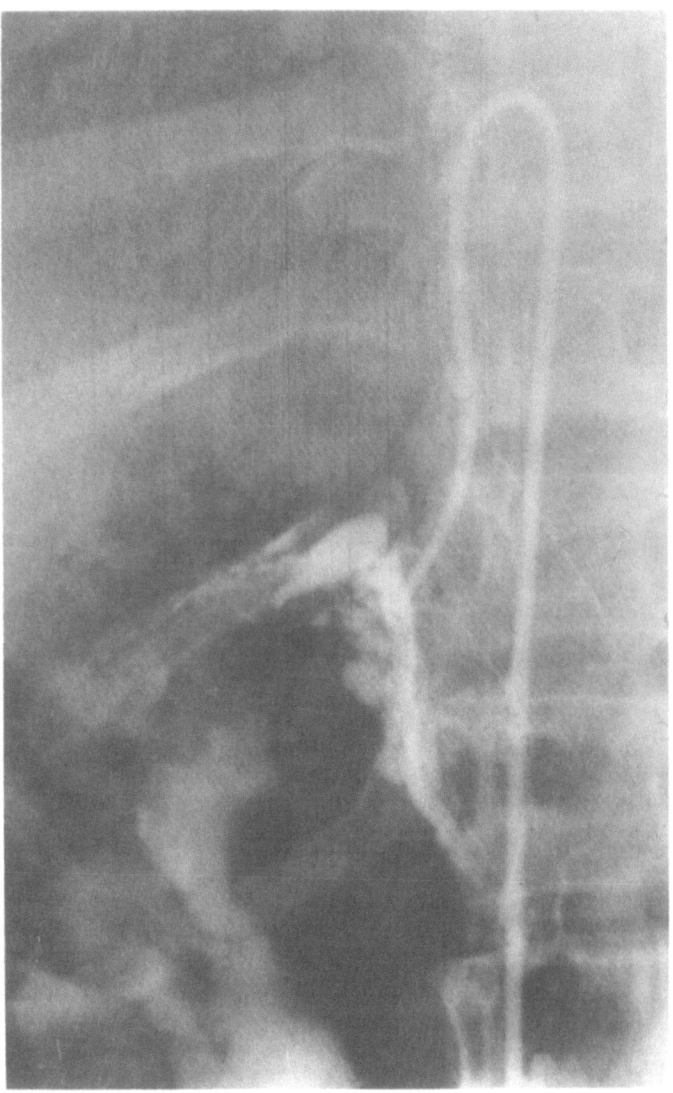

ovaries have parallel androgen secretion during the early follicular phase; the same applies to adrenal steroid output. Discordant bilateral levels have been reported by other investigators; nonparallel ovarian hormone production is to be expected in the presence of preovulatory follicles or a corpus luteum (27), whereas dissimilar adrenal values may result from unpredictable pulsation (28,29). The problems of data interpretation due to the episodic, circadian, and cyclic variations of glandular steroidogenesis can be overcome by serial sampling and uniform timing of the procedure.

Nontumorous Hyperandrogenemia

The type, frequency, and extent of hormonal changes vary considerably between androgenized patients. The degree of deviation does not correlate to either the severity of symptoms or the laparoscopic, angiographic, or histological findings.

The wide range of individual concentrations of T and DHEA-S measured in the peripheral vein as well as in the four glandular effluents is depicted in Fig. 1.20. There is considerable overlap of T and DHEA-S levels between

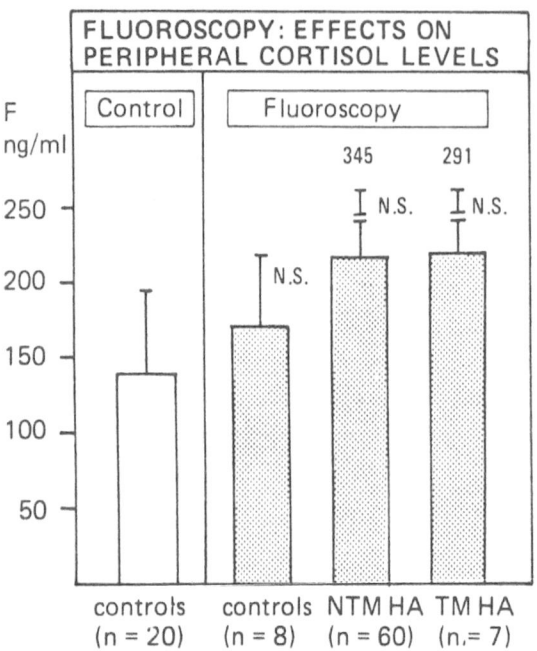

Figure 1.18. Peripheral cortisol (F) levels during the catheterization procedure of 75 women in comparison with a control group of normal outpatients ($n = 20$).

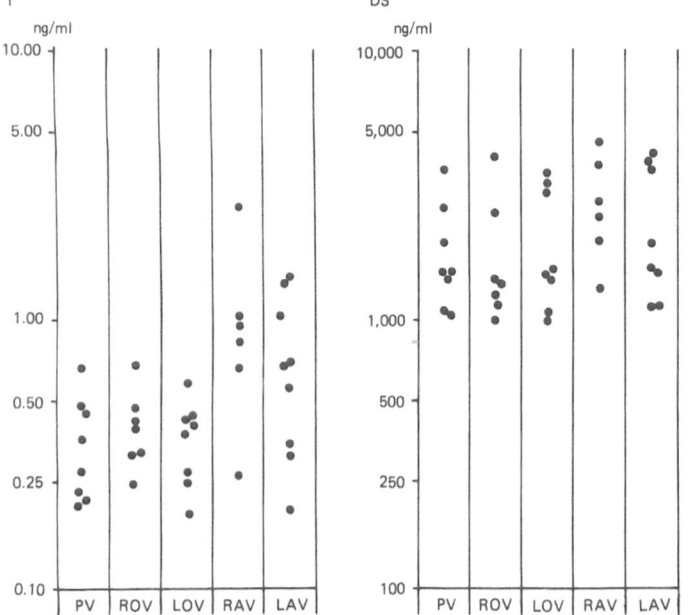

Figure 1.19. Individual peripheral and glandular vein levels of T and DHEA-S (OS) in eight normal volunteers during the early follicular phase. T, testosterone; DS, dehydroepiandrosterone sulfate.

healthy and hirsute women in every vessel. This observation also applies to the variations of DHT, $\triangle_4$-A, DHEA, and F levels. The upper 95% confidence limits of peripheral T and DHEA-S levels are 1.54 and 6,685 ng/ml, respectively. Compared to the normal cohort (early follicular phase) the mean levels of all steroids, except F, in peripheral blood were significantly elevated in women with nonneoplastic hyperandrogenism as a group ($p < 0.05$). Peripheral concentrations of T and DHEA-S during catheterization are above

Figure 1.20. Individual peripheral and glandular vein levels of T and DHEA-S (DS) in 60 patients with nonneoplastic hyperandrogenism. T, testosterone; DS, dehydroepiandrosterone sulfate.

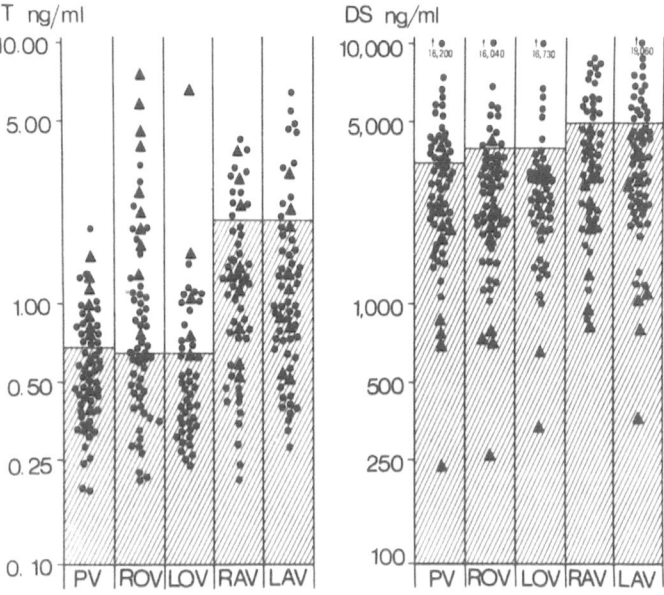

Figure 1.21. Individual (bars) and cumulative (connected dots) percentage incidence of elevated peripheral vein steroids in 60 patients with nonneoplastic hyperandrogenemia (> mean + 2 standard deviations of eight normal control subjects). (Reproduced, from ref. 18, with the permission of the publisher, the American Fertility Society.)

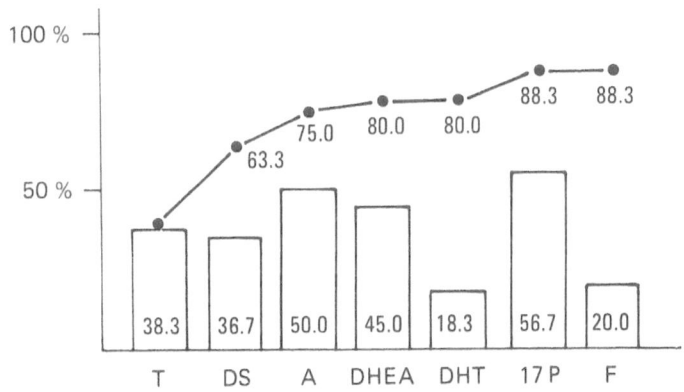

normal in about one-third of nontumorous androgenic women, whereas $\triangle_4$-A, DHEA, and 17-OHP were increased in about half of the patients (Fig. 1.21). Peripheral hyperandrogenemia is evident in only 65%, when hormone analysis is restricted to the measurement of peripheral T and DHEA-S; however, almost 90% of patients show abnormalities when all seven steroids are taken into consideration.

The steroid gradients in hirsute patients reflecting glandular secretion are demonstrated in Table 1.6. During the early follicular phase, all hormone assays are released bilaterally in parallel fashion by the gonads and adrenals. The ovaries and adrenals of these patients as

a group produce significant quantities of T, DHT, $\triangle_4$-A , DHEA, and 17-OHP (significance of differences between glandular and peripheral vein levels, $p < 0.001$); DHEA-S and F are secreted by the adrenals only. The observed negative OPGs of DHEA-S and F imply gonadal utilization and metabolism; however, they may also be artifacts due to episodic fluctuations. Our findings document the direct ovarian and adrenal secretion of DHT in hirsute women and confirm the preliminary results presented by Maroulis (30). In absolute terms, adrenal steroid release is significantly greater than gonadal steroid output during the early follicular phase; this applies to all seven

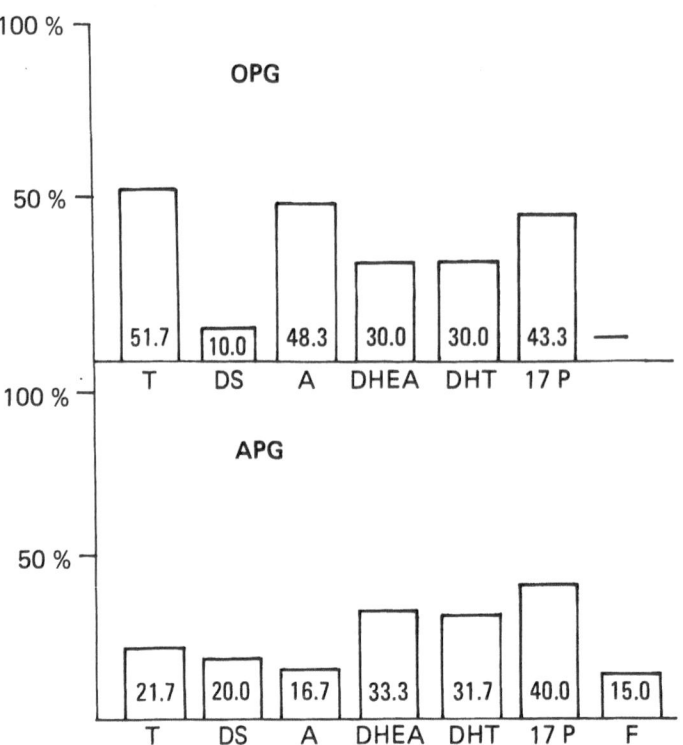

Figure 1.22. Individual percentage incidence of elevated OPGs and APGs in 60 patients with nonneoplastic hyperandrogenemia. (Reproduced from ref. 19, with the permission of the publisher, the American Fertility Society.)

hormone assays ($p < 0.001$). Compared to the group of healthy women, the mean OPGs for T, Δ_4-A, DHEA, and 17-OHP, and the APG for 17-OHP surpass the upper limit of normal; yet these differences are significant only in regard to gonadal output of 17-OHP ($p < 0.05$).

In contrast, evaluation of each individual case shows that glandular hypersecretion of at least one androgen, (T, DHT, Δ_4-A, DHEA, or DHEA-S) is present in 80% (Fig. 1.22). This, however, does not always result in an increase of peripheral levels. This may be due to dilutional effects as well as to a rise of metabolic clearance rates in hirsute women (1). Moreover, the aberrations are often minor and restricted to a limited number of patients and/or a single hormone. For instance, direct ovarian release of DHEA-S can be present in individual cases and therefore not be reflected in the overall group results.

The differentiation between ovarian, adrenal, and combined ovarian-adrenal hyperandrogenism of nonneoplastic origin is made on the basis of previous catheterization findings in healthy women. Excess ovarian and/or adrenal androgen output is assumed in a given individual, if one or more of the respective T, DHT, Δ_4-A, DHA, and DHEA-S gradients exceed the upper 95% confidence limit of normal secretions (Table 1.6). Combined hypersecretion can be expected in 41% of patients and is the most frequent cause of hyperandrogenism. Purely ovarian (27%) or adrenal overproduction (12%) is identified less often; normal glandular androgen output is found in 20% of hirsute patients.

The relative incidence of ovarian and/or adrenal involvement in the etiology of nonneoplastic hyperandrogenism is still a debated issue. Regardless of the diagnostic approach, the distribution pattern reported in the literature varies extremely (9,31–33; Table 1.7). Abraham and Manlimos (33) have been among the advocates of a predominantly adrenal site of androgen hypersecretion. Their classification was based on the results of long-term dexamethasone suppression tests. However, it has been documented directly that glucocorticoids may significantly reduce not only adrenal but also ovarian androgen secretion (2). Kir-

Table 1.7. Relative percentage frequency of ovarian, adrenal, and combined ovarian-adrenal nonneoplastic hyperandrogenism reported in the literature.

Authors	$D_{\bar{x}}^a$	Subjects(n)	Ovarian	Adrenal	Combined	Other
Cruikshank et al. (1971)	FT	130	58	12	30	–
Abraham and Manlimos (1978)	FT	97	22	50	21	7
Kirschner and Jacobs (1971)	SC	44	95	5	–	–
Stahl et al. (1973)	SC	20	–	40	45	15
Present study	SC	60	27	12	41	20

From Ref. 3, with permission.
[a] FT, function test; SC, selective cathetarization

schner and Jacobs (9) suggested a preponderance of ovarian hyperandrogenism on the basis of catheterization data. Their study was restricted to the measurement of effluent T, Δ_4-A, and F levels and result comparison with healthy control subjects. Their calculation of androgen secretion rates was based on several assumptions that were later shown to be erroneous (23), including parallel secretion of F and adrenal androgens, normal F output during radiography of premedicated patients, and constant peripheral conversion of androgen precursors. In addition, they only differentiated between ovarian and adrenal sources, neglecting the possibility of combined dysfunction.

The present investigation relies on established normal steroid gradients. It indicated that excessive glandular androgen release often has a mixed ovarian-adrenal origin, which only becomes evident when a broad spectrum of steroids is analyzed. The close interaction between gonads and adrenals is underlined by numerous reports in the literature (34–36) documenting (a) the induction of ovulation by glucocorticoid therapy, (b) the stimulation of adrenal steroidogenesis by estrogen administration, and (c) the coexistence of both adrenal and ovarian nonneoplastic as well as neoplastic hyperandrogenism. The validity of our results regarding incidence rates is limited by the small number of control subjects, single effluent sampling in patients as opposed to serial sampling in healthy volunteers, and a definition of "normal" based exclusively on early follicular phase data.

Polycystic Ovary Syndrome

It is still a matter of controversy whether the presence of polycystic ovaries constitutes a nosological entity or a nonspecific morphologic substrate associated with hyperandrogenism. Hirsute women should undergo laparoscopy to rule out a macroscopically visible ovarian neoplasm. The changes suggestive of polycystic ovary syndrome are a thickened and whitish cortex, multiple subcapsular cysts, and gross gonadal enlargement. There is no correlation between morphological, clinical, and endocrine changes; a PCO-specific hormonal pattern is not identifiable (37).

Analysis of gradient data obtained by selective catheterization reveals that combined ovarian-adrenal androgen hypersecretion is present in 46% of PCO cases; purely ovarian (21%) or adrenal (12%) overproduction are not as frequent. This pattern of distribution concerning etiology does not differ significantly from that observed in patients without laparoscopic signs of PCO (37). Gradient evaluation in each individual case showed that glandular hypersecretion of at least one androgen is present in 80% (Fig. 1.23). Again, the percentage incidence of elevated OPGs and APGs does not deviate substantially from those found in a group of 60 patients with nontumorous hyperandrogenism (19). From these data it is concluded that PCO is not a nosological entity, but rather a nonobligatory sign of hyperandrogenism. Laparoscopy is, therefore, without clinical relevance in these patients with nonneoplastic hyperandrogenemia.

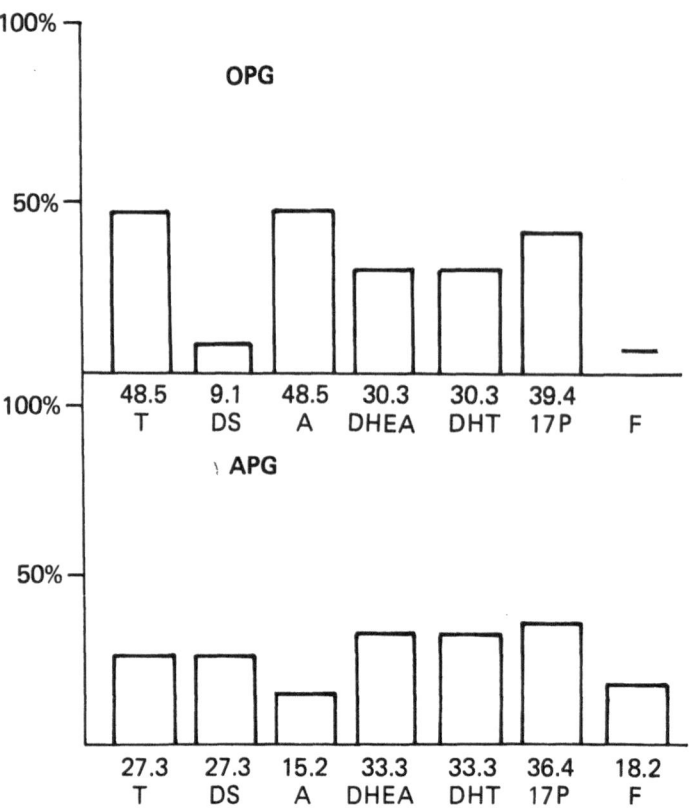

Figure 1.23. Individual percentage incidence of elevated ovarian and adrenal peripheral vein gradients (OPG, APG) in 33 patients with polycystic ovaries. (Reproduced from ref. 37, with the permission of the publisher, Thieme Verlag.)

Figure 1.24 illustrates the nonspecific suppression of ovarian and adrenal secretion of T and DHEA-S by dexamethasone in two cohorts with and without PCO. Qualitatively similar results apply to the other steroid measurements. These data clearly indicate that glucocorticoid suppression tests cannot reliably discriminate between ovarian and adrenal nontumorous hyperandrogenism due to extremely variable individual responsiveness.

Ovarian Hyperthecosis

Hyperthecosis has repeatedly been described as a tumor-like disease entity separate from PCO and characterized by a pathognomonic histology (stromal versus perifollicular theca cell hyperplasia and luteinization) as well as distinct clinical and endocrine features, e.g., obligatory signs of virilization and excess ovarian androgen secretion without significant adrenal contribution (38). This assertion remains a topic of debate.

Our present investigation includes patients with histologically proven hyperthecosis (39). The clinical and biochemical findings were as inconsistent as in PCO (40). Peripheral T levels varied between 0.4 and 2.5 ng/ml before and during catheterization. A specific hormone profile could not be identified.

Figure 1.25 shows the overlap of testosterone levels in peripheral and glandular effluent blood between healthy women and patients with hyperthecosis as well as androgen-secreting ovarian neoplasms. In four individuals, testosterone secretion fell within the tumorous range (3). Gradient analysis of all androgens indicates purely ovarian hypersecretion in six patients, but also additional significant adrenal involvement in four women. As in PCO, dexamethasone suppresses gonadal as well as adrenal androgen output. The minor differences between HYP and PCO represent only variable manifestation of the same condition of a disturbed androgen metabolism. A tumor, however, should be ruled out in patients with HYP.

Figure 1.24. Individual peripheral vein levels (PV), ovarian and adrenal peripheral vein gradients (OPG, APG) for testosterone (T) and, DHEA sulfate (DHEA-S) before and after intravenous dexamethasone in hirsute patients with and without polycystic ovaries (PCO). (Reproduced, from ref. 37, with the permission of the publisher, Thieme Verlag.)

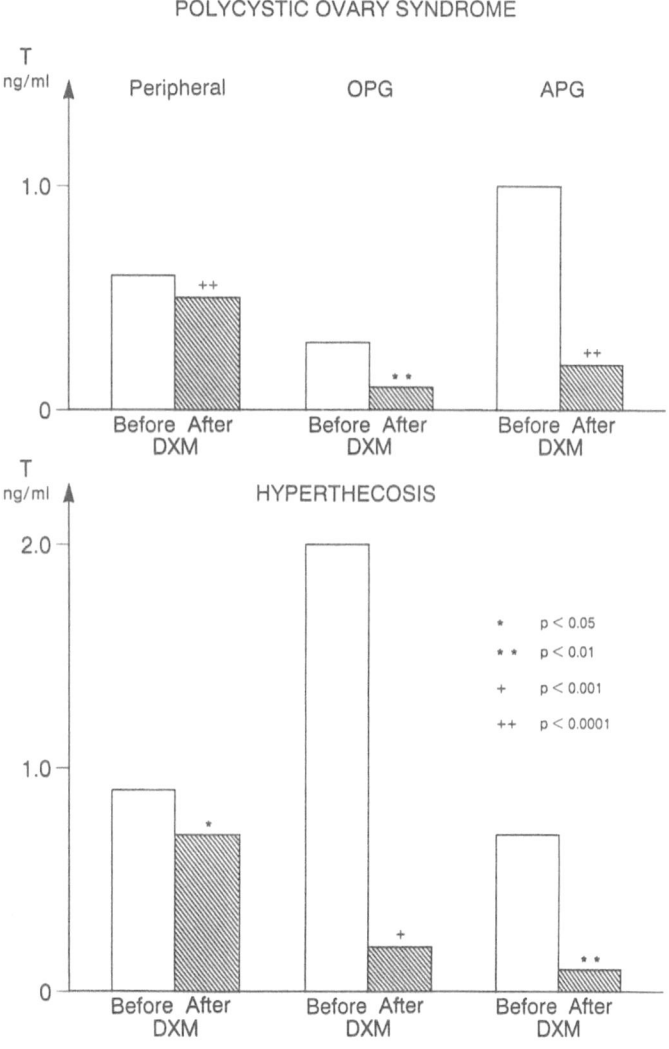

Tumorous Hyperandrogenemia

Androgen-secreting ovarian neoplasms is rare, but may be the underlying cause of virilism and related symptoms. Neoplastic hyperandrogenism should be ruled out in women with severe, sudden/late onset, and/or progressive hirsutism. Other signs of virilism (temporal balding, deepening of the voice, clitorimegaly, and male body habitus) are suspicious of tumorous hyperandrogenism. Selective catheterization has been used to study glandular secretion of several ovarian and adrenal androgen secreting tumors (3). Representative secretion patterns or criteria demarcating nontumorous and

tumorous hyperandrogenism, however, could not be established because these investigations constituted single case reports.

According to the literature it appears that virilizing adrenal tumors secrete predominantly either T or DHEA-S, although simultaneous elevated output of Δ_4-A and DHEA was also described. Ovarian vein sampling, however, was not performed in any of these cases investigated by preoperative catheterization. Thus, information concerning the potential involvement of ovarian hypersecretion is not available.

The presence of an adrenal adenoma in addition to hyperthecosis has been reported (41).

The nonspecific response of adrenal tumors to glucocorticoid suppression and gonadotropin stimulation has already been described (42–44). Standardized bilateral ovarian-adrenal vein catheterization has been found to be successful in preoperatively assessing glandular steroid release in seven occult virilizing gonadal neoplasms (3). The histology of the involved ovaries in our serious revealed three lipid cell, two Leydig cell, and two Sertoli-Leydig cell tumors measuring between 0.6 and 2.2 cm in diameter. Endoscopy and radiography failed to locate the functional lesions. Prior to catheterization, peripheral T surpassed the upper 95% confidence limit of the nontumorous group (1.5 ng/ml in all instances; in one patient it was below this critical value during catheterization). This may indicate unpredictable episodic T secretion by the ovarian lesion. Antecubital vein DHT exceeded the nontumorous range in two subjects. The peripheral concentrations of the other

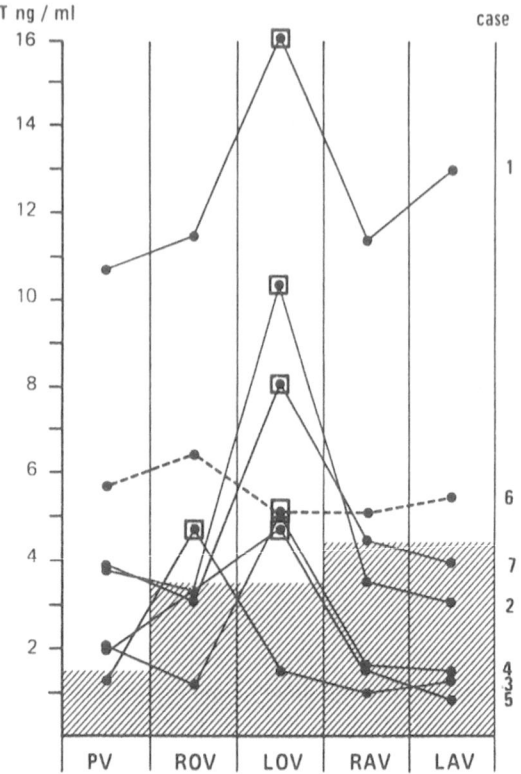

Figure 1.26. Individual peripheral and glandular vein testosterone levels in seven patients with neoplastic ovarian hyperandrogenemia. (Reproduced from ref. 3, with the permission of the publisher, the American Fertility Society.)

steroids fell within the nonneoplastic range in all instances.

Selective cannulation of ovarian veins was accomplished in six cases, displaying a unilateral increase of T in the effluent draining in neoplastic gonads (Fig. 1.26) which exceeded the upper 95% confidence limit of the nontumorous group (2.7 ng/ml). In the remaining patient, gradient analysis ruled out an adrenal tumor, but did not facilitate lateralization of a gonadal lesion due to unsatisfactory ovarian effluent sampling.

CATHETERIZATION: OVARIAN TUMORS (●)
HYPERTHECOSIS (▲)

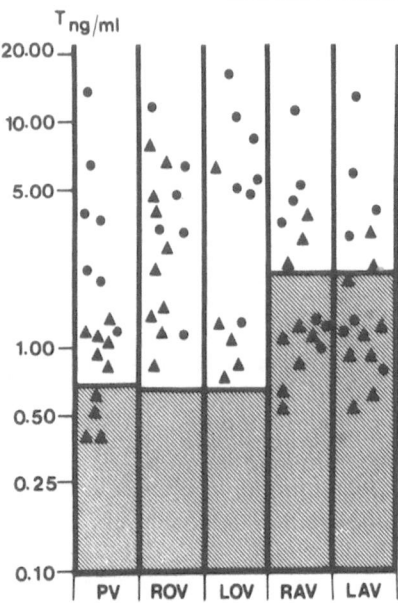

Figure 1.25. Individual peripheral and glandular vein levels of testosterone (T) in ten patients with hyperthecosis (denoted by triangles) and seven patients with androgen-secreting gonadal tumors (denoted by dots). (Reproduced, from ref. 40, with the permission of the publisher, Thieme Verlag.)

Conclusion

At the present time selective bilateral ovarian-adrenal catheterization (four-vessel sampling) appears to be the most sensitive method avail-

Table 1.8. Comparison of special parameters of the androgen metabolism in normal women (NW), and patients with polycystic ovaries (PCO), hyperthecosis (HYP), and androgen-secreting ovarian tumors (TM): mean ± standard deviation, range.

Parameter	NW $n = 8$	PCO $n = 33$	HYP $n = 10$	TM $n = 7$
T: peripheral (ng/ml)	0.36 ± 0.16	0.62 ± 0.33	0.89 ± 0.34	4.21 ± 3.23
	0.20 − 0.67	0.18 − 1.91	0.39 − 1.50	1.30 − 10.7
T: ovarian-peripheral	0.03 ± 0.50	0.23 ± 0.50	2.04 ± 2.11	4.28 ± 1.62
gradient (ng/ml)	−0.05 − 0.11	−0.11 − 0.96	0.27 − 6.60	2.7 − 6.6
DHEA-S: peripheral	1,860 ± 820	3,600 ± 1,870	1,800 ± 1,160	1,741 ± 704
(ng/ml)	1,100 − 3,590	160 − 8,580	250 − 4,020	960 − 3,050
Free T: peripheral	2.6 ± 2.3	8.7 ± 4.8	20.3 ± 9.3	126.8 ± 127.2
(pg/ml)	0.8 − 6.3	3.4 − 24.6	5.6 − 34.7	29.1 − 342.4

able for semiquantitative estimation of glandular androgen secretion. It is the only technique allowing separate analysis of each ovary and adrenal gland, respectively. The procedure is reliable and safe, provided that it is performed at centers with adequate experience under strict standardized conditions to reduce the interference of episodic, circadian, and cyclic variations of steroidogenesis. Stimulation and suppression tests cannot reliably differentiate between ovarian and adrenal, nontumorous and tumorous hyperandrogenemia, due to frequently occurring nonspecific pharmacodynamic effects. The evolutionary pathophysiology of glandular androgen hypersecretion must be regarded as a continuous process without sharp borderlines from normal to nontumorous conditions, such as polycystic ovaries and hyperthecosis, to neoplastic disease (Table 1.8). Hirsutism and related symptoms are most often caused by excess androgens of ovarian and/or adrenal origin. As demonstrated by selective catheterization of glandular effluents, combined hypersecretion occurs more frequently than either purely gonadal or adrenal overproduction. No correlation can be found between the type, frequency, and extent of hormonal changes and the clinical, laparoscopic, angiographic, or histologic findings.

The preoperative verification and localization of a virilizing neoplasm is of utmost importance. It may reduce the need for an operative exploration and may help in selecting the appropriate surgical approach.

References

1. Maroulis GB. Evaluation of hirsutism and hyperandrogenemia. *Fertil Steril* 1981;36:273–305.
2. Moltz L, Schwartz U, Hammerstein J, Sörensen R. Hyperandrogenism: nonspecificity of dynamic function tests. In: Xth World Congress of Gynecology and Obstetrics, San Francisco Abstract 1982;2129:581.
3. Moltz L, Pickartz H, Sörensen R, Schwartz U, Hammerstein J. Ovarian and adrenal vein steroids in seven patients with androgen-secreting ovarian neoplasms: selective catheterization findings. *Fertil Steril* 1984;42:585–593.
4. Abrams HL, Siegelmann SS, Adams DF, Sanders R, Finberg HJ, Hessel SJ, McNeil BJ. Computed tomography versus ultrasound of the adrenal gland: prospective study. *Radiology* 1982;143:121–128.
5. Mitty HA, Yeh HC. *Radiology of the Adrenals with Sonography and CT*. Philadelphia: Saunders; 1982:56–57.
6. Chan FL, Wang C. Imaging for adrenal tumors. *Baillieres Clin Endocrinol Metab* 1989;3:153–189.
7. Moltz L. Rationeller Einsatz endokrinologischer und radiologischer Verfahren bei der Differentialdiagnose von Androgenisierungserscheinungnen der Frau. *Geburtshilfe Frauenheilkd* 1982;42:321–326.
8. Moltz L, Pickartz H, Sörensen R, Schwartz U, Hammerstein J. A Sertoli-Leydig cell tumor and pregnancy—clinical, endocrine, radiologic, and electron microscopic findings. *Arch Gynecol* 1983;233:295–308.
9. Kirschner MA, Jacobs JB. Combined ovarian and adrenal vein catheterization to determine

the sites of androgen over-production in hirsute women. *J Clin Endocrinol Metab* 1971;33:199–209.

10. Moltz L. Differential-diagnostic clarification of androgen-producing tumors. In Hammerstein J, Lachnit-Fixson U, Neumann F, Plewig G, eds. *Androgenization in Women.* Exc Med, Int Congr Ser No. 493, North Holland: Elsevier; (1980),1979:114–124.

11. Soules MR, Abraham GE, Bossen EH. The steroid profile of a virilizing ovarian tumor. *Obstet Gynecol* 1978;52:73–78.

12. Sörensen R, Moltz L, Schwartz U. Technical difficulties of selective venous blood sampling in the differential diagnosis of female hyperandrogenism. *Cardiovasc Intervent Radiol* 1986;9:75–82.

13. Haggar AM, Froelich JW. MR imaging strategies in primary and metastatic malignancy. *Radiol Clin North Am* 1988;3:689–696.

14. Sörensen R, Moltz L. Diagnostik bei progredientem Hirsutismuns. Kathetertechnik und Ergebnisse *Fortschr Röntgenstr* 1981;135:257–266.

15. Lecky JW, Wolfman NT, Modic CW. Current concepts of adrenal angiography. *Radiol Clin N Am* 1976;14:309–352.

16. Sörensen R, Moltz L. Technical Aspects and anatomical difficulties of adrenal and gonadal phlebography and blood sampling. Exc Med, Amsterdam, International Congress, series No. 550. 1980;78–88.

17. Lamarque JL, Bruel LN, Lopez P, Michel LJ, Rouanet JP, Senac JP, Bruno C, Roquefeuil C. Les complications de l'angiographie surrenalienne. *Ann Radiol* 1979;22:401–408.

18. Moltz L, Sörensen R, Schwartz U, Hammerstein J. Ovarian and adrenal vein steroids in healthy women with ovulatory cycles—selective catheterization findings. *J Steroid Biochem* 1984;20:901–905.

19. Moltz L, Schwartz U, Sörensen R, Pickartz H, Hammerstein J. Ovarian and adrenal vein steroids in patients with nonneoplastic hyperandrogenism: selective catheterization findings. *Fertil Steril* 1984;42:69–75.

20. Horton R, Romanoff E, Walker J. Androstenedione and testosterone in ovarian venous and peripheral plasma during ovariectomy for breast cancer. *J Clin Endocrinol Metab* 1966;26:1267–1276.

21. McNatty KP, Makris A, DeGraziac, Osathanondh R, Ryan KJ. The production of progesterone, androgens and estrogens by granu-

losa cells, thecal tissue, and stromal tissue from human ovaries in vitro. *J Clin Endocrinol Metab* 1979;49:687–699.

22. Genazzani AR, Magrini G, Facchinetti F, et al. Behaviour and origin of plasma androgens throughout the menstrual cycle. In: Martini L, Motta M, eds. *Androgens and Antiandrogens.* New York: Raven Press; 1977:247–261.

23. Vermeulen A, Rubens R. Adrenal virilism. In: James VHT, ed. *The Adrenal Gland.* New York: Raven Press; 1970:259–282.

24. Abraham GE, Chakmakjian ZH. Serum steroid levels during the menstrual cycle in a bilaterally adrenalectomized women. *J Clin Endocrinol Metab* 1973;37:581–592.

25. Ito T, Horton R. Dihydrotestosterone in human peripheral plasma. *J Clin Endocrinol Metab* 1970;31:362–366.

26. Maroulis GB, Abraham GB. Concentration of androgens and cortisol in the various zones of the human adrenal cortex. In: Genazzani A, Thijssen JHH, Siiteri P, eds. *Adrenal Androgens.* New York: Raven Press; 1980:49–53.

27. Wentz AC, White RI, Migeon CJ, Hsu TH, Barnes HV, Jones GS. Differential ovarian and adrenal vein catheterization. *Am J Obstet Gynecol* 1976;125:1000–1007.

28. Nicolis GL, Babich AM, Mitty HA, Gabrilove LJ. Observation on the cortisol content of human adrenal venous blood. *J Clin Endocrinol Metab* 1974;38:638–645.

29. Eisenberg H. Radiologic techniques in tumor localization. In: De Groot LJ, Cahill Jr GF, Odell WD, et al., eds. *Endocrinol,* vol 3. New York: Grune & Stratton, 1979:2125–2143.

30. Maroulis GB, Lindstrom R, Abraham GE, Marshall JR. Testosterone and dehydrotestosterone secretion by the adrenal and ovary in hirsute patients. *Endocrine Society Meeting Abstract* 1975;471:286.

31. Cruikshank DP, Yannone ME, Chapler FK. Arrhenoblastoma associated with adrenal androgenic hyperfunction. *Obstet Gynecol* 1974; 43:535–543.

32. Stahl NL, Teeslink CR, Beauchamps G, Greenblatt RB. Serum testosterone levels in hirsute women: a comparison of adrenal, ovarian, and peripheral vein values. *Obstet Gynecol* 1973;41:650–654.

33. Abraham GE, Manlimos FS. The role of the adrenal cortex in hirsutism. In: James VHT, Serio M, Giusti G, Martini L, eds. *The Endocrine Function of the Human Adrenal Cortex.* London: Academic Press; 1978:325–355.

34. Goldzieher JW. Polycystic ovarian disease. *Fertil Steril* 1981;35:371–379.

35. Korth-Schütz 5, Levine LS, Merkatz LR, New MI. An unusual case of Cushing's syndrome, hilus cell tumor and polycystic ovaries. *J Clin Endocrinol Metab* 1974;38:794–878.

36. Lobo RA, Goebelsmann U. Adult manifestation of congenital adrenal hyperplasia due to incomplete 21-hydroxylase deficiency mimicking polycystic ovarian disease. *Am J Obstet Gynecol* 19;138:720–727.

37. Moltz L, Sörensen R, Römmler A, Schwartz U, Hammerstein J. Polyzystische Ovarien: eigenständiges Krankheitsbild oder unspezifisches Symptom? *Geburtshilfe Frauenheilkd* 1985;45:107–114.

38. Karam K, Haji S. Hyperthecosis syndrome. *Acta Obstet Gynecol Scand* 1979;58:73–78.

39. Scully RE. Ovarian tumors with endocrine manifestations. In: De Groot LJ, Cahill Jr GF, Odell WD, et al., eds. *Endocrinology*, vol. 3. New York: Grune & Stratton; 1979:1473–1488.

40. Schwartz U, Moltz L, Pickartz H, Sörensen R. Die Hyperthecose—eine tumorähnliche Ovarialveränderung bei androgenisierten Frauen. *Geburtshilfe Frauenhkeilked* 1986;46:391–397.

41. Trost BN, Koenig MP, Zimmerman A, Zachmann M, Müller J. Virilization of a postmenopausal woman by a testosterone-secreting Leydig cell type adrenal adenoma. *Acta Endocrinol* 1981;98:274–282.

42. Matthews JI, Fariss BL, Chertow BS, Howard WB. Adrenal adenoma with variable response to dexamethasone suppression and metyrapone stimulation. *J Clin Endocrinol Metab* 1972;34:902–906.

43. Larson BA, Vanderlaan WP, Judd HL, McCullough DL. A testosterone-producing adrenal cortical adenoma in an elderly woman. *J Clin Endocrinol Metab* 1976;42:882–887.

44. Mack E, Sarto GE, Crummy AB, et al. Virilizing adrenal angioneuroma. *JAMA* 1978;239:2273–2274.

2

Selective Venous Sampling for Adrenal Hormone Excess

—— Reingard Sörensen ——

Adrenal Glands

Introduction

Indications for adrenal imaging are the detection of metastatic disease tumors of hormone excess, or hormone deficiency of greater than 1 cm in diameter. The lesions can be detected by ultrasound, computed tomography (CT), or magnetic resonance imaging. If those modalities cannot locate the source of excess hormone production, selective venous sampling followed by determination of plasma hormone levels will solve the problem.

Ultrasonography

Adrenals can be visualized by ultrasound, and lesions in adults are successfully examined in 92% of the cases on the right side and in 71% on the left. The overall detection rate of masses is more than 90% (1). This depends on the examiner's experience, the size of the patient, and the position of the patient's intestine (2,3). There is a high false-positive rate of 27 to 39% described in the literature (4).

Adrenal Scintigraphy

There are special radiopharmaceuticals available to assist in examining the adrenal medulla and cortex by scintigraphy. For scanning of the cortex 13l-I-6β-iodomethyl-19-norcholesterol (NP59) is employed. Other substances are 131-I-19 iodocholesterol (19-C) and selenium-75 selenomethyl cholesterol. Dexamethasone suppression may improve the accuracy of scanning. The techniques are able to locate adrenal tumors in Cushing's syndrome (5) and in primary aldosteronism (6). There are, however, false-positive and false-negative results and the examination by CT was also found to be less expensive (7). Radiopharmaceuticals for the adrenal medulla have been used to localize intra- and extraadrenal pheochromocytomas. Usually metaiodobenzylguanidine (MIBG) containing 0.5 mCi of 131-iodine is injected intravenously and the patient is scanned on day 1, 2, and 3. MIGB molecules compete with adrenaline for cellular uptake and thus can be employed to localize tumors. 123-I has been found to be more accurate than 131-I, with better detection efficiency and better dosimetry. It also allows single photon emission computed tomography (8–10). There is a high false-negative rate and radiation exposure is high as well (11). Normal adrenal tissue does not store this isotope but 90% of pheochromocytomas do.

Computed Tomography

The most effective imaging technique for adrenal pathology is computed tomography (Fig. 2.1). Its high resolution is able to image

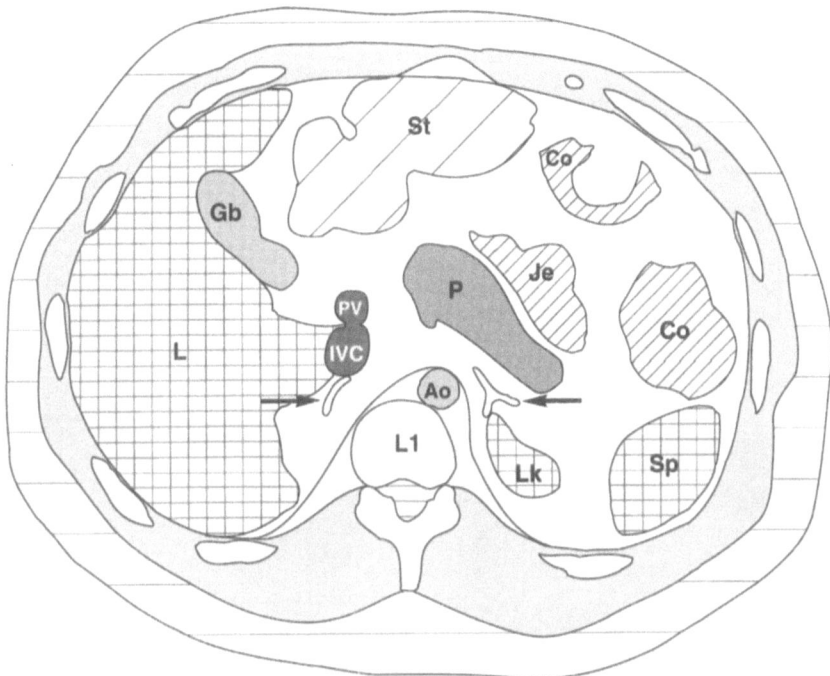

A

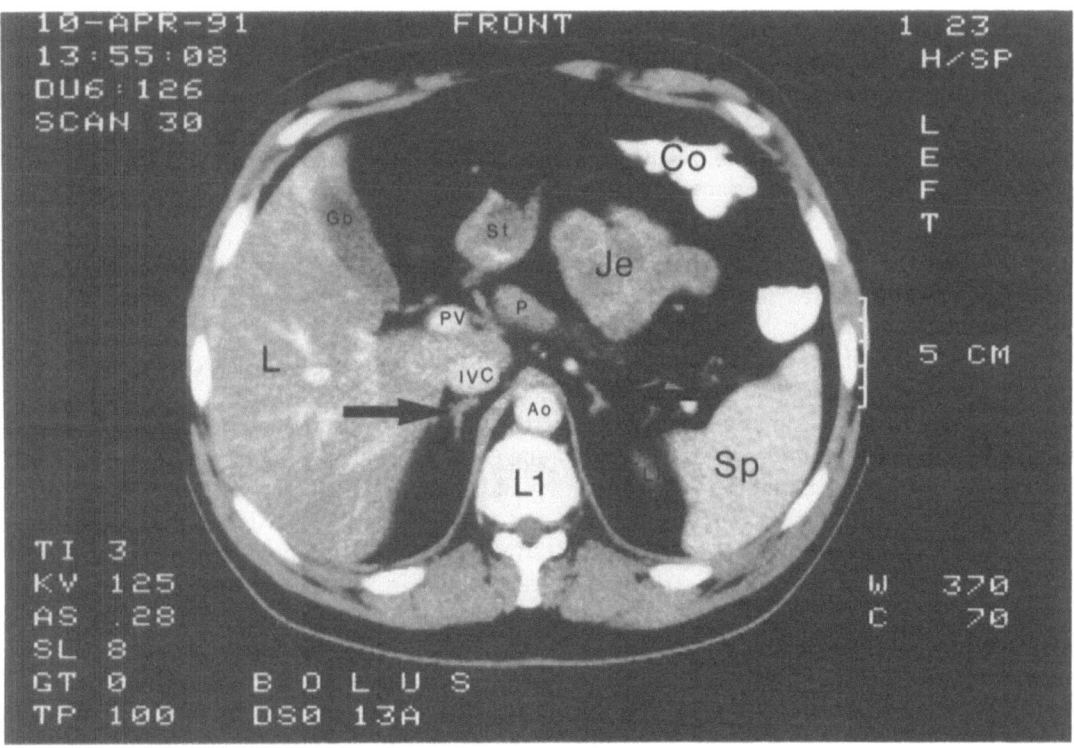

B

Figure 2.1. **A**: Pattern of computed tomography of the abdomen at level L1. L, liver; Sp, spleen; Gb, gallbladder; Co, colon; Je, jejunum; St, stomach; P, pancreas; LK, left kidney; Ao, aorta; PV, portal vein; IVC, inferior vena cava. Left and right adrenal (arrows). **B**: Computed tomography of the abdomen with normal adrenal glands. L, liver; Sp, spleen; Gb, gallbladder; Co, Colon; Je, jejunum; St, stomach; P, pancreas; Lk, left kidney; Ao, aorta; PV, portal vein; IVC, inferior vena cava. Left and right adrenal (arrows).

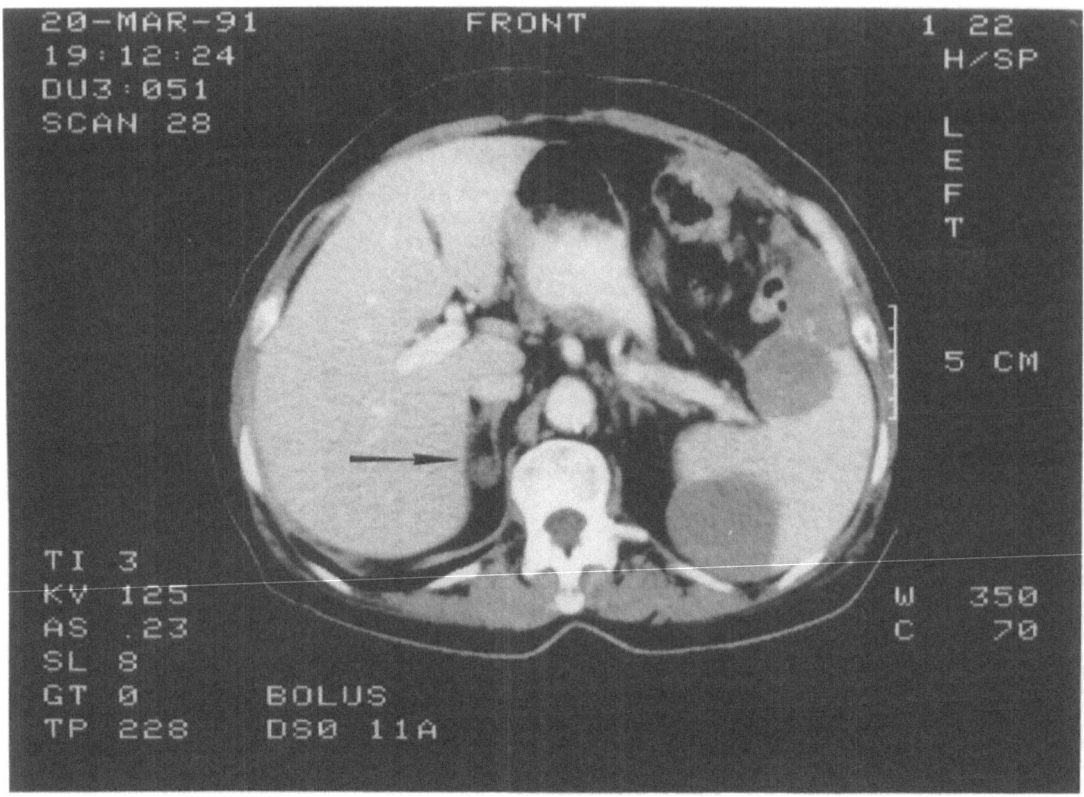

Figure 2.2. Computed tomography of the abdomen with a small nodule of the right adrenal gland (arrow). The patient has a lymphoma and lesions in the spleen.

both adrenal glands and their relationship to their surrounding structures in almost all adults (12). False-negative examinations will occur if the tumor is smaller than 1 cm in diameter and if it is within the tissue of the adrenal gland (Fig. 2.2). False-positive examinations are rare and are usually due to interpretation errors from mistaking varices, splenic vessels, gastric fundus, splenic lobulations, or pancreas for an adrenal mass (13,14). Contrast media might be helpful for the differentiation of structures; however, it cannot distinguish benign from malignant disease. The accuracy of computed tomography in combination with ultrasonography (US) in detecting adrenal nodular lesions is 60 to 90% (2,3,15–23). Adenomas smaller than 1 cm in diameter are difficult to diagnose and it is not always possible to distinguish between small adenomas and bilateral nodular hyperplasia (6,7,21,24–30). The examination of an adenoma can usually be performed

quickly, noninvasively, with little radiation exposure, and without preparation of the patient.

Magnetic Resonance Imaging

It is possible to use magnetic resonance imaging (MRI) for diagnosing lesions of the adrenal glands and for tissue characterization of adrenal tumors (Fig. 2.3). MRI is able to demonstrate normal anatomy of the adrenal glands very well (Fig. 2.3). Hyperfunctional tumors—aldosteronomas, Cushing adenomas, and virilizing/feminizing lesions—are generally low in signal intensity on T1- and T2-weighted images. It is not possible to distinguish functioning lesions from nonfunctioning lesions on the basis of the T2 signal intensity (31,32). The resolution necessary to separate adenomas from multinodular hyperplasia usually requires CT. Nodules may measure only several millimeters in diameter but they are of great importance

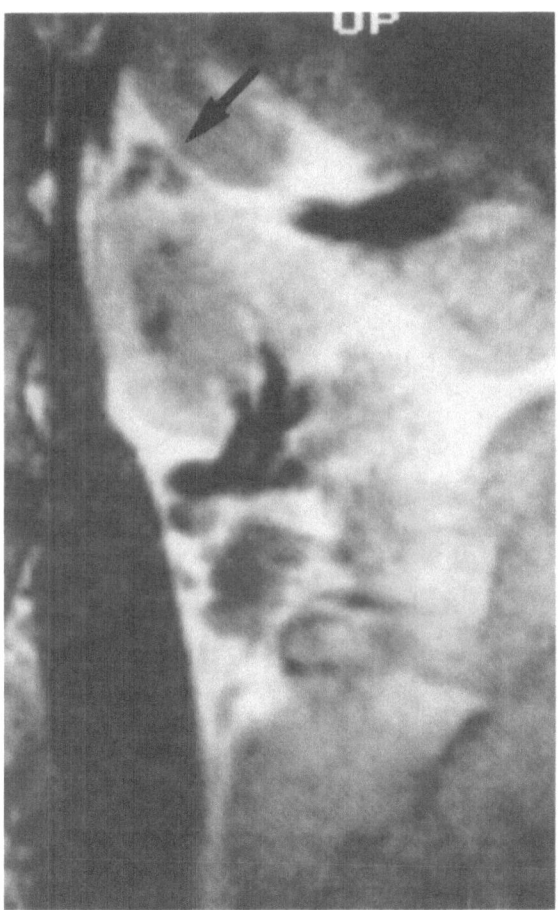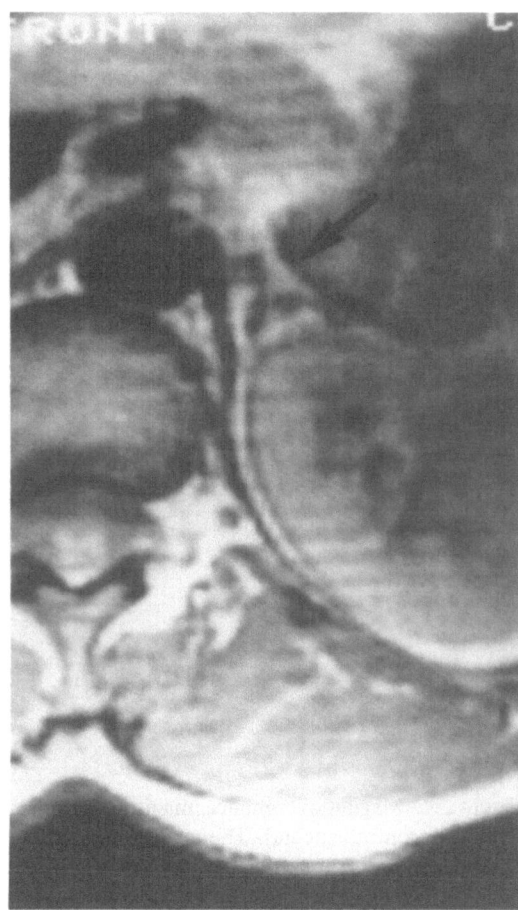

Figure 2.3. Magnetic resonance imaging of normal adrenal glands. (Courtesy of Hermann König, M.D., Klinikum Steglitz Berlin.)

because they may be associated with an extra-adrenal source of excessive hormone production and those patients are not candidates for surgical adrenalectomy.

MRI has shown some utility in the diagnosis of adrenal hemorrhage and Addison's disease. The appearance of myelolipomas is characteristic, but CT usually suffices for this diagnosis. MRI is more useful in confirming the presence of pheochromocytomas, especially small or multifocal pheochromocytomas (Fig. 2.4). Considering the large territory at risk for pheochromocytomas (the entire sympathetic chain), MRI is still not considered a primary tool in the evaluation of ectopic disease. Paragangliomas, glomus tumors, and neuroblastomas have similar imaging characteristics, and

MRI has proved useful in detecting and staging these lesions.

Many reports have addressed the usefulness of MRI in distinguishing between benign and malignant adrenal tumors (33–38). Most authors, however, have concluded that, although relatively specific (for example, of lesions with "benign" characteristics, 90 to 95% will prove to be benign), T2-weighted imaging is insensitive (for example, of lesions with "malignant" characteristics, only 70 to 80% will prove to be metastases). Benign adenomas are usually low in signal intensity on T2-weighted images relative to liver or fat. At higher field strengths, calculated T2 values produce comparable separation of the two entities. MR imaging has been proved insufficiently reliable for clinical

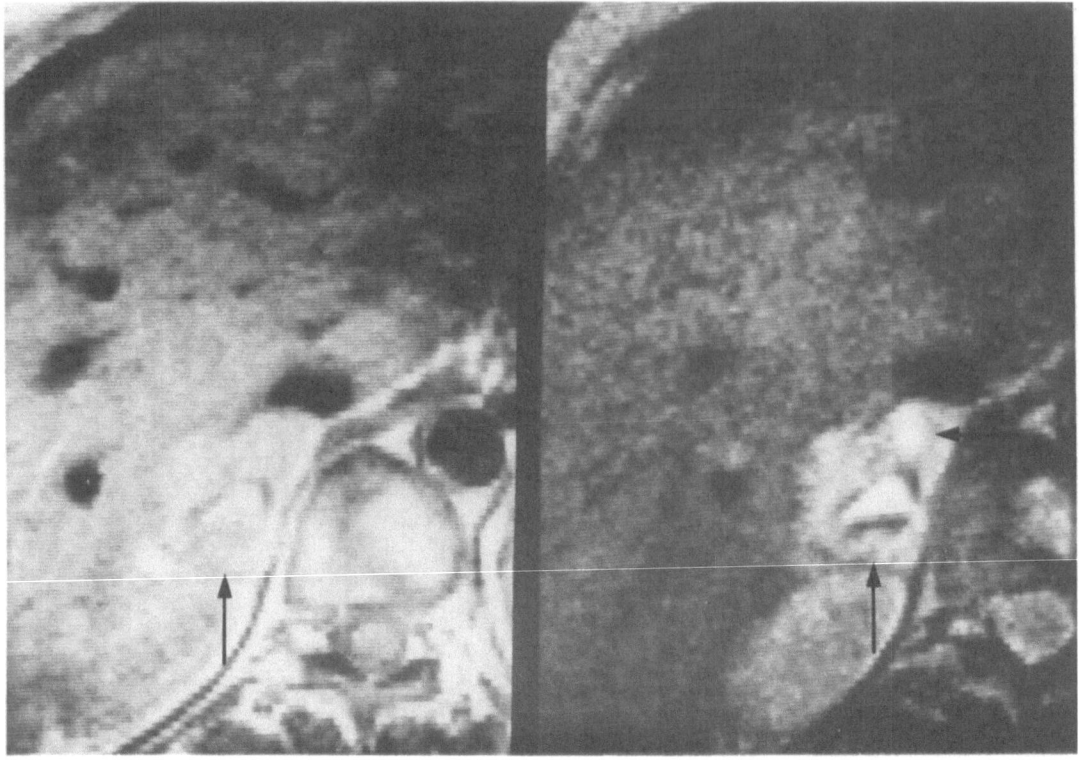

Figure 2.4. Magnetic resonance imaging of a tumor of the right adrenal gland (SED: TR 1,6; TE 22; 90; SD 5 mm, no contrast media). The patient has a proven pheochromocytoma of the right adrenal gland with a ventral and a dorsal cystic structure (arrows). The dorsal cyst is partially filled with hemosiderin due to previous hemorrhage. (Courtesy of H. König, M.D., Klinikum Steglitz, Berlin.)

use, and when distinguishing a benign adrenal lesion from a malignant one in the initial staging percutaneous biopsy is still required. In patients at low risk for adrenal malignancy, a low-signal-intensity adrenal lesion is most compatible with a benign adenoma.

Venous Sampling

Nodules are very common in the normal adrenal gland. They are usually not hormone-active. Phlebography should not be done for reasons that have been discussed previously; although displacement of parenchymal veins can be seen to suggest a tumor (Fig. 2.5). The accuracy of this examination is known to be only 50 to 80%. Small adenomas are easily overlooked and bilateral hyperplasia is difficult to diagnose, because in spite of hyperplasia the adrenal glands can be normal in size and shape

(24,26,28,29). Venography has side effects, whereas CT, US, and MRI do not. Selective bilateral catheterization of the adrenal veins in combination with blood sampling concentration provides a highly specific test. Its accuracy is described as being between 75 and 100%.

Selective venous sampling has become a rare event because of the high quality noninvasive imaging systems. Almost all adrenal tumors are localized noninvasively. If a tumor is too small to be seen or if it has to be determined that a tumor, incidentally found, could be responsible for the excessive hormone production, venous sampling remains the method of choice.

For a discussion of venous anatomy, see Anatomy and Anatomical Variations in Moltz and Sörensen (Chapter 1). For a discussion of technique, see Catheterization in Moltz and Sörensen (Chapter 1).

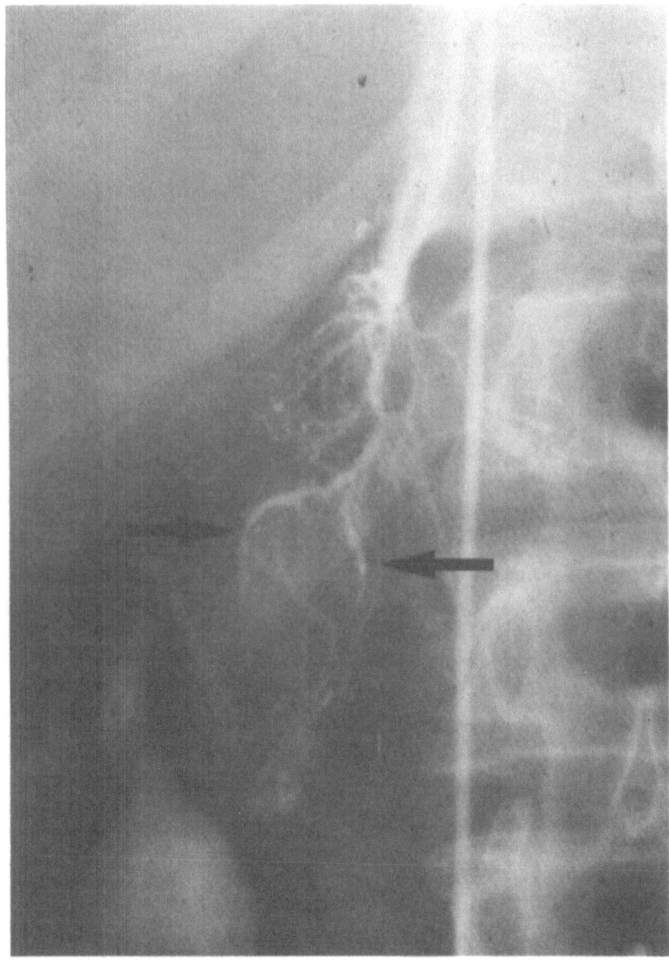

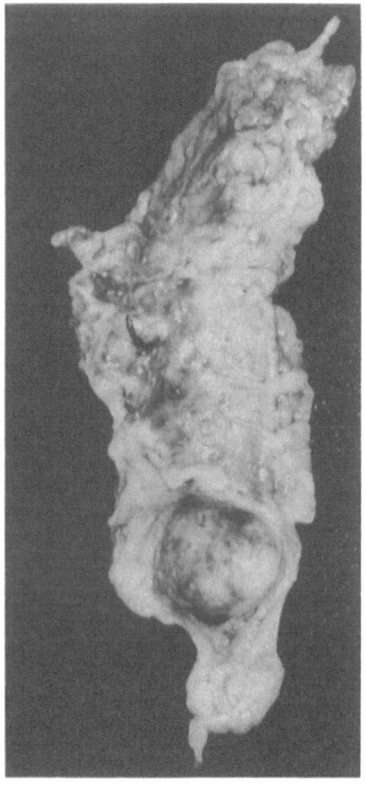

B

Figure 2.5. Retrograde phlebography of a small adenoma of the right adrenal gland. **A:** There is displacement of the venous structures. The veins are draped around the lesion (arrows). **B:** Surgical specimen of an adenoma.

A

Diseases of the Adrenal Cortex

Hypercortisolismus

Cushing's Syndrome

The cause of excess production of glucocorticoids can either be exogenous or endogenous. Exogenous Cushing's syndrome is the result of steroid therapy. There are two causes of endogenous Cushing's syndrome: autonomous adrenal tumors and cortical hyperplasia. Autonomous tumors of the adrenal cortex can be benign or malignant (adenomas, carcinomas). There is an increase of secretion of cortisol by these tumors. Unregulated excretion of adrenocorticotropic hormone (ACTH) can be the cause of adrenal hyperplasia. Patients with adrenal hyperplasia can have macronodules that may be diagnosed with computed tomography. In about 70% of patients with endogenous Cushing's syndrome the disease is caused by adrenal hyperplasia.

Cushing's Disease

Cushing's disease is caused by increased secretion of ACTH by different sources. In 75% of patients with Cushing's disease a microadenoma of the pituitary gland is diagnosed; 25% are found to have either an adenoma of the adrenal cortex or they show signs of ectopic ACTH production by a malignant tumor (39).

Bilateral adrenal hyperplasia (Fig. 2.6) is

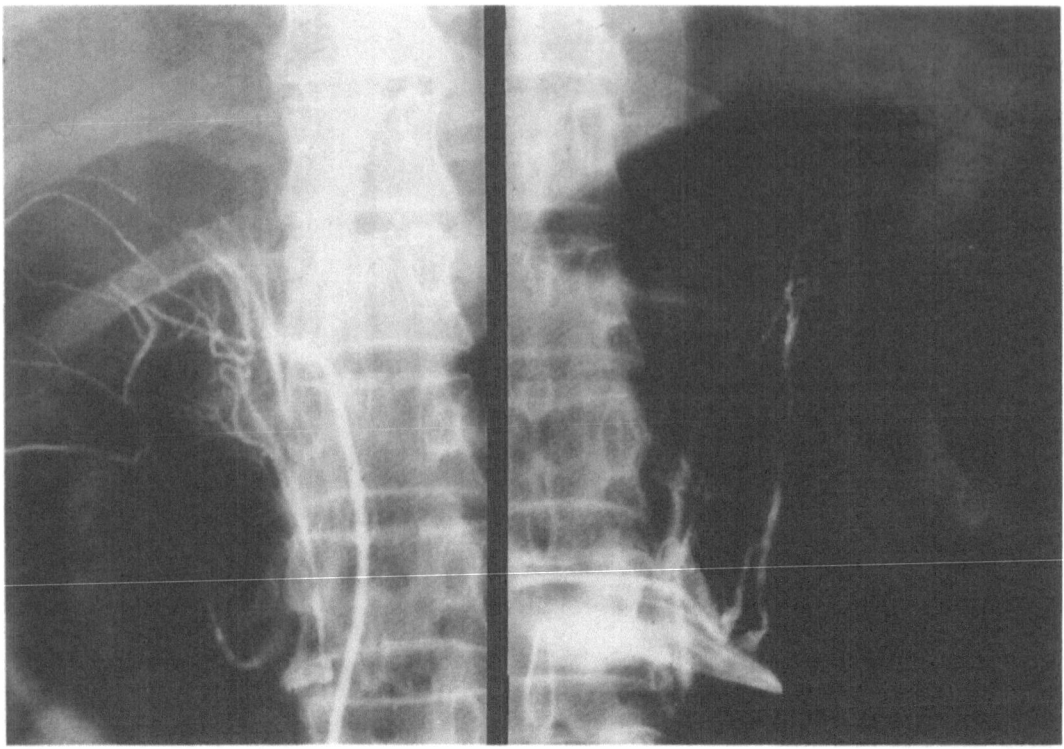

Figure 2.6. Adrenal hyperplasia. Retrograde phlebography of bilateral adrenal hyperplasia with very large adrenal veins in a patient with Cushing's disease caused by a microadenoma of the pituitary gland.

caused by a pituitary adenoma in most of the cases (75%). Ectopic ACTH syndrome can also cause bilateral hyperplasia and is the result of excessive production of ACTH or its precursors of nonpituitary origin. A variety of tumors may produce ACTH and are responsible for excretion of ACTH. This "ectopic ACTH syndrome" is seen in patients with small cell carcinoma of the lung (oat cell carcinoma), with tumors of the neuroectodermal tissue, thymomas, islet cell tumors of the pancreas, carcinoids of the lung, medullary thyroid cancers, pheochromocytomas, and ovarian tumors (39–41). A benign adrenal cortical adenoma may be the cause of endogenous Cushing's disease in approximately 20% of the cases; a carcinoma is responsible for this condition in 10%. Macronodular hyperplasia refers almost always to an ACTH-producing microadenoma of the pituitary gland (Fig. 2.7A,B). The macronodules are 1 to 3 cm in diameter. Primary pigmented nodular adrenocortical disease occurs

in children or young adults and is very rare. The hyperplastic cells within the pigmented nodules of the adrenals produce cortisol. The disease is treated by bilateral adrenalectomy.

Clinical Workup

If Cushing's syndrome is diagnosed biochemically, the source of excess hormones has to be located prior to treatment. Patients with pituitary hypercorticolism show suppression of 17-ketosteroids in their urine following the administration of dexamethasone in 40 to 50% of the cases.

A microadenoma of the pituitary gland can rarely be seen on a conventional tomogram. Computed tomography will almost always locate the source of hormone production. Dexamethasone does not suppress urine 17-ketosteroids in patients with ectopic ACTH production. The exception is a carcinoid tumor of the lung (20). To distinguish ectopic ACTH

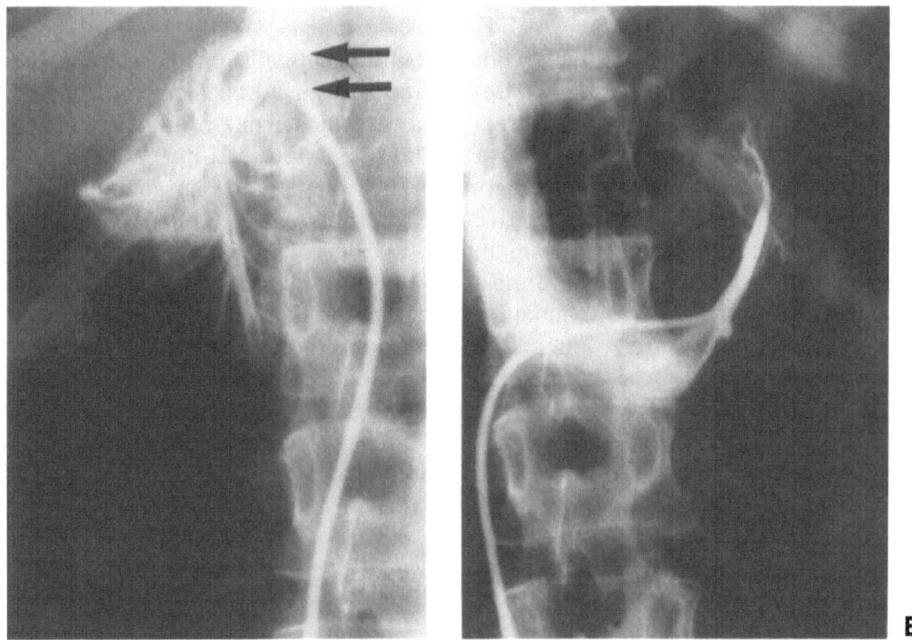

A

B

Figure 2.7. Macronodular hyperplasia. **A:** Retrograde phlebography of the right adrenal gland. The organ is very large and a nodule (arrows) is demonstrated by displacement of venous structures in the upper pole of the gland. **B:** Phlebography of the left adrenal gland. The organ is normal in size and shape. No nodularity is seen on phlebography; however, at surgical exploration several small nodules were found (**C**, arrow).

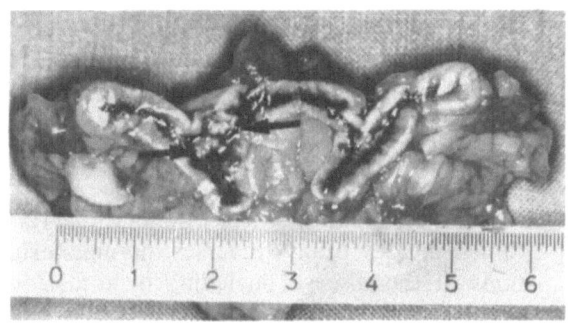

C,D: Surgical specimens of both right and left adrenal glands in a patient with Cushing's disease and macronodular hyperplasia. **C:** A very large right adrenal gland. A nodule was found at surgery according to the retrograde phlebogram.

C

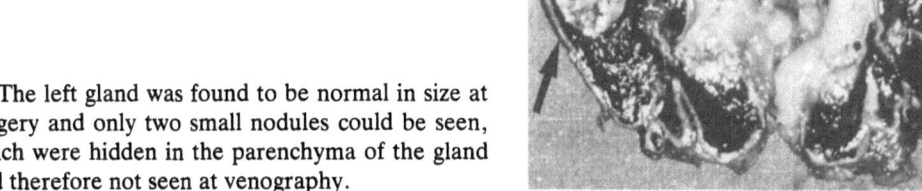

D: The left gland was found to be normal in size at surgery and only two small nodules could be seen, which were hidden in the parenchyma of the gland and therefore not seen at venography.

D

production from autonomous functioning adenomas of the adrenal gland, plasma ACTH levels should be determined. In patients with adenomas of the adrenal cortex, ACTH is suppressed evenly. Ectopic production causes normal and high ACTH levels in plasma. CT of the adrenals will demonstrate the tumor unless it is < 1 cm in diameter. Hormone-active tumors of the adrenal gland are usually small. If they exceed 7 cm in diameter they are most likely malignant (42). If noninvasive imaging techniques cannot find the source of increased hormone secretion, selective venous sampling is necessary.

Primary Hyperaldosteronism, Conn's Syndrome

Aldosterone is the most potent mineralocorticoid produced by the adrenal glands. It causes sodium retention and potassium loss. In the kidney, aldosterone is responsible for the transfer of sodium from the lumen of the distal tubule into the tubular cells in exchange for potassium and hydrogen. The same effect occurs in the salivary glands, sweat glands, and cells of the intestinal mucosa, and in the exchange between intra- and extracellular fluids.

Aldosterone secretion is regulated by the renin-angiotensin mechanism, and to a lesser extent by ACTH. Renin, a proteolytic enzyme, is stored in the juxtaglomerular cells of the kidney. Reduction in blood volume and flow in the afferent renal arterioles induces secretion of renin. Renin causes transformation of angiotensinogen to angiotensin I in the liver, which is converted to angiotensin II. Angiotensin II causes the secretion of aldosterone, cortisol, and desoxycorticosterone. The sodium and water retention resulting from increased aldosterone secretion increases the blood volume and reduces renin secretion. Aldosterone is measured by radioimmunoassay. In humans, aldosterone accounts for 50 to 60% of mineralocorticoid activity, with cortisol providing 30 to 40% and cortisone and others less than 10% (43–47).

Aldosterone-producing tumors of the adrenal cortex are usually benign nodules responsible for almost 80% of patients with primary hyperaldosteronism (Fig. 2.8). Primary hyperaldosteronism is due to an adenoma of the glomerulosa cells of the adrenal cortex or, rarely, to an adrenal carcinoma or to hyperplasia. Aldosterone-producing adenomas react not to angiotensin II but to ACTH (42). In 70 to 80% of patients, an adenoma is the cause of symptoms. Adenomas are bilateral in 2%; 20 to 30% of patients are considered to have idiopathic hyperaldosteronism (20,24,27,48–55); less than 1% of all hypertensive patients are found to have an aldosteronoma.

Bilateral adrenal hyperplasia accounts for only 20% of the cases with primary hyperaldosteronism. Adrenal cortical carcinoma very rarely produces symptoms of primary hyperaldosteronism (15).

Clinical Workup

Hypersecretion of aldosterone results in hypernatremia, hyperchlorhydria, hypervolemia, and a hypokalemic alkalosis manifested by episodes of weakness, paresthesias, transient paralysis, and tetany. Diastolic hypertension and a hypokalemic nephropathy with polyuria and polydipsia are common. Aldosterone excretion on a high sodium intake (> 10 gm/day) is usually > 200 μg/day if a tumor is present. Depriviation of sodium causes potassium retention. Personality disturbances hyperglycemia and glycosuria are occasionally seen. The only manifestation may be mild to moderate hypertension. The application of spironolactone (200 to 400 mg/day orally) reverses the manifestations of the disease, including hypertension, within 5 to 8 weeks and serves as a test. Measurement of the plasma renin activity is helpful to diagnose increased aldosterone secretion. This is usually carried out by determining the plasma renin activity in the morning with the patient recumbent, giving furosemide 80 mg orally, and then repeating the renin determination after the patient has remained upright for 3 hours. Normal individuals will have a marked increase in renin in the upright position, whereas the patient with hyperaldosteronism will not. About 20% of patients with essential hypertension, who do not necessarily have aldosteronism, have a low renin that does

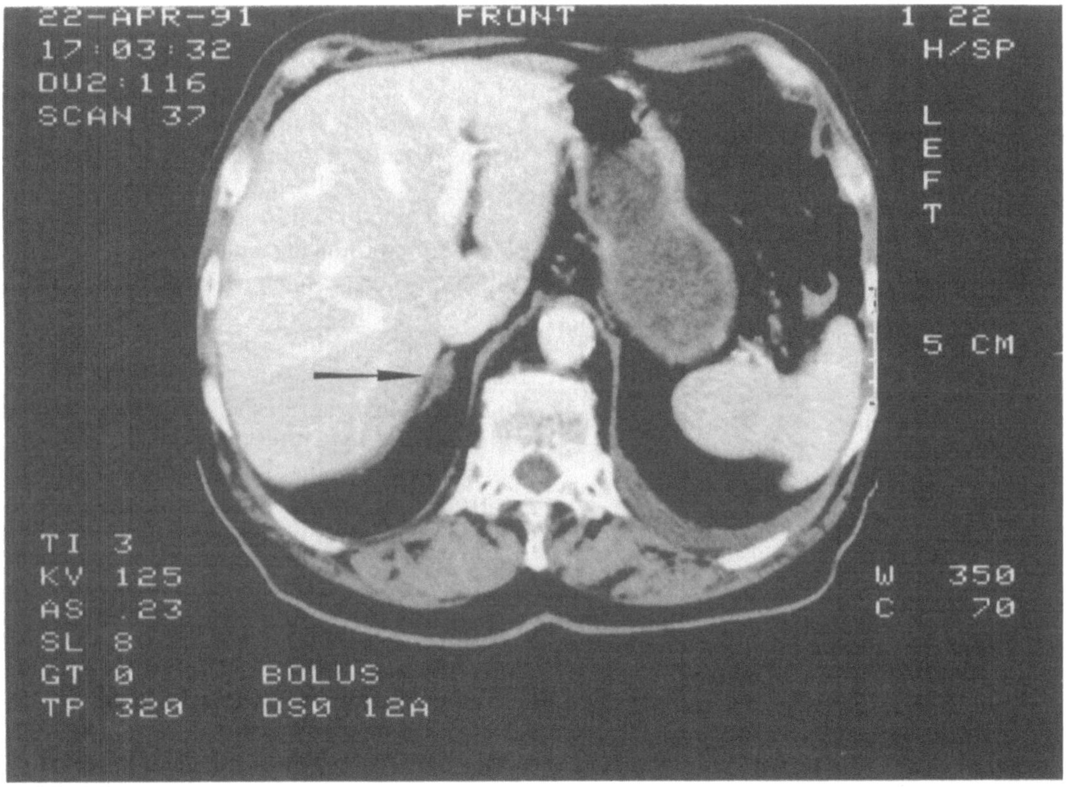

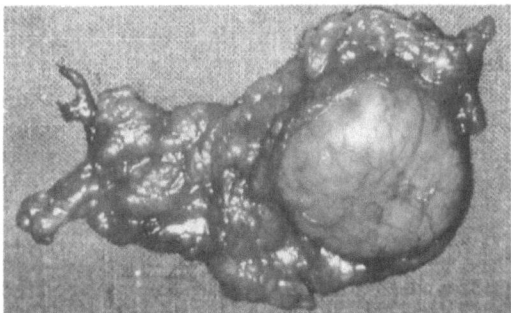

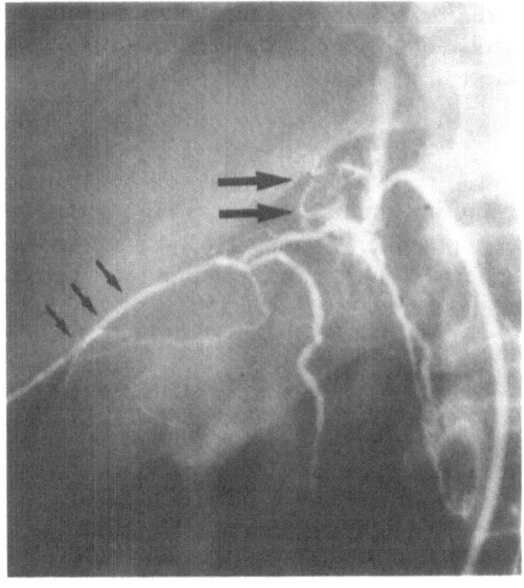

Figure 2.8. Aldosteronoma of the right adrenal gland in a patients with Conn's syndrome. **A:** CT shows a small nodule of the right adrenal gland (arrow). **B:** At retrograde venography a round small lesion can be identified by draping of venous structures (arrow). Several capsular veins are also demonstrated by retrograde filling (three arrows). **C:** At surgery a round small Conn adenoma was found corresponding to the CT and the phlebographic findings.

not respond to the upright position. Measurement of plasma aldosterone, either peripherally or following catheterization of the adrenal veins, may be helpful. The diagnosis is dependent upon demonstrating elevated secretion of aldosterone, either in urine or blood. CT will demonstrate a small adenoma in these cases (Fig. 2.8).

Secondary aldosteronism is an increased production of aldosterone by the adrenal cortex caused by stimuli originating outside the adrenal glands. This condition mimics the primary disease and is related to hypertension and edematous disorders such as cardiac failure, cirrhosis of the liver with ascites, and nephrotic syndrome. Secondary aldosteronism seen with the accelerated phase of hypertension is believed to be due to renin hypersecretion secondary to renal vasoconstriction. Aldosteronism is also seen in patients with hypertension due to obstructive renal artery disease by atheromas or by stenoses caused by the reduced blood flow into the affected kidney. Hypovolemia, which is common in edematous disorders, particularly during diuretic therapy, stimulates the renin-angiotensin mechanism with hypersecretion of aldosterone. Secretion rates may be normal in cardiac failure, but because hepatic blood flow and aldosterone metabolism are reduced the circulating level of the hormone is elevated.

Among patients with adenomas, hypokalemia may be expected in 90% or more if repeated samples are taken while patients are being kept on a low sodium diet. If the plasma renin activity (PRA) is low and the plasma aldosterone level is high or normal, an infusion of sodium chloride should be administered. If the plasma potassium level returns to normal and the plasma aldosterone level is suppressed, a primary hyperaldosteronism can be ruled out.

Invasive Diagnostic Procedures

Selective blood sampling procedures for the localization of excess hormone release have been described extensively in Moltz and Sörensen (Chapter 1).

Treatment

Once the diagnosis of aldosteronism is biochemically established, a tumor should be looked for noninvasively and, if necessary, by an invasive procedure followed by surgery. The prognosis is good when a solitary adenoma can be defined. Following the removal of an aldosterone-producing adenoma, the blood pressure decreases in all patients. Complete remission of the disease occurs in 70% of the cases. If adrenal hyperplasia is the cause for the hyperaldosteronism, about 70% of the patients remain hypertensive, although there is reduction of hypertension in most patients. Aldosteronism in these patients can usually be controlled by spironolactone. Bilateral adrenalectomy is rarely necessary.

Adrenogenital Syndrome

Adrenogenital syndrome is an inborn error of the adrenal enzyme system that blocks or impairs the synthesis of cortisol or aldosterone. Each different enzyme deficiency results in a different form of congenital adrenal hyperplasia. The clinical manifestations are determined by the degree of deficiency of cortisol, aldosterone, and by the biological properties of the biochemical intermediates that are secreted.

Feminizing Tumors

Feminizing tumors are rare as well and occur in men, prepubertal girls, and postmenopausal women. Clinical manifestation is gynecomastia.

Androgen-Producing Tumors

Androgen-producing tumors are described in Moltz and Sörensen (Chapter 1). Androgen-producing tumors are rare. They are benign or malignant, and occur in males or females at any age. Virilization is due to tumor present at a later age than in those with congenital hyperplasia. Clinical manifestations are amenorrhea, hirsutism, enlargement of the clitoris, and deepening of the voice.

Diseases of the Adrenal Medulla

Hypercatecholaminism and Pheochromocytoma

Pheochromocytomas are tumors of the chromaffin cells of the adrenal medulla. Their excessive and fluctuating production of catecholamine produces hypertension. They are found in 0.1% of the hypertensive population (56–59). It is important to diagnose these tumors because they are a vital threat to the patient (hypertensive crisis) and they are curable by surgery. Less than 5% are malignant. Extraadrenal pheochromocytomas (paragangliomas) are more likely to be malignant. Pheochromocytomas can be part of the syndrome of familial multiple endocrine adenomatosis—type II (Sipple's syndrome), and may be found along with or associated with medullary thyroid carcinoma and parathyroid adenomas. A type III syndrome has been described that includes pheochromocytoma, mucosal (oral and ocular) neuroma, and medullary thyroid carcinoma. There is a significant association (10%) with neurofibromatosis (von Recklinghausen's disease) and it may be found with hemangiomas, as in von Hippel-Lindau disease (56,60–66). The multiple endocrine neoplasia (MEN) syndrome, type IIa, includes medullary carcinoma of the thyroid and parathyroid hyperplasia as well as pheochromocytoma. MEN syndrome type IIb comprises pheochromocytoma, medullary carcinoma of the thyroid, and mucocutaneous manifestations including mucosal neuromas, intestinal ganglioneuromatosis, and a marfanoid habitus. All manifestations of the syndrome may not occur at the same time. The history of a previous abnormality should be obtained. These abnormalities are inherited in an autosomal-dominant fashion.

There is also a syndrome of familial pheochromocytoma not associated with other endocrine tumors.

Pheochromocytomas are found wherever chromaffin cells are located, within the sympathetic ganglia, and most likely in the adrenal medulla (90%). In about 80% of the cases, pheochromocytomas are located in the adrenal medulla, but may also be found in other tissue derived from neural crest cells. They appear equally in both sexes, are bilateral in 10% of the cases (20% in children), and are usually benign (95%). They occur at any age; the maximum incidence is between the third and fifth decades.

Extraadrenal tumors are found from the carotid bifurcation to the urinary bladder, most of them within the paravertebral ganglia, in the organ of Zuckerkandl at the aortic bifurcation, or in dermoid cysts. The second most common location of extraadrenal tumors is the mediastinum. Multiple lesions occur in 10%. Bilateral adrenal tumors are found in familial MEN syndrome (64). Bilateral hyperplasia of the medulla is probably the precursor of pheochromocytoma (62).

Pheochromocytomas can vary in size but the avarage diameter is 5 to 6 cm. The tumor is usually well encapsulated (Fig. 2.9). It may be considered to be benign if it has not invaded the capsule and if no metastases are found.

Tumors are located in the adrenal medulla (90%). Pheochromocytomas associated with MEN II syndromes are always intraadrenal. Pheochromocytomas found in MEN II patients are usually multicentric and involve both adrenal glands in more than 80% of cases. They are usually benign, but in approximately 13% demonstrate malignant behavior.

Extraadrenal pheochromocytomas (paragangliomas) are found along the sympathetic chain in the retroperitoneum. Sporadic pheochromocytomas are located outside the adrenal gland in as many as 25% of cases.

Clinical Workup

Clinical symptoms are related to catecholamine release and include headache, palpitations, anxiety, and hot flushes (67,68). The symptoms appear paroxysmally and are combined with hypertension. The episodes usually last only a few minutes, but sometimes they continue for hours. Measurements of catecholamines, total metanephrine, and vanillylmandelic acid in the urine are routine examinations to establish the diagnosis (61). The most prom-

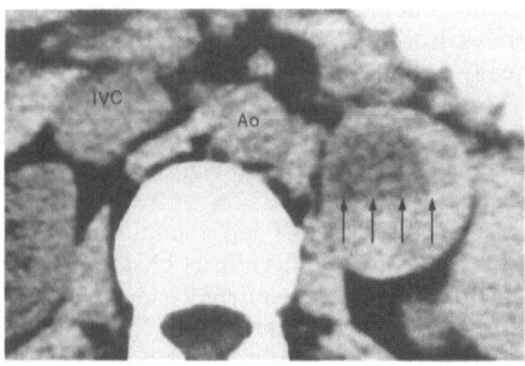

A

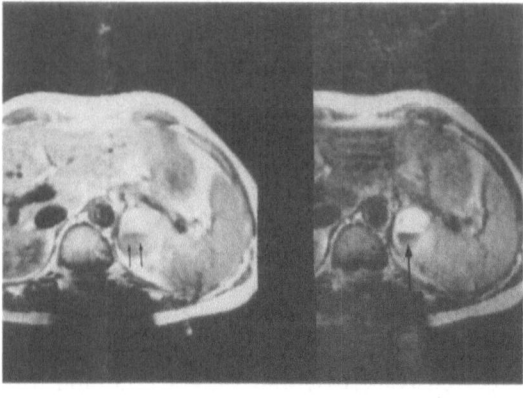

B

Figure 2.9. **A:** Computed tomography of a proven pheochromocytoma of the left adrenal gland following an infusion of contrast media. There is evidence of hemorrhage into a cystic structure with layering of contrast media. (Courtesy of H. König, M.D., Klinikum Steglitz, Berlin.)

B: Magnetic resonance image of a pheochromocytoma of the left adrenal gland (same patient; TR 1,6; TE22; 90; SD 5 mm, no contrast media). There is layering of blood from a previous hemorrhage into the cyst (hemosiderin) and the contents of the cyst. (Courtesy of H. König, M.D., Klinikum Steglitz, Berlin.)

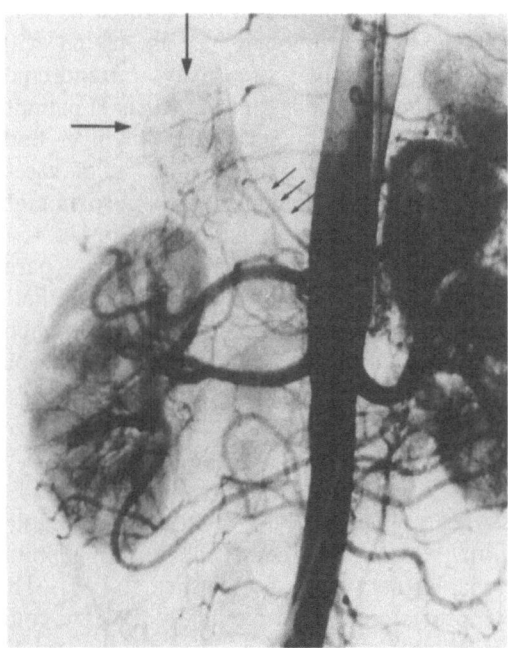

C

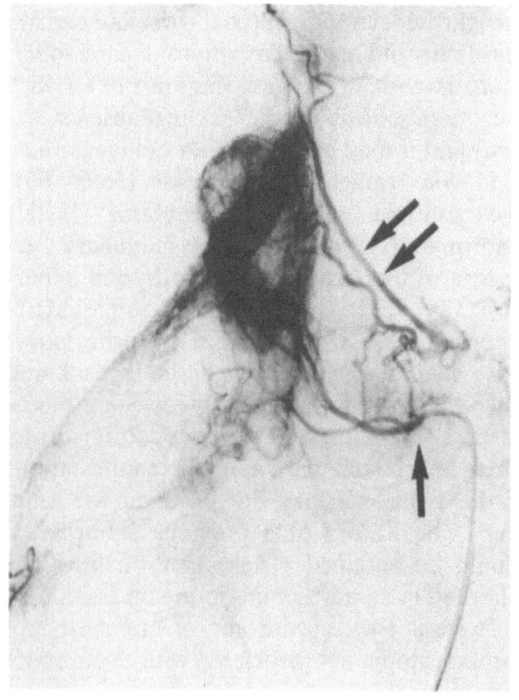

D

C,D: Arteriography of a pheochromocytoma of the right adrenal gland. **C:** Aortography, subtraction film: a vascular mass is demonstrated replacing the right adrenal gland. **D:** Selective injection into the middle adrenal artery. There is retrograde filling of the inferior phrenic artery via the superior adrenal artery. The tumor is well demonstrated.

inent feature is hypertension, which may be paroxysmal (45%) or persistent (50%) and rarely is absent. It is due to secretion of one or more of the catecholamine hormones or precursors: norepinephrine, epinephrine, dopamine, or dopa. Additionally, tachycardia, diaphoresis, postural hypotension, tachypnea, flushing, cold and clammy skin, severe headache, angina, palpitation, nausea, vomiting, epigastric pain, visual disturbances, dyspnea, paresthesias, constipation, and a sense of impending doom are common; some or all of these symptoms and signs may occur in any patient. Paroxysmal attacks may be provoked by palpation of the tumor, postural changes, abdominal compression or massage, induction of anesthesia, emotional trauma, β-adrenergic blocking agents, and, rarely, micturition.

Physical examination except for the common finding of hypertension, usually is normal, unless performed during a paroxysmal attack. The severity of retinopathy and cardiomegaly is often less extensive than might be expected for the degree of hypertension present.

If a pheochromocytoma is suspected, the diagnosis can be made by measuring elevated levels of serum or urine catecholamines. Urinary metanephrines or vanillylmandelic acid (VMA) are elevated in over 90% of patients when 24-hour urine collections are measured. Epinephrine, norepinephrine, and dopamine can be measured by liquid chromatography, which further aids in the diagnosis. Several separate determinations should be made because of the episodic hormone secretion found in these patients. Furthermore, patients taking medications such as methyldopa or mandelamine may have falsely high catecholamine levels. The urinary metabolic products of epinephrine and norepinephrine are the metanephrines and VMA. Normal persons excrete only very small amounts of these substances in the urine. Measurements of catecholamines, total metanephrine, and VMA in the urine are routine examinations to establish the diagnosis (61).

Normal values for 24 hours are: free epinephrine and norepinephrine <100 μg; total metanephrine <1.3 mg; and VMA <10 mg. In pheochromocytoma and neuroblastoma,

there is an intermittent increased urinary excretion of epinephrine, norepinephrine, and their metabolic products. Excretion of these compounds may be measured in the same urine specimen. The methods of detection of VMA and metanephrines depend upon the conversion to vanillin, the extraction of vanillin into toluene, and the final spectrophotometric determination of vanillin at 360 my. These values may be exceeded in patients being treated with rauwolfia alkaloids, methyldopa, or catecholamines, or following the ingestion of foods containing large quantities of vanilla, especially if renal insufficiency is present. Catecholamines (mainly epinephrine and norepinephrine) are measured fluorometrically after extraction and absorption on alumina gel. Interference from epinephrine-like drugs, antihypertensiva (e.g., methyldopa), and other drugs that produce fluorescence (tetracycline, quinine) must be considered in the evaluation of abnormal results. Radioenzymatic procedures are also available.

Plasma catecholamines determinations are usually of no value unless they are collected during a paroxysm or following a drug such as glucagon that is known to provoke the release of catecholamines.

Because of their hyperkinetic state these patients may have an elevated basal metabolic rate (BMR) in spite of being euthyroid. Although the BMR is rarely measured, these patients appear hyperkinetic. Blood volume is reported to be constricted. Hyperglycemia, glucosuria, or overt diabetes mellitus may be present with elevated fasting levels of plasma free fatty acid and glycerol. Plasma insulin concentrations are inappropriately low for the simultaneously collected plasma glucose values.

Provocative tests with histamine or tyramine are hazardous and should not be used. Glucagon (0.2 to 1 mg injected rapidly I.V.) will provoke a rise in blood pressure exceeding 35/25 mm Hg within 2 minutes in normotensive patients with pheochromocytoma. Phentolamine mesylate must be available to terminate any hypertensive crisis.

If a patient with pheochromocytoma is hypertensive, 5 mg of phentolamine injected intravenously will cause a fall in blood pressure (BP) exceeding 35/25 mm Hg within 2 minutes. False-positive results occur in patients with uremia, stroke, and malignant hypertension, and in those taking certain pharmacologic agents. A modification of this test has been developed that takes advantage of catecholamine inhibition of insulin release. An intravenous infusion of 10% glucose and water is given (2 ml/min) 30 minutes prior to injection of phentolamine (blood is sampled twice for measurement of glucose and insulin prior to the injection). Following the administration of phentolamine, each time the BP is measured, blood is again sampled. A pheochromocytoma is present if there is a significant fall in BP, a fall in glucose exceeding 18 mg/dl, or a rise in insulin exceeding 13 μU/ml.

A new test using oral clonidine has been described. Forty-eight hours after discontinuation of all drug therapy that acts on the sympathetic nervous system, the patient is treated with 0.3 mg of clonidine. Blood is drawn for plasma catecholamine determinations prior to and 3 hours following the administration of the drug. The normal response is a decrease of plasma norepinephrine to normal (<400 ng/ml) and a decrease of at least 40% of the basal plasma level. Patients with pheochromocytoma maintain elevated plasma catecholamines.

Noninvasive Imaging

The lesion usually can be diagnosed by US, CT, and MRI (Fig. 2.3, 2.4, 2.9) if it is not smaller than 1 cm in diameter.

Pheochromocytomas are usually hyperintense on T2-weighted images at low and middle field strengths. High-signal-intensity adrenal masses are not "pathognomonic" for pheochromocytomas, because necrotic metastases, cysts, and acute inflammation can produce hyperintensity of adrenal MRI images. However, when elevated urinary or serum catecholamine levels are present, a hyperintense adrenal or extraadrenal mass invariably represents a pheochromocytoma. For most adrenal pheochromocytomas, CT is adequate to suggest the diagnosis in the presence of elevated serum and urine catecholamine levels. When

the masses are bilateral and particularly when they are ectopic, MRI can be quite useful in localizing the ectopic site.

Radiopharmaceuticals have been used to localize pheochromocytomas with nuclear imaging techniques. Usually metaiodobenzylguanidine (MIBG) containing 0.5 mCi of 131-iodine is injected intravenously and the patient is scanned on days 1, 2, and 3. Normal adrenal tissue does not store this isotope but 90% of pheochromocytomas do. Extraadrenal tumors may be visualized by scintigraphy with 131-iodine MIBG (69).

Invasive Imaging

Arteriography and venography should be done only if patients are treated with phenoxybenzamine prior to the procedure in order to prevent the provocation of a hypertensive crisis. Aortography with subtraction and venous blood sampling from all branches of the superior and inferior vena cava can be helpful to locate the tumor (Figs. 2.8, 2.9).

Treatment

Surgery is the treatment of choice. The patient should be treated with β-adrenergic blocking agents until the surgical procedure is performed (phenoxybenzamine 40 to 160 mg/day and propranolol 30 to 60 mg/day, and an infusion of trimethaphan camsylate or sodium nitroprusside). When adrenergic blocking agents are used, the alpha-compounds should be started first. Metyrosine may be used alone or in combination with α-adrenergic blocking agents (phenoxybenzamine); the optimally effective dosage of metyrosine should be given for at least 5 to 7 days prior to surgery.

Malignant Tumors of the Adrenal Gland

Primary adrenal cortical carcinoma is an uncommon malignancy. Men and women are affected equally, but functional tumors are more common among females. The age range is 1 to 80 years. Adrenal cortical carcinomas are more common on the left side. They occur up to 10% bilaterally. Usually they are quite

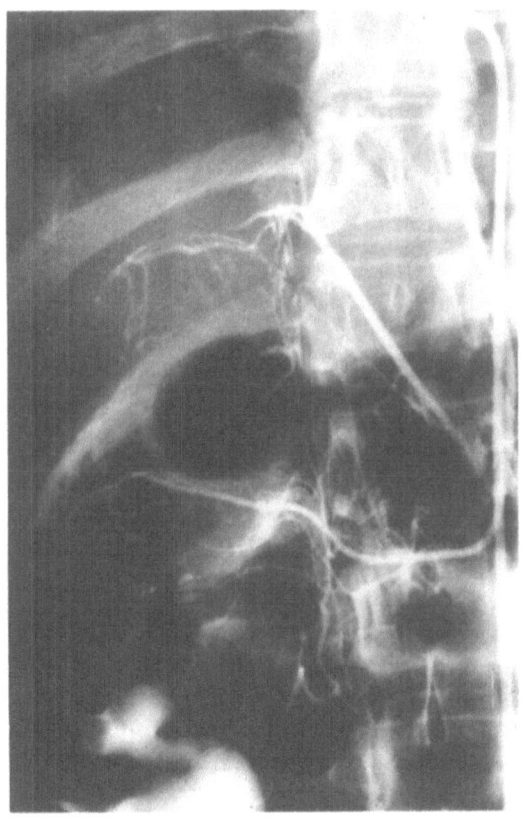

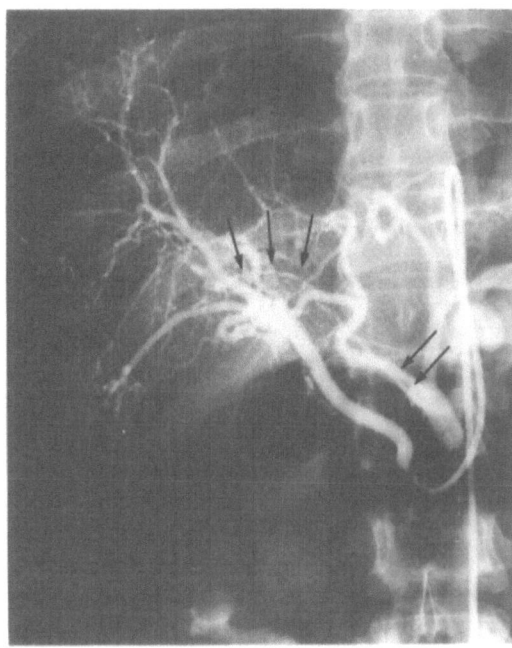

B

A

Figure 2.10. Arteriography of an adrenal carcinoma. **A:** Injections into a renal capsular artery. There is retrograde filling of the middle and superior adrenal arteries by multiple tumor vessels in the region of the right adrenal gland. **B:** Injection into the right hepatic artery shows retrograde filling of a middle hepatic artery and of an occluded celiac trunk. Multiple tumor vessels are seen in the liver due to direct invasion of the adrenal carcinoma partially supplied by the inferior phrenic artery (arrows).

large at presentation. Symptoms are abdominal pain or a palpable mass. Malignant tumors of the adrenal gland can have signs of hormone overproduction; 50% are functional and may be detected by the manifestations of excess hormone production (35,36). Cushing's syndrome is the most frequent symptom, followed by virilization and feminization. Aldosteronism is rarely due to a carcinoma. Patients with increased cortisol levels without an increase in androgen production are more likely to have an adenoma. Androgen excess—dehydroepiandrosterone (DHEA), dehydroepiandrosterone sulfate (DHEA-S), androstenedione, and testosterone—occurs more likely in malignant lesions. They can be found by examination of peripheral blood samples, by radioimmunoassay (RIA), and by analyzing metabolites of

DHEA and DHEA-S that are excreted in the urine (17-ketosteroids).

The hormone production of carcinomas of the adrenal cortex cannot be suppressed by dexamethasone or stimulated by ACTH. CT usually gives the diagnosis of a larger lesion. Carcinomas of the adrenal gland rarely are an indication for venous blood sampling. There may be, however, an indication for arteriography, to demonstrate for the surgeon the extent of the disease (Figs. 2.10 and 2.11).

Incidentalomas

"Incidentalomas" are small adrenal nodules, 1 to 3 cm in diameter, incidentally diagnosed by computed tomography, magnetic resonance imaging, or ultrasound (42,70). They are found

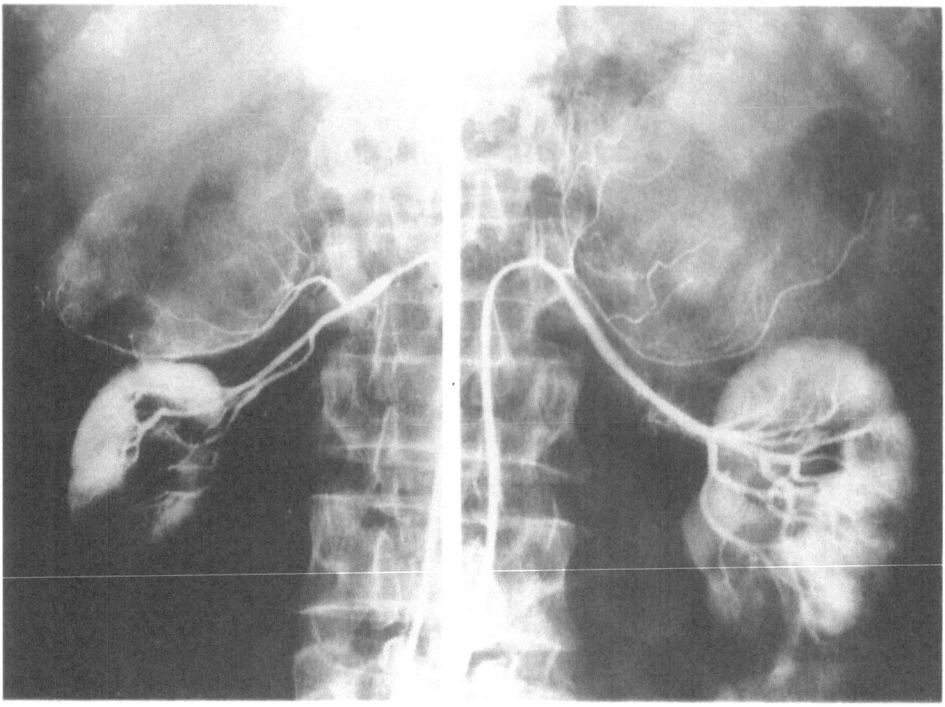

Figure 2.11. Arteriography of bilateral adrenal metastases. Injection into both renal arteries with filling of the inferior adrenal arteries. The patient has a sarcoma.

in approximately in 1% of patients during computed tomography (1,34). One to 9% of nonfunctioning adrenal nodules are incidentally detected in large autopsy series (71). If they are hormone active, venous sampling should verify the diagnosis and this should be followed by surgery. If they are not producing hormones, a follow-up CT 3 months later can determine growth. If a nodule is less than 4 cm in size and has not grown at reexamination, it is not likely that the tumor is a carcinoma. If there has been no change in size, no further therapy is necessary.

Incidentalomas in patients with a history of cancer need to be examined more carefully. If they are bilateral they are usually assumed to be metastases except in patients with pheochromocytoma (1). MRI may solve this problem by tissue characterization. CT-guided biopsy can be obtained for tissue diagnosis (72).

Conclusion

Venous sampling of the adrenal glands is the method of choice to locate excess hormone production, if a tumor cannot be demonstrated by noninvasive imaging systems. Sampling is also a reliable examination in lesions seen with other imaging modalities, if it is unknown whether they are responsible for the excess hormone release or not. In skilled hands it is a simple procedure and can be performed on an outpatient basis.

References

1. Chan FL, Wang C. Imaging for adrenal tumors. *Bailliéres Clin Endocrinol Metab* 1989;3:153–189.
2. Sample WF. Adrenal ultrasonography. *Radiology* 1978;127:461.
3. Yeh HC. Sonography of the adrenal glands: normal glands and small masses. *AJR* 1980;135:1167.
4. Abrams JE, Siegelmann SS, Adams DF et al. Computed tomography versus ultrasound of the adrenal glands: a prospective study. *Radiology* 1982;143:121–128.
5. Barbarino A, DeMarinis L, Liberale I, Mincini E. Evaluation of steroid laboratory tests and adrenal gland imaging with radiocholesterol in the aetiological diagnosis of Cushing's syndrome. *Clin Endocrinol* 1979;10:107–121.
6. Gross MD, Shapiro B, Gretkin RJ, Freitas JE. Scintigraphic localization of adrenal lesions in primary aldosteronism. *Am J Med* 1984;77:839.
7. Guerin CK, Wahner HW, Gorman CA, Carpenter PC, Sheedy PF. Computed tomographic scanning versus radioisotopic imaging in adrenocortical diagnosis. *Am J Med* 1983;75:653.
8. Lynn MD, Shapiro B, Sisson JC, et al. Pheochromocytoma and the normal adrenal medulla: improved visualization with I-123 MIBG scintigraphy. *Radiology* 1985;156:789–792.
9. Bomanji J, Conry BG, Britton KE, Reznek RH, Imaging neural crest tumours with ^{123}I-metaiodobenzylguanidine and x-ray computed tomography: a comparative study. *Clin Radiol* 1988;39:502–506.
10. Sisson JC, Frager MS, Valk TW, et al. Scintigraphic localization of pheochromocytoma. *N Engl J Med* 1981;305:12–17.
11. Swensen SJ, Brown ML, Sheps SG, et al. ^{131}I-MIBG in the evaluation of suspected pheochromocytoma. *Mayo Clin Proc* 1985;60:299–304.
12. Reynes CJ, Churchill R, Moncada R, Love L. Computed tomography of adrenal glands. *Radiol Clin North Am* 1979;17:91–104.
13. Chang A, Glazer HS, Lee JKT, Ling D, Heiken JP. Adrenal gland: MR imaging. *Radiology* 1987;153:123–128.
14. Johnson CM, Sheedy PF II, Welch TJ, Hattery RR. CT of the adrenal cortex. *Semin Ultrasound CT MR* 1985;6:241–260.
15. Dunnick NR, Schaner EG, Doppman JL, Strott CA, Gill JR, Javadpour N. Computed tomography of adrenal tumors. *AJR* 1979;132:43.
16. Elie G, Le Treut A, Dilhuydy MH, Brueneton JN, Calabet A. Computed tomography examination of the adrenal tumors in adults. *J Radiol* 1980;61:597.
17. Haertel M, Probst P, Bollmann J, Zingg E, Fuchs WA, Computertomographische Nebennierendiagnostik. *ROFO* 1980;132:31.
18. Hofer B, Triller J, Haertel M. Sonographisch-phlebographische Diagnostik der Nebenniere. *ROFO* 1978;129:686.
19. Hübener KH, Grehn ST, Schulze K. Indikation zur computertomographischen Nebennierenuntersuchung: Leistungsfähigkeit, Stellenwert und Differentialdiagnostik. *ROFO* 1980;132:37.
20. Korobkin M, White EA, Kressel HY, Moss AA. Computed tomography in the diagnosis of adrenal disease. *AJR* 1979;132:231.
21. Meek DR, Duncan JG, McAreavey D. Computed tomography in the localization of aldosteronesecreting adrenal adenomas. *Clin Endocrinol* 1981;15:593.
22. Mödder UR, Lang R, Rosenberg J, Friedmann G. Computed tomography in the diagnosis of adrenal disease. *Dtsch Med Wochenschr* 1980;105:478.
23. Scherer K, Mischke W. Wertigkeit der Ultraschalluntersuchungen bei Tumoren und Hyperplasien der Nebenniere. *ROFO* 1978;128:609.
24. Bravo EL, Tarazi RC, Dustan HP, Fovad FM, Textor SC, Gifford RW, Vidt DG. The changing clinical spectrum of primary aldosteronism. *Am J Med* 1983;74:641.
25. Geisinger MA, Zeich MG, Bravo EL, et al. Primary hyperaldosteronism: Comparison of CT, adrenal venography and venous sampling. *AJR* 1983;141:299.
26. McAreavey D, Brown JJ, Cumming AMM, Davidson JK, Duncan JG, Fraser R, Lever AF, Meck D, Robertson JIS. Preoperative localization of aldosterone-secreting adrenal adenomas. *Clin Endocrinol* 1981;15:593.
27. Swales JD. Primary aldosteronism: How hard should we look? *Br Med J* 1983;287:702.
28. Weinberger MH, Grim CE, Hollifield JW, Kem DC, Ganguly A, Kramer NS, Yane HY, Wellman H, Donohue JP. Primary aldosteronism: Diagnosis, localization and treatment. *Ann Intern Med* 1979;90:386.
29. Weinberger MH. Primary aldosteronism: Diagnosis and differentiation of subtypes. *Ann Intern Med* 1984;100:300.
30. White EA, Schambelan M, Rost CR, Biglieri EG, Moss AA, Korobkin M. Use of computed tomography in diagnosing the cause of primary aldosteronism. *N Engl J Med* 1980;303:1503.

31. Remer EM, Weinfeld RM, Glazer GM, et al. Hyperfunctioning and nonhyperfunctioning benign adrenal cortical lesions: Characterization and comparison with MR imaging. *Radiology* 1989;171:681–685.

32. Choyke PL, Filling-Katz MR, Shawker TH, et al. Von Hippel-Lindau disease: Radiologic screening for visceral manifestations. *Radiology* 1990;174:815–820.

33. Reinig JW, Doppman JL, Dwyer AJ, Frank J. MRI of indeterminate masses. *AJR* 1986;147: 493–496.

34. Glazer GM, Woolsey EJ, Borrello J, et al. Adrenal tissue characterization using MR imaging. *Radiology* 1986;158:73–79.

35. Baker ME, Blinder R, Spritzer CE, et al. MR evaluation of adrenal masses at 1.5 T. *AJR* 1989;153:307–312.

36. Kier R, McCarthy S. MR characterization of adrenal masses: Field strength and pulse sequence considerations. *Radiology* 1989;171: 671–674.

37. Chezmar JL, Robbins SM, Nelson RC, Steinberg HV, Torres WE, Bernardino ME. Adrenal masses: Characterization with Tl-weighted MR imaging. *Radiology* 1988;166:357–359.

38. Chang A, Glazer HS, Lee JKT, Ling D, Heiken JP. Adrenal gland: MR imaging. *Radiology* 1982;163:123–128.

39. Huff TA. Clinical syndromes related to disorders of adreno-corticotropic hormones. In: Allen M, Mahesh V, eds. *The Pituitary: A Current Review*. New York: Academic Press; 1977:153.

40. Azzopardi J, Williams E. Pathology of nonendocrine tumors associated with Cushing syndrome. *Cancer* 1968;22:274.

41. Ratcliffe J, Knight R, Besser G. Tumor and plasma ACTH concentration in patients with and without the ectopic ACTH syndrome. *Clin Endocrinol* 1972;1:27.

42. Copeland P. The incidentally discovered adrenal mass. *Ann Intern Med* 1983;98:940.

43. Banks WA, Kastin AJ, Biglieri EG, Ruiz AE. Primary adrenal hyperplasia: A new subset of primary hyperaldosteronism. *J Clin Endocrinol Metab* 1984;3:783.

44. Drury PL, Al-Pujaili EAS, Edwards CRW. The renin-angiotensin-aldosterone system. In: O'Riordan JHL, ed. *Recent Advances in Endocrinology and Metabolism*, vol. 2. Edinburgh: Churchill Livingstone; 1982:157.

45. Drury PL. Disorders of mineralocorticoid activity. *Clin Endocrinol Metab* 1985;14:175.

46. Vaughan ED, Bühler FR, Laragh JH, Sealey JE, Baer L, Bard RH. Renovascular hypertension: renin measurement to indicate hypersecretion and contralateral suppression, estimate renal plasma flow, and score for surgical curability. *Am J Med* 1973;55:402.

47. Fraser IR, Beretta-Piccooli C, Brown JJ, et al. Response of aldosterone and 18-hydroxycorticosterone to angiotensin H in normal subjects and patients with essential hypertension. Conn's syndrome and non-tumorous hyperaldosteronism. *Hypertension* 1981;3 (suppl 1):187.

48. Beevers DG, Nelson CS, Padfield PL, et al. The prevalence of hypertension in an unselected population and the frequency of abnormalities of potassium, angiotensin II and aldosterone in hypertensive subjects. *Acta Clin Belg* 1974; 29:276.

49. Berglund G, Andersson O, Wilhelmsen L. Prevalence of primary and secondary hypertension: studies in a random population sample. *Br Med J* 1976;2:554.

50. Conn JW, Knopf RF, Nesbit RM. Clinical characteristics of primary aldosteronism from an analysis of 145 cases. *Am J Surg* 1964;107:159.

51. Davies DR, Ives DR, Shaw DG, Thomas BM, Watson L. Selective venous catheterization and radioimmunoassay of parathyroid hormone in the diagnosis and localization of parathyroid tumors. *Lancet* 1973;1:1079.

52. Davies DL, Beevers DG, Brown JJ, Cumming AMM, Morton JJ, Robertson JJS, Titterington M, Tree M. Aldosterone and its stimuli in normal and hypertensive man: Are essential hypertension and primary hyperaldosteronism without tumour the same condition? *J Endocrinol* 1979;81:79.

53. Hug MS, Pfaff M, Jaspersen D, Zicker JR, Kirschner MA. Concurrence of aldosterone, androgen, and cortisol secretion in adrenal venous effluents. *Clin Endocrinol Metab* 1976;42:230.

54. Tait JF, Tait SAS. Recent perspectives on the history of adrenal cortex. *J Endocrinol* 1979; 83:3.

55. Thibonnier M, Sassano P, Dufloux MA, Plouin PF, Corvol P, Menard J. Test diagnostique simple de l'hyperaldosteronisme. *Presse Med* 1983; 12:1461.

56. Beard CM, Sheps SG, Kurland LT, Carney JA, Lie JT. Occurrence of pheochromocytoma in Rochester, Minnesota 1950 through 1979. *Mayo Clin Proc* 1983;58:802.

57. Sutton H, Wyeth P, Allen AP, Thurtle OA, Hames TK, Cawley MID, Ackery D. Disseminated malignant pheochromocytoma: localiza-

tion with iodine-131-1abeled metaiodobenzyl-guanidine. *Br Med J* 1982;285:1153.

58. Valk TW, Frager MS, Gross MD, Sisson JC, Wieland DM, Swanson DP, Manager TJ, Beier-walles WH. Spectrum of pheochromocytoma in multiple endocrine neoplasia: a scintigraphic portrayal using 131-I-metaiodobenzylguanidine. *Ann Intern Med* 1981;94:762.

59. Van Heerden JA, Sheps SG, Hamberger B, Sheedy PF, Poston JG, Remine W. Pheochromocytoma: current status and changing trends. *Surgery* 1982;91:367.

60. Carney JH, Go VLW, Sizeniore GW, Hayles HB. Alimentary tract ganglioneuromatosis: a major component of the syndrome of multiple endocrine neoplasia ' type 2b. *N Engl J Med* 1976;295:1287.

61. Cryer PE. Physiology and pathophysiology of the human sympathoadrenal neuroendocrine system. *N Engl J Med* 1980;303:136.

62. De Lellis RH, Wolfe HJ, Gagel RF, et al. Adrenal medullary hyperplasia. *Am J Pathol* 1976;83:177.

63. Hamilton BP, Landsberg RJ. Measurement of urinary epinephrine in screening for pheochromocytoma in multiple endocrine neoplasia type II. *Am J Med* 1978;65:1027.

64. Lips KJM, Veer JVDS, Struyvenberg A, Alleman A, Leo JR, Wittebol P, Minder WH, Kooiker CJ, Geerdink RA, Van Waes PFGM, Hackeng WHL. Bilateral occurrence of pheochromocytoma in patients with the multiple endocrine neoplasia type 2a (Sipple's syndrome). *Am J Med* 1981;70:1051.

65. Shea SD, Tse TF, Clutter WE, Cryer PE. The human sympathochromaffin system. *Am J Physiol* 1984;247:E380.

66. Steiner AL, Goodman AD, Powers SR. Study of a kindred with pheochromocytoma, medullary thyroid carcinoma, hyperparathyroidism and Cushing's disease: multiple endocrine neoplasia, ype 2. *Medicine (Baltimore)* 1968; 47:371.

67. Bray GA, De Quattro V, Fisher AA, et al. Catecholamines: a symposium. *California Med* 1972;117:32.

68. Manger WM, Gifford RW. Hypertension secondary to pheochromocytoma. *Bull NY Acad Med* 1982;58:139.

69. Francis IR, Smid A, Gross MD, et al. Adrenal masses in oncologic patients: functional and morphologic evaluation. *Radiology* 1988;166: 353–356.

70. Siegelmann S, Fishman E, Gatwood S. CT of the adrenal gland. In: Siegelmann S, Gatwood O, Goldmann S, eds. *Computed Tomography of the Kidney and Adrenals*. Edinburg: Churchill Livingstone; 1984:223.

71. Hedeland H, Ostberg G, Hokfelt B. On the prevalence of adrenocortical adenomas in an autopsy material in relation to hypertension and diabetes. *Acta Med Scand* 1968;184:211–214.

72. Katz RL, Shirkhoda A. Diagnostic approach to incidental adrenal nodules in the cancer patient: results of a clinical, radiologic, and fine needle aspiration study. *Cancer* 1985;55:1995–2000.

3

Selective Simultaneous Bilateral Sampling from the Inferior Petrosal Sinuses

—— Hans H. Schild and T.R. Strack ——

Introduction

Cushing's disease is caused by adrenocorticotropic hormone (ACTH) and/or cortisol hypersecretion due to a variety of underlying diseases. About 70% of the patients have ACTH hypersecretion, originating from the pituitary gland in about 90% and from non-pituitary, ectopic sources in 10 to 15% of the cases (1). Primary adrenal adenomas and adrenal carcinomas with cortisol hypersecretion can be responsible for Cushing's syndrome in about 20% and 5 to 10%, respectively (2).

Successful treatment requires the precise localization of the source of ACTH/cortisol hypersecretion. In the case of a pituitary disease, eradication of the tumor should correct hypercortisolism and avoid postoperative endocrine deficiency at the same time (3–5).

Diagnostic Workup

Clinical Features

Major clinical features of hypercortisolism include a variety of signs and symptoms (3,6–9): centripetal obesity, hypertension (in part due to hypersecretion of catecholamines), diabetes mellitus, amenorrhea and hirsutism in females (by androgenic effects of some steroids), acne, osteoporosis and spinal compression fractures, muscular wasting, violaceous striae and general capillary fragility, impaired function of the immune system (impaired wound healing, decreased resistance to infection), and behavioral changes such as mania or psychosis.

The increased secretion of ACTH and related compounds results in increased pigmentation of the skin, especially over pressure points (knees, elbows, knuckles, belt and brassiere strap regions), in the areolae, genitalia, mucous membranes, and at the site of new scar formation. However, hypercortisolism nowadays is mostly detected in an early stage of the disease, when ACTH levels are not much elevated and, thus, hyperpigmentation is not very pronounced.

An underlying pituitary tumor may cause headache, and visual disturbances through pressure on the optic chiasm.

Tests and procedures, to help in the diagnostic workup of patients with suspected Cushing's disease are outlined below.

Laboratory Tests

Plasma concentrations of the adrenal hormones such as cortisol and their trophic factors, such as ACTH, may vary widely in normal individuals, and in both endocrine and nonendocrine disorders. More precise information is obtained by determining integrated assessments of hormone production, and the responses to appropriate stimulation and suppression tests.

Cortisol Measurement

Cortisol measurement can be achieved by either competitive protein binding assay, radioimmunoassay, high-performance liquid chromatography (HPLC), radioreceptor assay, or measurement of the "plasma free cortisol" not bound to the cortisol binding globulin, which can also be measured in the saliva with sufficient reliability (10–17).

All tests mentioned are now quite accurate and reliable. Commonly used drugs and medications usually do not interfere with the assessment of cortisol concentrations in plasma.

Cortisol levels follow a circadian rhythm with the highest levels in the morning ($10 \pm 4 \mu g/dl$) and low levels between 10 P.M. and 2 A.M. (less than 3 $\mu g/dl$) (18). (Concentrations measured by fluorometric assays are approximately 2 to 3 $\mu g/dl$ higher.)

In general, elevated cortisol levels, especially at night, should arouse suspicion of adrenal hyperfunction, but more specific testing of the hypothalamo-pituitary-adrenal axis is required to establish the diagnosis.

Dexamethasone Suppression Tests

Dexamethasone is used in the diagnosis of Cushing's syndrome to assess the integrity of negative feedback control by glucocorticoids of the hypothalamic-pituitary-adrenal axis. Dexamethasone is a synthetic steroid analogue with a greater affinity for the cortisol receptor than its natural competitor at the binding site, cortisol. The potency of dexamethasone is about 30 times higher. In normal individuals dexamethasone inhibits pituitary ACTH release and consequently adrenal cortisol secretion (Fig. 3.1A).

The simple *dexamethasone overnight test* is a reliable screening test for Cushing's syndrome and basically requires only one plasma specimen. For this test a single dose of 3 mg dexamethasone is administered at 11 P.M. and plasma cortisol is measured at 8 A.M. the following morning. A plasma cortisol level below 2 $\mu g/dl$ should exclude Cushing's syndrome. False-positive results may occur under a variety of circumstances: in obese patients (13%); acutely or chronically ill patients (25%) (19); in patients with severe depression, anorexia nervosa, anxiety, alcoholism, chronic renal failure, high estrogen states (pregnancy, oral contraceptives) (20); and in patients in whom phenytoin, barbiturates, and other anticonvulsants have induced an accelerated metabolism of steroids such as dexamethasone.

High-dose dexamethasone tests are helpful in differentiating Cushing's disease from the patients mentioned above, and from other types of hypercortisolism. This test depends on the characteristic finding, that the hypothalamic-pituitary-adrenal axis is suppressible with glucocorticoids in patients with an ACTH-secreting pituitary tumor (Fig. 3.1B), although higher than normal doses are required. Thus, ACTH and cortisol decrease when large amounts of dexamethasone are administered (19,21).

In contrast, in patients with hypercortisolism secondary to an adrenal tumor (Fig. 3.1C) or the ectopic ACTH-syndrome (Fig. 3.1D), high-dose dexamethasone characteristically fails to suppress cortisol hypersecretion, since it is not under the control of the hypothalamic-pituitary axis. However, a number of exceptions may still occur, as will be discussed below in detail. In practice, for high-dose dexamethasone testing we recommend the 8 mg overnight test, where a single dose of 8 mg dexamethasone is administered orally at 11 P.M., and cortisol is measured at 8 A.M. the following morning. It has been shown, that in 55 out of 60 patients with an ACTH-secreting pituitary tumor cortisol levels could be suppressed below 50% of the baseline value, whereas in no patient with ectopic ACTH syndrome or adrenal tumor could this degree of suppression be achieved (22).

Corticotropin Releasing Factor (CRF) Testing

The only stimulatory test used in the differential diagnosis of Cushing's syndrome is the CRF test. In general, patients with a pituitary

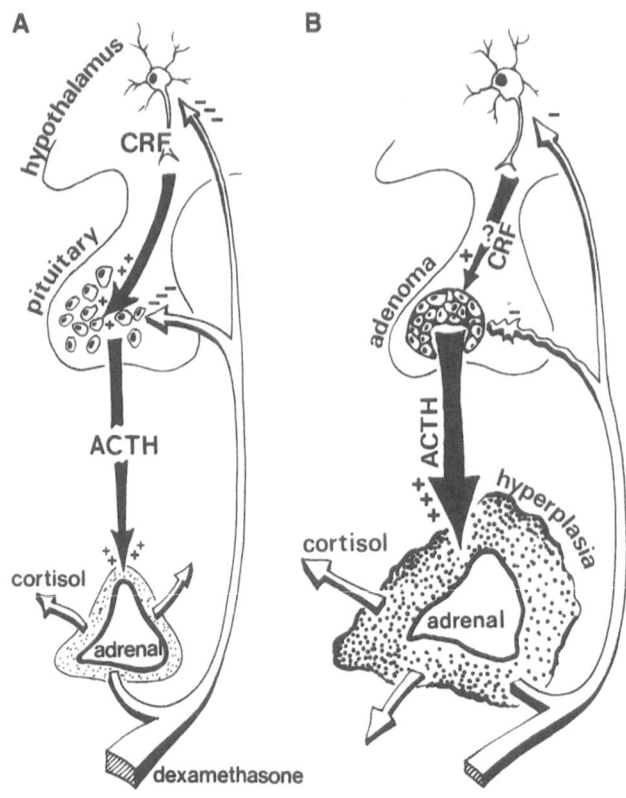

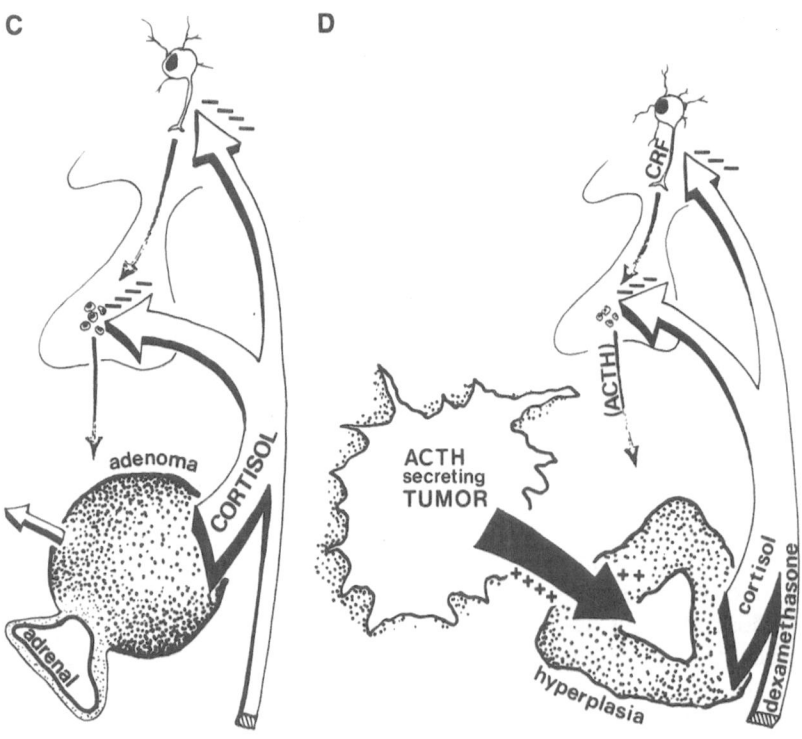

Figure 3.1. **A**: Hypothalamic-pituitary-adrenal axis in a healthy subject. CRF stimulates ACTH secretion from the anterior pituitary, and ACTH in turn enhances cortisol secretion from the adrenals. Cortisol and synthetic steroids such as dexamethasone exert a negative feedback on both the anterior pituitary and the hypothalamus. Because dexamethasone is approximately 30 times as potent as cortisol, complete suppression of the hypothalamic-pituitary axis can be accomplished at moderate doses already. **B**: In Cushing's disease a pituitary adenoma secretes inappropriate amounts of ACTH leading to hypersecretion of cortisol and diffuse or, in later stages, nodular hyperplasia of both adrenals. Although cortisol levels are increased, cortisol is not able to suppress ACTH secretion sufficiently. Dexamethasone, however, may partially reduce ACTH and hence cortisol levels. CRF hypersecretion as a possible cause of Cushing's disease and a pituitary adenoma or diffuse hyperplasia of the adrenocorticotrophic cell is still under debate.

C: The usually single adenoma of the adrenal gland leads to high cortisol levels that suppress spontaneous and CRF-stimulated ACTH concentrations.
D: The ectopic ACTH syndrome, usually caused by a bronchial carcinoma, leads to adrenal hyperplasia and hypercortisolism similar to the pituitary tumor. In contrast to the latter, pituitary ACTH levels are suppressed and cannot be stimulated by exogenous CRF, nor can dexamethasone suppress ectopic ACTH secretion, hence cortisol levels. Most nonpituitary tumors seem to lack steroid receptors exerting a negative feedback on hormone secretion.

tumor have normal or exaggerated plasma ACTH and cortisol responses to CRF; patients with ectopic ACTH syndrome or an adrenal tumor, on the other hand, do not respond to CRF, though numerous exceptions have been reported as well (23). For the test 100 μg ovine or synthetic human CRF are administered into a peripheral vein. ACTH and cortisol levels are measured after 15, 30, 45, and 60 minutes.

Radiological Procedures

Skull Films/Polytomography of the Sella

Enlargement of the sella, alterations of sella shape, thinning of the dorsum sellae, erosion of the sellar floor or of clinoid processes may indicate pituitary pathology. Only 10 to 15% of the patients with Cushing's disease, however, show findings on conventional radiographic examinations. False-negative and false-positive studies are frequent, and the area of abnormality even on tomography correlates poorly with the site of a microadenoma. In general, plain radiography and conventional sellar tomography are not helpful in the diagnostic workup of patients with Cushing's disease (24–28).

Abdominal Computed Tomography (CT)

Abdominal CT may demonstrate adrenal abnormalities in patients with Cushing's syndrome. Adrenal adenomas can be identified by state-of-the-art CT when they are larger than 0.5 to 1 cm in diameter. They normally present as unilateral round tumors of varying density (0–40–50 HE), which may rarely have calcifications (2). With adrenal hyperplasia CT may show

- homogeneous enlargement of the glands, so-called diffuse hyperplasia; if there is marked bilateral enlargement, this should suggest the possibility of ACTH production by an ectopic neoplasm
- small (<2 cm, micronodular form) or larger (>2 cm, macronodular form) nodules in cases of nodular hyperplasia
- normal glands in 50% of the cases with functional hyperplasia.

Adrenal carcinomas nearly always present as unilateral tumors of varying size and density (2,29).

Cranial CT

Pituitary Cushing adenomas may present as focal hypodensity, or focal bulge, with or without deviation of the pituitary stalk. Unfortunately, the majority of the ACTH-secreting tumors are microadenomas, i.e., less than 1 cm in diameter. Due to this small size and their enhancement characteristics after intravenous application of contrast medium, Cushing adenomas are difficult to detect with CT. Even state-of-the-art high-resolution CT with intravenous application of contrast medium only has an overall sensitivity between 17 and 58% for CT detection of pituitary Cushing adenomas (30–36).

Magnetic Resonance Imaging (MRI)

High-resolution MRI is the most sensitive imaging method for preoperative localization of ACTH-secreting adenomas [sensitivity of 71%, and specificity of 87% (37)]. The appearance of ACTH-secreting microadenomas on MRI is nonuniform. This is influenced by, among other factors, the physical characteristics of the tumor and the pulse sequence used. Diagnosis of small solid microadenomas may require I.V. administration of gadolinium-DTPA (Magnevist, produced by Schering AG, Berlin; distributed in the United States by Berlex), a contrast agent for MRI. However, even then tiny adenomas (1 to 3 mm in size) may still remain undetectable. Even though MRI is the best imaging procedure for diagnosis of pituitary microadenomas at the present time, its ultimate utility remains to be determined (37–41).

Blood Sampling

Blood sampling from several vascular regions has been described to be helpful in the diagnostic workup of patients with Cushing's syndrome (42–45). Sampling from the adrenal veins is described in Chapter 2. In this chapter sampling from the inferior petrosal sinus will be covered in detail.

Diagnostic Problems

Diagnostic problems may be encountered in several areas of the diagnostic workup in patients with Cushing's disease. As these problems may indicate further workup by inferior petrosal sinus sampling, they shall be discussed more in detail.

Problems with Hormone Measurements

ACTH is secreted episodically with a distinct diurnal rhythm. Plasma levels of ACTH in healthy adults may vary from less than 10 pg/ml to 80 pg/ml. Peak ACTH levels occur early in the morning and closely parallel those of cortisol; the lowest levels are measured at about midnight. In addition, ACTH levels can rise to 10 times the normal values during periods of stress such as venous puncture alone. Due to this high physiological variability of ACTH concentration in blood, it is difficult to separate normal from pathological ACTH levels. These difficulties are compounded by additional problems with ACTH measurements: because ACTH has relatively poor antigenicity and bears a close resemblance to other circulating peptides, the radioimmunoassay is difficult. Also, ACTH is prone to rapid destruction at room temperature by plasma peptidases, and on glass surfaces (46). Therefore, careful sample collection and preparation are essential. Specimens should be collected with EDTA/aprotinin in plastic tubes on ice, centrifuged in the cold within 1 hour of collection, and then frozen at −20°C until assayed.

The antibody should react with the biologically active 1–24 sequence of human ACTH in order to reduce detection of biologically inactive fragments. The latter point may be of special interest in malignant disease when larger size forms of ACTH ("big ACTH") have been observed, which represent incompletely processed precursor molecules (46).

Problems with Endocrinologic Testing

With endocrinologic testing problems are encountered in several areas. Interpretation of peripheral ACTH and cortisol levels may be difficult in patients with periodic or episodic hormonogenesis who may have either a pituitary adenoma (Cushing's disease), the ectopic ACTH syndrome, or adrenal tumors (47–49). Thus, these patients may show normal suppression with the low-dose dexamethasone test, if it is performed during certain periods. When studied at other times, secretion of ACTH and cortisol may be nonsuppressible, or even may show a paradoxical increase during high-dose dexamethasone administration (48).

Urinary 17-hydroxycorticosteroid excretion fails to be suppressed in approximately 10 to 30% of patients who received low-dose dexamethasone (1 to 3 mg). In the presence of measurable ACTH levels this may falsely suggest an ectopic ACTH syndrome (19,22,50). This frequency of nonsuppressibility is decreased by the use of the overnight 8 mg high-dose dexamethasone suppression test. This may be of special importance in patients with nonsuppressible function who have nodular hyperplasia of the adrenals. No less than 75% of these patients have nonsuppressible function with the low-dose dexamethasone suppression test (50).

Plasma ACTH levels may be undetectable, normal, or elevated and may vary dramatically in the same patient. In patients who do not show suppression with high-dose dexamethasone, in whom ACTH levels are not markedly elevated, and who do not have an obvious ectopic tumor, even higher doses of dexamethasone (16 or 32 mg over 2 to 4 consecutive days) should be administered. If steroid suppression occurs with higher doses of dexamethasone, the diagnosis of Cushing's disease may be more likely. Also, the diagnosis of Cushing's disease may be suggested by the demonstration of bilateral diffuse or nodular hyperplasia of the adrenals by CT scan.

Although the ectopic ACTH syndrome is usually easily diagnosed by elevated ACTH levels and nonsuppressible steroid hypersecretion in the presence of an extrapituitary tumor, there are some cases in which the tumor is occult. In these, steroid secretion may even be dexamethasone suppressible (51). The occult tumors are usually bronchial carcinoids. In these cases, the plasma ACTH levels can be in the range of those seen with Cushing's disease, and can lead to inappropriate pituitary therapy. Although it is not possible to make the differentiation with certainty in all cases, some features should arouse suspicion of the presence of ectopic ACTH syndrome: male sex, rapid onset, severe hypercortisolism, hypokalemia, weight loss.

If the ectopic ACTH syndrome is suspected, but no tumor obvious, selective venous sampling of ACTH and other tumor markers [e.g. calcitonin, carcinoembryonic antigen (CEA), etc.] may be helpful. In the absence of a pituitary-peripheral ACTH gradient, the ectopic ACTH syndrome is likely, and further selective venous sampling may help to localize the ACTH secreting ectopic tumor.

Problems with Radiological Procedures

As a rule, pathological processes can be detected by radiological procedures when they cause a change in the size, contour, or density (with or without application of contrast media) of a normal structure.

Whether a pathological process secretes hormones or is functionally inactive cannot be determined by radiological imaging methods. Incidental findings, such as nonfunctioning adenomas also called incidentalomas, may be the cause of false-positive diagnosis. These can be seen in the adrenals in 5% of all abdominal CT studies (2); in the pituitary they have been reported in up to 30% of the population at autopsy (52–54). All findings thus have to be interpreted in the clinical context, which is also true for the results of endocrinological tests. When in a given clinical setting radiological methods show a tumor in the pituitary or in another location, this points to a specific diagnosis.

Major problems arise in those patients with ACTH-hypersecretion, in whom radiological findings are negative or questionable. These patients may have a pituitary microadenoma or an occult tumor in a different location with ACTH secretion, e.g., bronchogenic carcinoma, pheochromocytoma, thymoma, carcinoid (especially bronchial carcinoid), or medullary thyroid carcinoma (50,55–59). Selective venous sampling may help in these cases to establish the diagnosis, and eventually lateralize a pituitary adenoma.

Indications for Inferior Petrosal Sinus (IPS) Sampling

IPS sampling can be performed to

1. differentiate pituitary from ectopic ACTH hypersecretion in those patients in whom the source of ACTH hypersecretion is in doubt. In a clinical context, these may be patients with Cushing's syndrome and a nonsuppressible dexamethasone test, or nodular adrenal hyperplasia, or an occult ACTH-secreting tumor;
2. localize/lateralize a pituitary adenoma in patients with normal CT and MRI findings in order to enable elective surgery.

With a pituitary source of ACTH hypersecretion, blood from at least one inferior petrosal sinus should have a twofold higher ACTH-concentration than that from a simultaneous peripheral sample (51,60,61). Thus, IPS sampling may be helpful when a source of ACTH hypersecretion cannot be identified by less invasive diagnostic methods.

Under normal circumstances there is ipsilateral venous drainage of the pituitary blood. The majority of ACTH-secreting microadenomas is located laterally in the pituitary (62).

Hormonal concentration differences in samples from both inferior petrosal sinuses may thus point to the side of the pituitary where an adenoma resides. A hormonal concentration being more than 1.4 times higher in one IPS is considered significant (63). Also, small microadenomas, which are not detected by any imaging method, can be lateralized by means of IPS sampling. If no discernible microadenoma is seen at the time of transsphenoidal pituitary surgery, resection of the specific side indicated by the sampling may be sufficient, and result in a cure of Cushing's disease. Thus, IPS sampling may avoid total resection of the pituitary gland and postoperative endocrine deficiency.

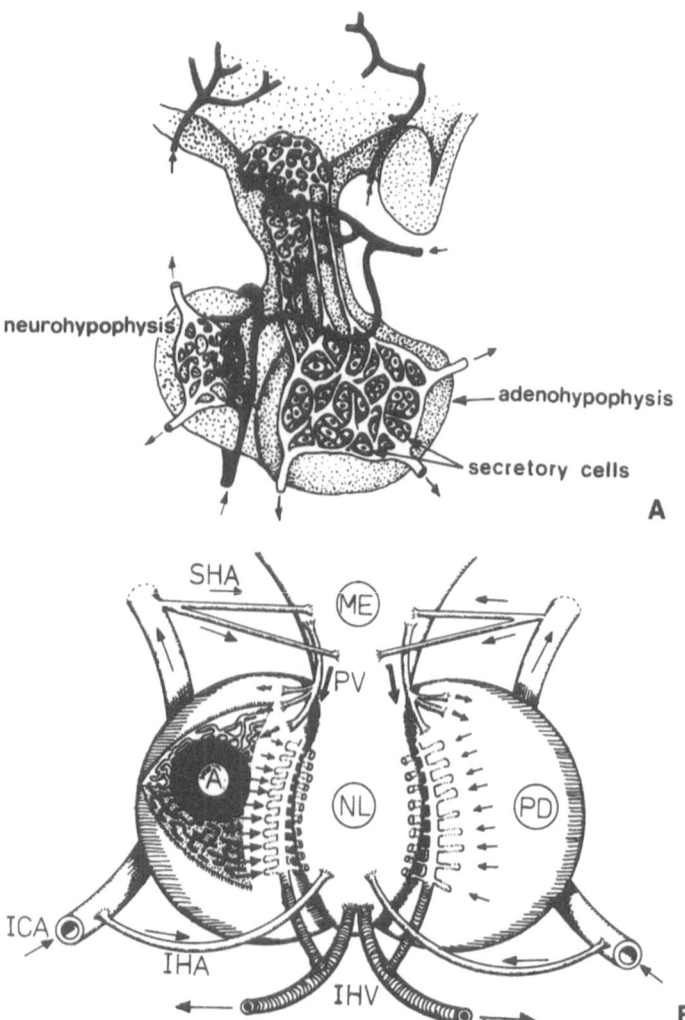

neurohypophysis

adenohypophysis

secretory cells

A

Figure 3.2. **A** and **B**: Schematic representation of the pituitary blood supply. Blood enters the median eminence (ME) through superior hypophyseal arteries (SHA) and the neural lobe (NL) through inferior hypophyseal arteries (IHA), which originate from the internal carotid arteries (ICA). The blood from the SHA passes through the primary capillary plexus of the pars distalis (PD). The inferior hypophyseal veins (IHV) drain both the neuro- and adenohypophysis to the left and right cavernous sinuses, respectively. Thus, adenomas (A) can be localized by side-to-side comparison of hormone levels in the pituitary effluents.

SHA

ME

PV

A

NL

PD

ICA

IHA

IHV

B

Anatomy

Venous drainage of the pituitary itself is a very complex matter and shall not be discussed here in detail (for information see Fig. 3.2, and ref. 64–71,150). For practical purposes we summarize as follows (72–101):

Blood leaves the anterior lobe of the pituitary by numerous small hypophyseal veins. They empty into lateral adenohypophyseal veins, which converge into the confluent pituitary veins on the surface of the gland. These then course laterally to join the ipsilateral cavernous sinuses.

The cavernous sinuses are paired, roughly quadrangular structures, immediately lateral to

the pituitary fossa (Fig. 3.3). The dural coverings of the cavernous sinuses thus form the lateral walls of the sella turcica.

Right and left cavernous sinuses are interconnected by additional sinuses. The most important and most constant are:

sinus intercavernosus (sive coronarius) anterior: the anterior intercavernous sinus is located between the anterior surface of the anterior pituitary lobe, and the anterior sella margin, in or directly below the diaphragma sellae; it can be found in 76 to 85% of the cases

sinus intercavernosus (sive coronarius) posterior: in most cases the posterior intercavernous sinus is larger than the anterior

Figure 3.3. Schematic drawing of the anatomical relationships of the cavernous and inferior petrosal sinuses in lateral (**A**) and axial (**B**) view. The inferior petrosal sinus drains directly into the internal jugular vein, which is the case in 45% of the population (92). Variations of the drainage pattern are illustrated in Fig. 3.4. P, pituitary gland; CS, cavernous sinus; ICS, intercavernous sinus; IPS, inferior petrosal sinus; SPS, superior petrosal sinus; PP, pterygoid plexus; PB, plexus basilaris; JV, internal jugular vein; 1, v. ophthalmica superior; 2, sinus sigmoideus; 3, sinus transversus; 4, sinus sphenoparietalis.

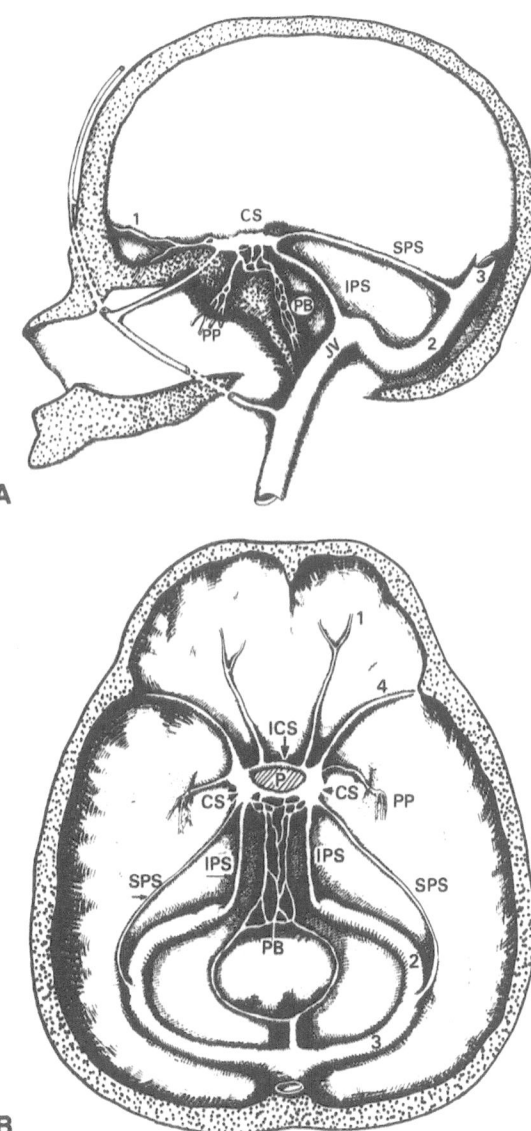

intercavernosus sinus. It runs behind the posterior pituitary lobe, and in front of the posterior clinoid plate, and is observed in only 32% of the cases

sinus intercavernosus inferior: the inferior intercavernous sinus is located in front of the sulcus, which delineates the border between anterior and posterior lobe of the pituitary. The sinus may be a single channel, often, however, it consists of multiple channels. With a diameter of 1 mm or less, it is smaller than the anterior or posterior intercavernosus sinus.

Located in the center of the skull, the cavernous sinuses have multiple affluents and effluents (Fig. 3.3):

1. At the ventral aspect:
   • the inferior and superior ophthalmic veins, which run through the respective orbital fissures. The superior ophthalmic vein communicates with the facial veins via the angular vein. So the sinus cavernosus can be outlined during transfrontal orbital phlebography.
   • the sphenoparietal sinus,

- sylvian veins, which sometimes communicate with the cavernous sinuses directly.
2. At the lateral aspect:
- venous plexuses, which connect the cavernous sinus with the pterygoid plexus via different foramina in the skull base [foramen ovale, f. lacerum, f. rotundum, f. venosum (Vesalii)].
3. At the dorsal aspect:
- the superior petrosal sinus (SPS), which is located at the attachment of the falx to the petrous pyramid. It enters the posterior superior angle of the cavernous sinus, and connects this structure with the transverse/ sigmoid sinuses. The SPS is 45 to 60 mm in length, and 1 to 4 mm in diameter at its end. Blood flow in the SPS can be bidirectional; normally, however, it is from dorsal to ventral.
- the inferior petrosal sinus (IPS), which runs along the lower border of the pyramids towards the ventromedial part of the jugular foramen. The IPS then leaves the skull through the pars nervosa of this foramen, and usually enters the internal jugular vein immediately below the skull base. The average length of the IPS is 23–28 mm, and at its end it has most often a diameter of 2–4 mm. The final part of the IPS runs in a plane, which has an average angle of 115° with the sagittal plane, and an average angle of 24° (left) respective 28° (right) with the transverse plane.

During its course the IPS receives tributaries, e.g. from the medulla, pons, and internal auditory meatus, and the anterior condylar/condyloid vein. The latter communicates with the venous plexus of the canalis hypoglossalis, and may be mistaken for the IPS, especially when prominent.

Normal anatomy with the IPS joining the internal jugular vein immediately below the skull base is found in less than half of the patients. In rare cases, the junction may be intracranial (73), or the IPS may communicate with the sigmoid sinus (98b).

The frequent variations (92) (frequency in parentheses) are (Figs. 3.3 and 3.4):
a. IPS drains directly into the internal jugular bulb, as described above (45%)

b. IPS drains into a communicating vein, that unites the internal jugular bulb with the deep cervical venous plexus (about 24%). More exactly, in this type of drainage, the IPS anastomoses, directly or indirectly, with the anterior condylar vein, which communicates with the vertebral venous plexus (94).
c. IPS is not a single vessel but consists of a plexiform vascular network. This plexus communicates with the internal jugular bulb, and directly or via the anterior condylar vein also with the vertebral venous plexus (about 24%).
d. IPS running along the basilar plexus, communicating directly with the deep cervical/vertebral venous plexus via the anterior condylar vein; there is no communication of the IPS with the internal jugular vein. The frequency of this type of drainage, in which the IPS cannot be catheterized, is reported between 0.6% (150) and 7% (92).

Occasionally variations between the two sides in the same patient can be observed.

- the basilar plexus, which is spread on the clivus. It extends down to the foramen magnum with the surrounding marginal sinus, and continues as internal and external vertebral venous plexus. The basilar plexus has varying anastomoses with the cavernous sinuses. In addition, there are one or more venous channels, leading to the medial wall of the IPS. These channels are important, since they may be confused with the IPS at catheterization.

Functional Anatomical Aspects

ACTH secretion by the pituitary causes a high hormonal concentration in the blood of its venous drainage. On the way to the heart, ACTH concentration diminishes through increasing venous admixture. This dilution varies and is unpredictable.

Studies of pituitary blood flow direction in the pig and monkey failed to demonstrate mixing of venous blood from the two sides of the anterior pituitary (63,101). Thus, ACTH secreted by a laterally located microadenoma

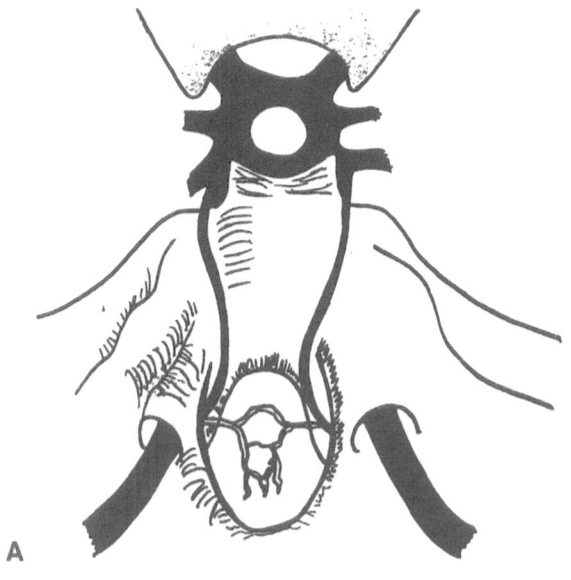

A

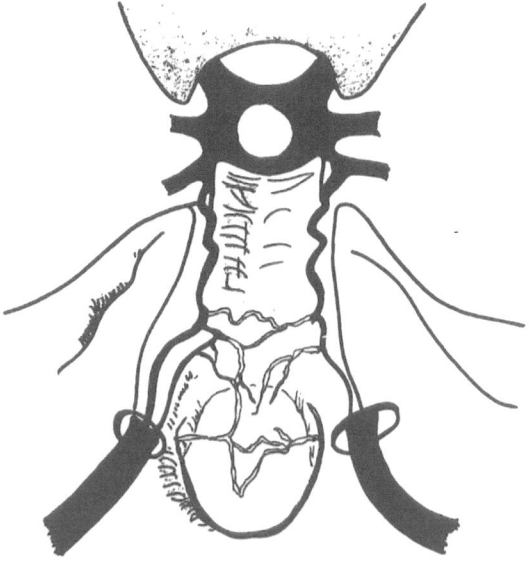

B

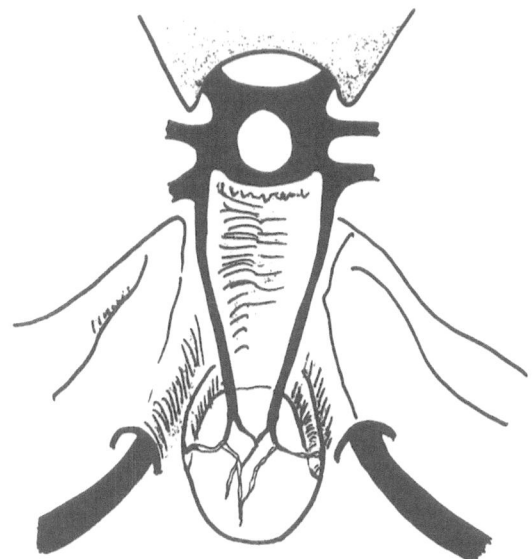

C

Figure 3.4. Anatomical variations of the inferior petrosal sinuses and their relative frequency (92). Direct communication with the internal jugular vein is observed in about 45% of the cases, and is illustrated in Fig. 3.3. **A**: IPS drains into communicating vein that unites the internal jugular bulb with the deep cervical plexus (24%). **B**: IPS is poorly formed and exists as a venous plexus (24%). **C**: IPS drains directly into the deep cervical venous plexus (7%).

may not reach the opposite IPS in a sufficient amount to produce a gradient with the peripheral blood (101). Though theoretically possible, intermixing of blood at the level of the IPS via the basilar venous sinus/plexus is also insignificant (101).

It is important to note that ACTH is secreted episodically in normal subjects as well as in patients with Cushing's disease. Moreover, its half-life in plasma is very short: 7 to 13 minutes (102). As a consequence, simultaneous bilateral central (IPS) and peripheral samples should

be drawn. Otherwise temporary peaks or lows can cause misleading results.

The following practical conclusions may be drawn:

1. With a pituitary source of ACTH, this hormone must have a higher concentration in IPS blood than in peripheral blood.
2. If there is no mixing of blood from both sides of the pituitary, blood from the side of an ACTH-producing adenoma should have a higher ACTH concentration; a side-to-

side ratio of more than 1.4 is considered to be significant (63).

3. Blood drawn from the IPS opposite to the side of an ACTH-secreting adenoma should have a lower ACTH concentration; due to suppression of contralateral ACTH-secreting cells ACTH levels may be about the same as in peripheral venous samples.

4. With stimulation of ACTH secretion from a pituitary adenoma, the ipsilateral hormonal concentration should increase, thus side differences in hormonal concentration should become more pronounced.

5. With an ectopic source of ACTH hyper-secretion, the hormonal concentration in IPS blood from both sides should be
   • about the same as in a peripheral sample, or
   • below that, when the peripheral sample was taken from the venous drainage of an ectopic ACTH-producing tumor.

6. If, for technical reasons, IPS sampling is feasible only on one side, an ACTH concentration equaling peripheral values may be due to
   • ectopic ACTH secretion, or
   • a contralateral pituitary adenoma.
   Therefore, the procedure is of no diagnostic use in this case. If, however, ACTH concentration is at least twofold higher than in a peripheral sample, a pituitary source of ACTH is established (57). A lateralization of a pituitary adenoma, however, is still not possible under these circumstances.

7. If IPS sampling is technically or anatomically impossible, blood should be drawn from the jugular bulbs and the internal jugular vein. If ACTH concentration
   • in one of the samples is higher than in a peripheral sample, a pituitary source for the hormone can be assumed. A lateralization, however, is impossible.
   • in both samples are of the same magnitude as the peripheral hormonal concentration no conclusions can be drawn, since admixture of venous blood is unpredictable.

8. Bilaterally higher ACTH concentrations in the IPS than in a peripheral sample may be due to
   • diffuse hyperplasia of the adrenocortico-troph cells
   • a medially located microadenoma (a situation that has not been reported yet).

It must be strongly emphasized, that later-alization of an adenoma requires:

bilateral correct catheter placement into the IPS

similar pituitary venous drainage on both sides. Side to side differences in drainage patterns may have anatomical reasons, or result from previous surgical interventions.

a microadenoma. Large adenomas, which can be detected with other radiological procedures, may alter the hemodynamic situation of the venous drainage in an unpredictable way.

a significantly higher hormonal concentration on the adenoma side (at least the concentration should be 1.4-fold higher than that from the opposite side).

Catheterization

Catheterization Technique (74,98,99)

Catheters

Catheters without side holes are used. These should have a slight angle at about 1 to 1.5 cm below the catheter tip (e.g., vertebral artery catheters) to conform to the anatomical situation. Catheters of French 5 diameter have sufficient torque control in most cases, and permit good blood flow during aspiration. Catheters of smaller diameter may be difficult to manipulate or may cause problems with sufficient blood aspiration.

Contrast Media

We routinely use nonionic contrast media.

Access

The common femoral veins are used for access. Both catheters may be placed in the same femoral vein. With a bilateral approach we use the right catheter for sampling on the left side

Figure 3.5. Schematic drawing showing both sampling catheters entering the inferior petrosal sinuses via the respective internal jugular veins (JV). P, pituitary gland.

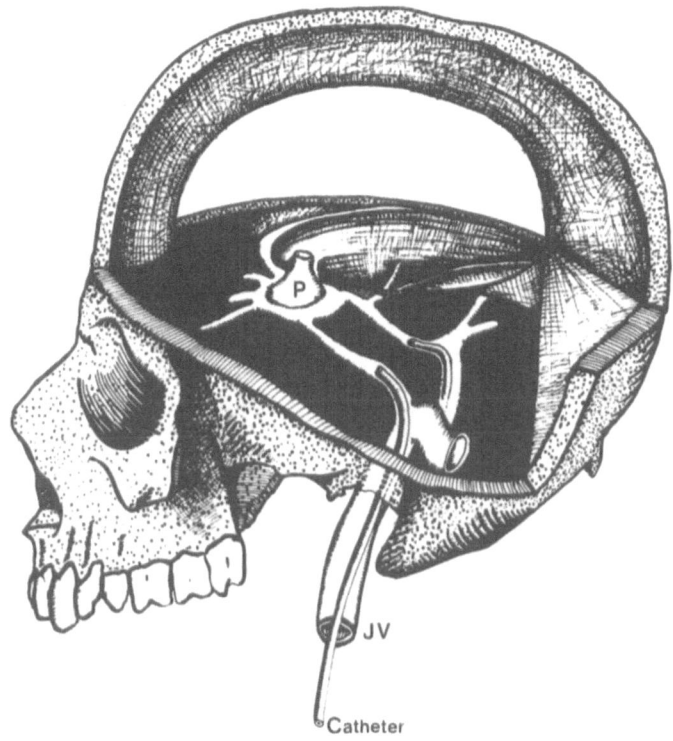

JV

Catheter

and vice versa. This allows for easier manipulation on the left side of the neck (the left catheter otherwise has to negotiate more curves). Using a sheath permits for peripheral blood sampling/drug administration via the side port.

Procedure

After having placed both catheters in the inferior caval vein, we administer 4,000 to 5,000 units of heparin (about 50 IU per kg body weight) to reduce the risk of thrombosis, which is known to be higher in patients with Cushing's disease. The right atrium is then passed using a J-guide wire, and both catheters are placed into the respective internal jugular veins. Passing the venous valves near the confluens with the subclavian veins often requires varying respiratory maneuvers, and may also be facilitated using a Terumo guide wire. The catheter tips are then directed in the anteromedial direction and advanced, using fluoroscopy guidance and contrast medium injections. Fluoroscopy should avoid the orbits as much as possible; preferentially it should be performed in a laterolateral direction.

DSA allows easy and fast localization of the catheter, which may otherwise be difficult due to the overlying skull base. Force and amount of contrast media injection can also be kept to a minimum with DSA. This is important, since forceful injections in proximity to the hypophysis may cause artificial changes in hormonal levels.

Advancing in the cranial direction, the catheters most often enter the jugular bulb or the sigmoid sinus. Only rarely will they directly enter an inferior petrosal sinus, which is frequently of large diameter in this case. Manipulations of the catheter should be performed carefully using a soft guide wire, and avoiding any forceful and brisk movements. With contrast media injection and DSA the anatomical situation will be demonstrated (Figs. 3.5–3.9). It is important to identify the IPS clearly.

At this time, it may become obvious that the patient has one of those anatomical variations that do not allow for unilaterally or bilaterally

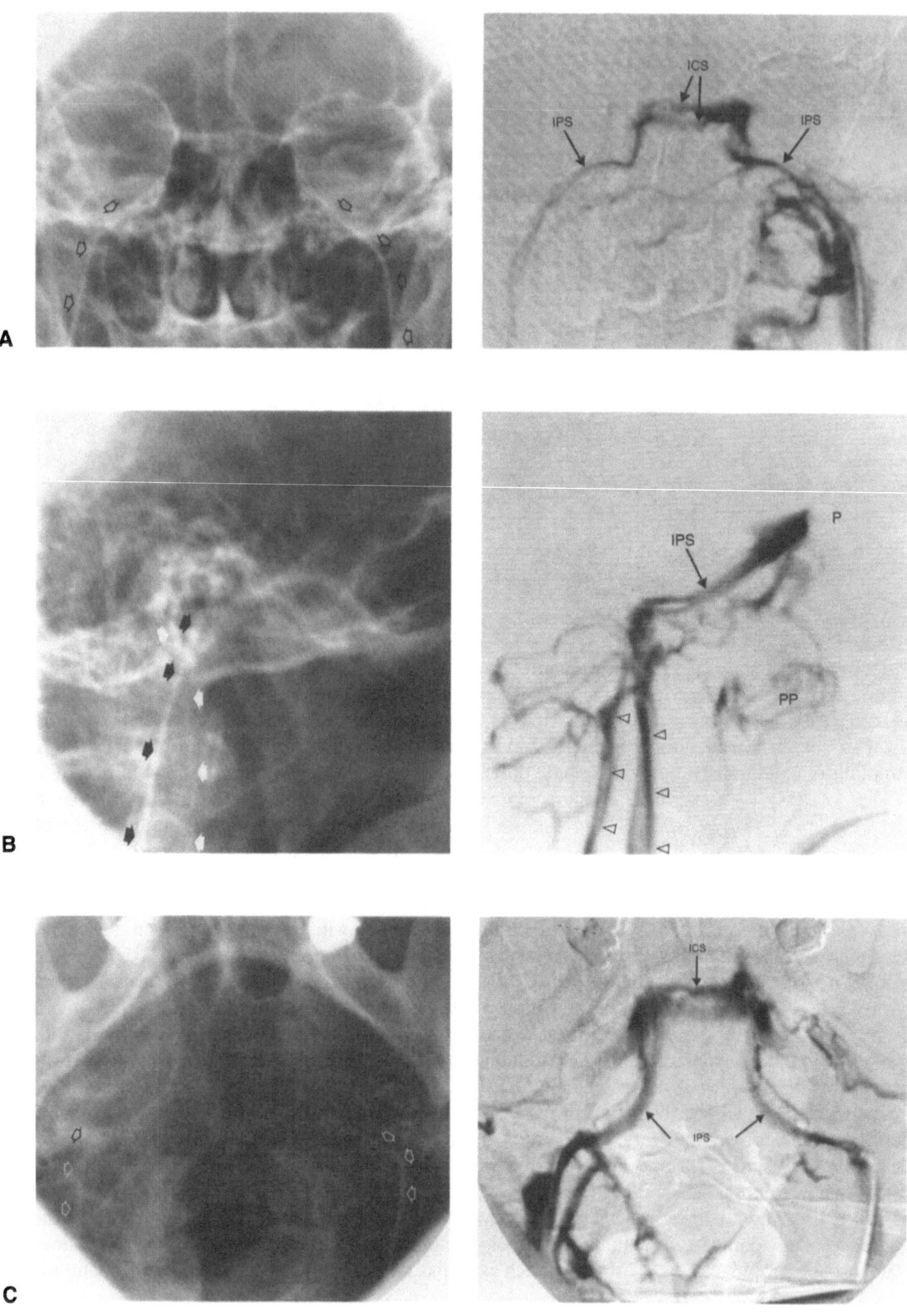

Figure 3.7. Catheterization with injection of contrast medium into right IPS. The left IPS fills via cavernous and intercavernous sinuses. The catheter tip on the left is still at the end of the IPS and should be advanced slightly further.

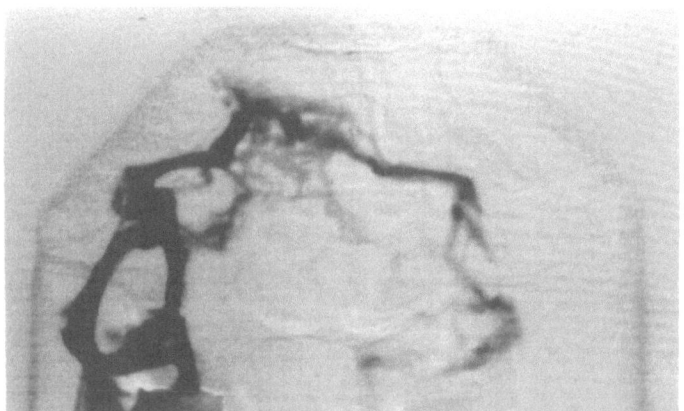

Figure 3.8. Catheterization of IPS: right cavernous and intercavernous sinuses are displaced (arrow) by a large pituitary adenoma. Note: contrast medium outlines the left superior ophthalmic vein.

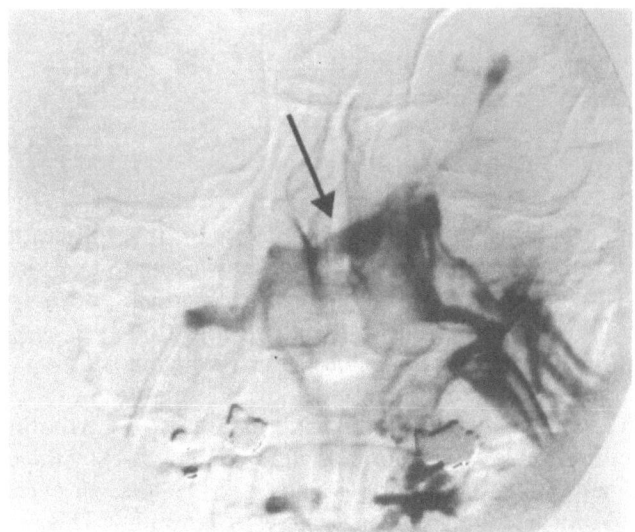

correct catheter placement. In these cases, samples should be still obtained from one IPS (if possible) and from the internal jugular veins, as this sampling may still allow differentiation between central and ectopic ACTH-hypersecretion. Lateralization of a pituitary adenoma, however, is not possible anymore, as outlined above.

If contrast injection shows a normal anatomical situation, it is possible to intubate the IPS in most cases. With the catheter close to or in the IPS, contrast injection may outline this sinus, the ipsilateral and contralateral cavernous sinuses, the opposite IPS, and sometimes the orbital veins. This depends on the injected amount of contrast, and force of injection. Outlining the opposite IPS may help with otherwise difficult contralateral intubations.

Ideally, catheter tips should be placed symmetrically close to the junction of the vertical and horizontal segment of the IPS. Care must be taken not to intubate clival veins/basilar

←————————————————————————

Figure 3.6. Catheterization of the IPS (catheters marked by arrows) in different projections, masks (left) and subtraction pictures (right). **A**: anterior view. **B**: Lateral view. **C**: Submento-occipital view. IPS, inferior petrosal sinus; ICS, intercavernous sinus; P, pituitary gland; PP, pterygoid plexus.

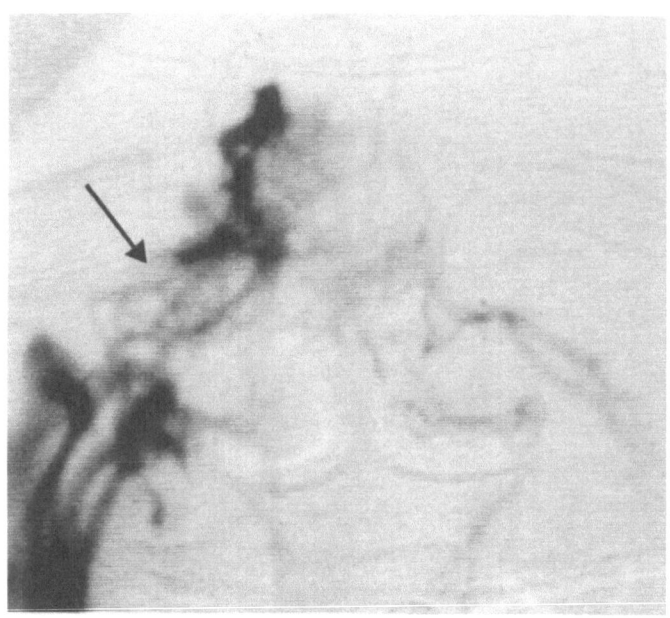

Figure 3.9. Catheterization of IPS: the IPS cannot be selectively intubated, as it is not a single channel but a plexiform vascular network (the arrow points to the internal carotid artery).

venous plexus of the posterior fossa or the anterior condylar vein. If the catheter has inadvertently entered one of these larger medially directed dural branches, contrast injection will not outline the cavernous sinus. Wedging of the catheters must be avoided, as this might divert draining blood to the contralateral IPS. Neither guide wires nor catheters should be advanced into the cavernous sinus!

With correct placement, samples from both catheters as well as a peripheral venous sample are withdrawn slowly and simultaneously as a baseline study. To enhance side-to-side differences in hormonal concentrations (this is described in detail below), corticotropin releasing factor (CRF) and/or perhaps thyrotropin releasing hormone (TRH) is injected through the peripheral venous access. Additional sampling is performed 2, 5, 10, and 15 minutes after injection of releasing hormones.

Each sample has a volume of about 5 ml. They are collected in chilled plastic tubes containing EDTA/aprotinin on ice.

As a routine, we also perform sampling from the major veins (subclavian veins, superior caval vein, inferior caval vein above and below the adrenals, as well as the adrenals) when withdrawing the catheters from the IPS. After

the catheters are removed, the patient rests in bed for 8 hours.

Side Effects and Complications of Catheterization

Irritation of the periostium of the jugular fossa by the catheter may cause transient discomfort or even pain in the area of the ipsilateral ear. This as a rule is of no clinical significance.

Sometimes patients report a sensation of noise on injection of contrast. This may be due to irritation of the venae labyrinthi and v. aqueductus vestibuli, which communicate with the IPS. Once in a while patients complain about slight headache during the procedure. This is of short duration and does not require any specific treatment. Up to now we did not see any severe complications during or after IPS, nor have such complications been reported in the literature.

Possible risks may be inferred from reported complications of phlebography of the cavernous sinus. This procedure was performed for diagnostic purposes rather often before the advent of CT and MRI. Cavernous sinus phlebography required more forceful injections of larger amounts of contrast medium, than selective sampling using DSA. Also, it was performed using less sophisticated catheters and guide wires. Despite these circumstances, complications have been reported only rarely. In two cases, extradural contrast injection was observed causing temporary headache (78,96,100). In an experimental postmortem study it was impossible to perforate the dura with a catheter (92).

One patient who developed hiccup and a partial lateral medullary syndrome has also been reported. This was probably due to rupture of a pontine vein from vigorous attempts to produce contrast medium filling of the cavernous sinus (92).

Endocrinological Background for IPS Catheterization

Selective pituitary venous sampling aims to detect significant differences of ACTH levels in the venous effluent. The sensitivity of this technique critically depends on the accuracy and specificity of the ACTH assay used and the correct positioning of the catheters. However, both prerequisites may not be fulfilled to a satisfactory level.

To make differences in hormonal concentration more obvious, a stimulatory agent that would preferentially act on the pituitary tumor was sought. A prime candidate was corticotropin releasing factor (CRF) which had been chemically defined in 1981 (103). The biological activity of human CRF (hCRF) has been extensively studied (103–107). Later, CRF was found in the paraventricular nucleus of several species (23,108) and in the basal telencephalon, hypothalamus, and brainstem, and scattered CRF-containing cells were detected throughout most areas of the cerebral cortex. CRF in vitro releases all peptide components derived from the proopiomelanocortin (POMC) molecule, among them ACTH (109). The mode of action on pituitary cells by CRF is not completely elucidated; available data, however, suggest that CRF stimulates adenosine 3′,5′-cyclic monophosphate (cAMP) formation in a manner similar to other releasing hormones (110–112). CRF increases peripheral plasma ACTH concentrations within 15 minutes following peripheral venous injection, although the magnitude of this rise is less than seen in other tests employed for detecting the integrity of the ACTH reserve.

The only other hypophyseal hormone that is stimulated by CRF in normal pituitary tissue is beta-endorphin (113,114).

In Cushing's disease there is normal responsiveness or hyperresponsiveness of ACTH and cortisol to CRF administration. With 100 μg biosynthetic human CRF injected intravenously, ACTH levels in peripheral plasma usually increase by 40 pg/ml above baseline. The normal or hyperresponsiveness to CRF in patients with ACTH-secreting tumors indicates a preservation of CRF receptors in the adenoma (115). This assumption is further supported by the first clinical results, which show a good correlation between high basal and CRF-stimulated ACTH levels and pituitary tumor localization (46,116,117). However, some patients do not respond to hCRF.

In the ectopic ACTH syndrome, ACTH secretion does not increase further in response to CRF (118,119). In adrenal tumors, basal ACTH levels are suppressed, and do not respond to CRF. Numerous exceptions, however, have been described (120–124).

Patients and Method

We diagnosed Cushing's syndrome in 12 patients with typical clinical and biochemical features of the disorder. Eleven patients proved to have pituitary-dependent hypercortisolism. All patients with Cushing's disease had nonsuppressible cortisol levels with the low-dose dexamethasone test (3 mg); five patients were partially suppressible with 8 mg dexamethasone, whereas six patients stayed nonsuppressible with high-dose dexamethasone.

In 10 of those 11 patients with a pituitary disease, skull x-ray films demonstrated a normal sella turcica, and thin slice state-of-the-art CT revealed a normal-appearing pituitary gland. In addition we studied one patient with an adrenal tumor and one healthy volunteer. Informed consent was obtained from all patients.

Blood (5 ml for each sample) was withdrawn simultaneously from both catheters and a peripheral vein for measurement of ACTH and prolactin concentrations. Blood samples obtained for measurement of ACTH were placed in chilled plastic tubes containing EDTA and aprotinin. The plasma was separated by centrifugation and stored at $-20°C$ until assay could be performed. ACTH was measured by double antibody assay reacting with the 1–24 amino acid sequence of human ACTH. Normal range of peripheral ACTH levels in healthy adults is 20 to 80 pg/ml. Intravenous stimulation with CRF was performed with 100 µg hCRF, and in 7 patients 200 µg TRH was injected intravenously 60 minutes after CRF application.

Results

Technical Results

Since 1985 we have performed selective IPS sampling in 36 patients. Our early results with the first 15 patients have been reported elsewhere (99). From an angiographic-technical point of view (e.g., success, problems, complications of catheterization) all of our patients are included in this chapter. Otherwise the presented results are limited to 13 patients, in whom selective sampling precisely followed a strict protocol, which included stimulation of the pituitary with CRF, and, in part, with TRH.

Due to anatomical variations, we were not able to selectively intubate the IPS bilaterally in 3 cases out of 36 (see Figs. 3.4 and 3.9); in 2 of these only one IPS could be catheterized.

In our second patient, sampling was erroneously performed out of the anterior condylar veins (this mistake was due to limited experience, and the fact that we performed sampling under normal fluoroscopy in our first four patients; thereafter we performed sampling under DSA guidance). In one case, sampling by an unexperienced angiographer was technically incorrect.

Complications were not observed. Occasionally, patients had a slight, temporary headache during the procedure.

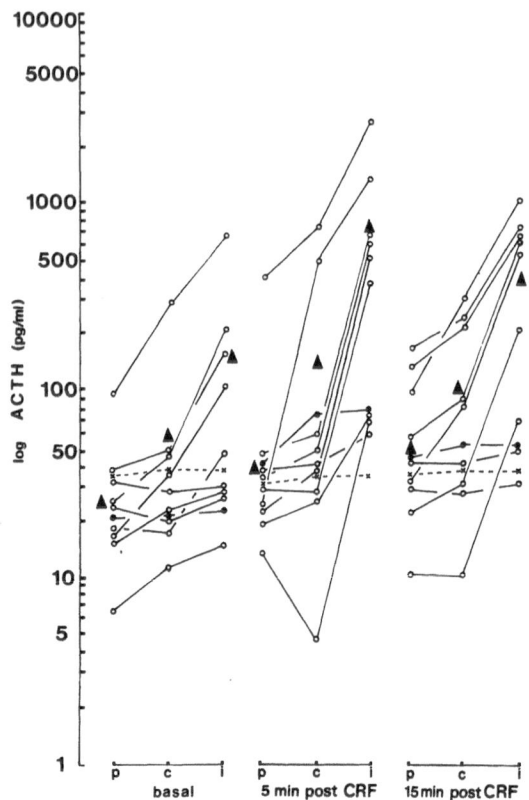

Figure 3.10. Plasma ACTH levels of 10 patients with a pituitary microadenoma (open circles), one patient with an adrenal tumor (crosses), and one healthy subject (closed circles). The mean values are depicted as triangles. p, peripheral; c, contralateral; i, ipsilateral.

Endocrinological Results

In 6 of the 11 patients with pituitary microadenomas, baseline plasma ACTH concentrations in the inferior petrosal sinus ipsilateral to the tumor were markedly higher than in the contralateral sinus; side-to-side ratios ranged from 1.5 to 6.8 (Fig. 3.10). Peripheral ACTH levels showed an average of 30.1 ± 8.5 pg/ml (SEM) (range: 4.0 to 97.0 pg/ml), contralateral central ACTH concentrations averaged 48.7 ± 27.9 pg/ml (range: 4.3 to 290.0 pg/ml), and ipsilateral central ACTH levels were 142.5 ± 72.4 pg/ml (range 15.5 to 632.0 pg/ml) at baseline.

After administration of hCRF 10 out of 11 patients with a pituitary adenoma showed higher ipsilateral ACTH levels, the side-to-side ratios varying between 1.7 and 19.0. Five minutes after CRF, contra- and ipsilateral ACTH levels showed their respective peaks: 137.2 ± 62.5 pg/ml (range: 11.4 to 374.0 pg/ml), and 935.6 ± 251.7 pg/ml (range: 52.5 to 2,340 pg/ml). Peripheral ACTH had an average concentration of 36.8 ± 16.6 pg/ml (range: 4.0 to 126 pg/ml) at the same time.

Peripheral prolactin levels were normal in all nine patients in whom measurements were obtained: at baseline, on the average, 7.7 ± 2.3 ng/ml (range: 1.9 to 9.5 ng/ml). Central prolactin levels already showed higher values on the tumor side: 39.9 ± 20.7 ng/ml (range: 5.0 to 149.2 ng/ml). On the contralateral side, prolactin averaged 14.5 ± 6.2 ng/ml (range: 2.2 to 46.7 ng/ml). After CRF, prolactin levels rose in eight out of nine patients: after 5 minutes peripheral levels had an average of 29.2 ± 12.9 ng/ml (range: 2.7 to 96.6 ng/ml), whereas ipsilateral levels even climbed to 201.7 ± 76.7 ng/ml (range: 9.7 to 482.4 ng/ml), and contralateral levels rose more moderately to 40.3 ± 19.6 ng/ml (range: 2.4 to 145.0 ng/ml) (Fig. 3.11).

Side-to-side ratios of prolactin paralleled those of ACTH, even after CRF administration: at baseline the same 6 out of 11 patients had ratios ranging from 1.7 to 8.1 with higher values on the tumor side; after CRF, however, eight out of nine demonstrated a higher hormonal concentration on the adenoma side, side-to-side ratios varying from 1.4 to 70.5 (Fig. 3.11).

One volunteer without Cushing's syndrome showed equivalent stimulation of ACTH on both sides at 5 minutes post-CRF (on the left side from 32.8 to 61.9 pg/ml, on the right side from 23.8 to 74.7 pg/ml), but exhibited no stimulation of prolactin levels after CRF (Figs. 3.10 and 3.12).

One patient with an adrenal adenoma had ACTH levels varying between 29.5 and 38.7 pg/ml peripherally and centrally without any response to CRF.

Seven patients received intravenous TRH 60 minutes past CRF. Plasma ACTH rose from 780 ± 357 pg/ml to a maximum of 2,025 ± 1,414 pg/ml on the side of an adenoma but only from 133 ± 59 pg/ml to 165 ± 72 pg/ml on the contra-

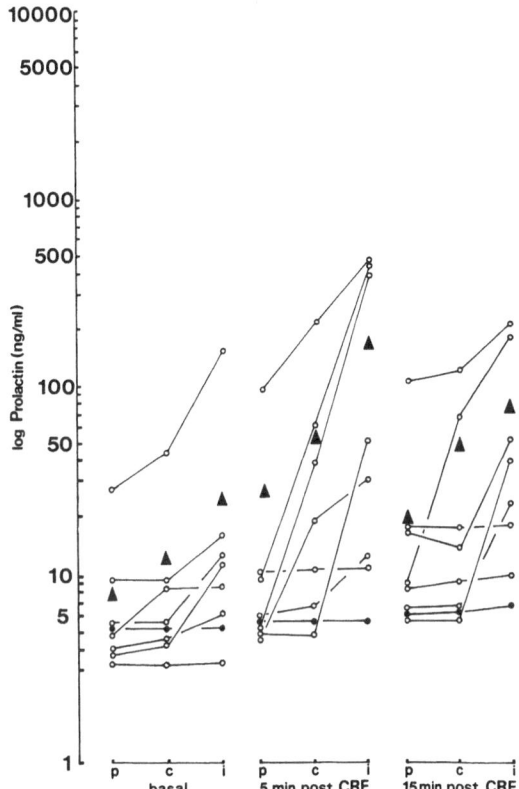

Figure 3.11. Plasma prolactin levels of seven patients with Cushing's disease (open circles) and one healthy subject (closed circles). The mean values are depicted as triangles. p, peripheral; c, contralateral; i, ipsilateral.

lateral side (Fig. 3.12). Plasma prolactin levels also increased to markedly higher levels on the tumor side: from 105 ± 53 ng/ml to 747 ± 168 ng/ml as compared to 28 ± 14 ng/ml and 68 ± 15 ng/ml, respectively, on the contralateral side (Fig. 3.13).

All eleven patients with suspected pituitary disease underwent elective microsurgery, and in all patients the tumor could be localized on the side predicted by the selective catheterization and stimulation of ACTH and prolactin by CRF or TRH.

Histologic examination confirmed the presence of an ACTH-containing microadenoma in all patients in whom Cushing's disease was suspected preoperatively by the high-dose dexamethasone test, and the selective bilateral catheterization with CRF or combined CRF/

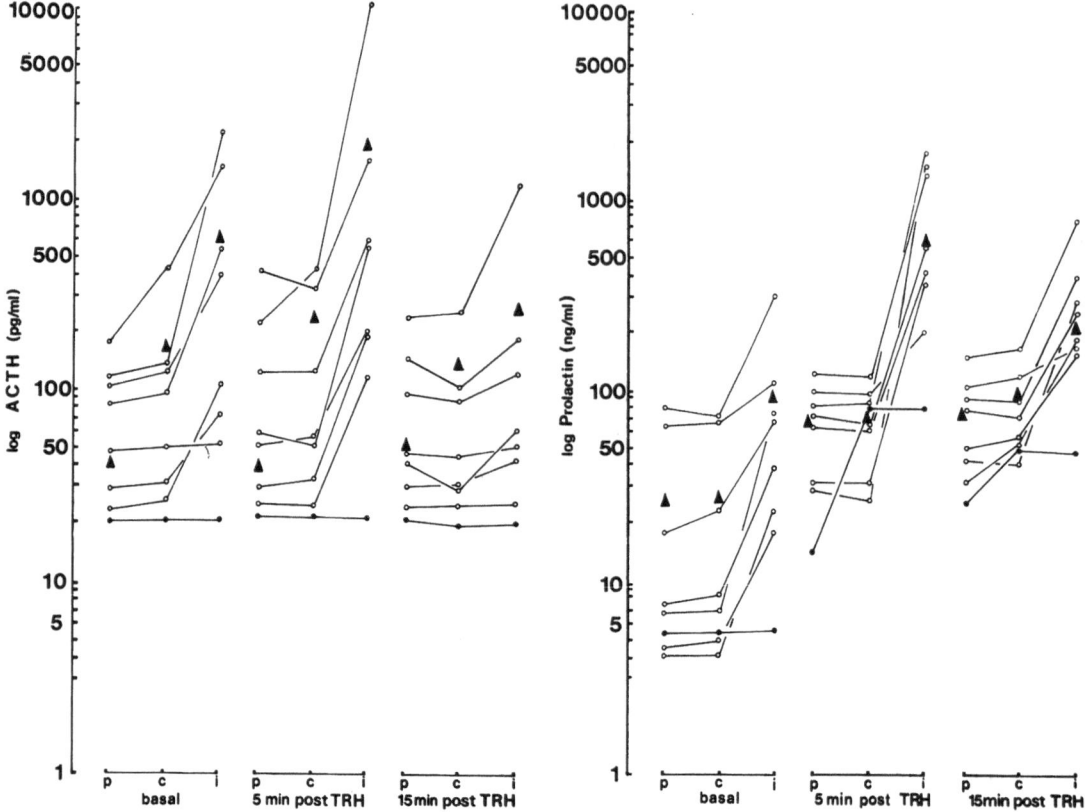

Figure 3.12. Plasma ACTH levels of seven patients with Cushing's disease (open circles) and one healthy subject (closed circles) following bolus injection of 200 μg TRH. The mean values are depicted as triangles. p, peripheral; c, contralateral; i, ipsilateral.

Figure 3.13. Plasma prolactin levels of seven patients with Cushing's disease (open circles) and one healthy subject (closed circles) following bolus injection of 200 μg TRH. The mean values are depicted as triangles. p, peripheral; c, contralateral; i, ipsilateral.

TRH stimulation. In the patient with adrenal mass, the disease was cured by removal of the respective adrenal gland.

Clinical and biochemical remission of hypercortisolism occurred postoperatively in all patients with pituitary disease, and pituitary function was normal, except for transient hypofunction of the hypothalamic-pituitary-adrenal axis, which was expected after successful removal of the ACTH-secreting pituitary microadenomas.

Discussion

Selective catheterization of the inferior petrosal sinus (IPS) with blood sampling and measurement of plasma ACTH may be of help in differentiating central from ectopic ACTH hypersecretion, and in localizing pituitary microadenomas (57,61,74,99,116,125,126).

Differentiation of central from ectopic ACTH-hypersecretion is impossible by laboratory/endocrinological tests in about 20% of the cases (1,21,126). The following facts should be kept in mind if one attempts IPS sampling for this reason:

ectopic ACTH-hypersecretion most often is due to a bronchial carcinoma;

next in frequency are carcinoid tumors, especially bronchial carcinoids, which may be very small (as may be pituitary adenomas); they can be suspected, when an arterial sample has a higher ACTH-concentration than a simultaneous venous sample (127–140).

If central ACTH-concentration in the IPS is at least two times higher than peripheral values, a pituitary source of ACTH can be assumed.

Under normal circumstances there is ipsilateral drainage of the pituitary blood (101). As most ACTH-secreting adenomas are situated laterally in the pituitary gland, blood from ipsilateral pituitary effluents should have a higher ACTH-concentration, than contralateral samples. As contralateral ACTH-producing cells may be suppressed, samples from the contralateral IPS often show hormonal levels similar to a peripheral sample. When concentration in one IPS is at least 1.4 times higher than in the opposite IPS, an ipsilateral pituitary source is likely.

Correct technique and catheter placement are the first major prerequisites for successful and reliable IPS sampling, as is the case with sampling elsewhere. Catheter tips should be positioned in the horizontal parts of both IPS, if possible central to affluents from the basilar plexus, which enter the IPS from the medial side. Unawareness of these anatomical structures may lead to malpositioning of the catheters, with false sampling.

Also, care must be taken to disturb hemodynamics as little as possible. The patient's head should be in a straight position, not turned to the side. Wedging of a catheter should be avoided, as this may cause preferential contralateral pituitary drainage. Forceful injections of contrast medium (and physiologic saline) can cause temporary alterations in hormonal levels. Therefore, sampling should start a few minutes (we wait about 5 minutes) after the last injection. Aspiration of blood should be gentle and with equal force on both sides.

It is essential to perform sampling simultaneously from both IPSs as well as a peripheral vein. Otherwise, well-known spontaneous fluctuations in hormonal secretion of ACTH may give rise to misleading results.

If for technical reasons only one IPS can be catheterized, and blood samples show peripheral ACTH-levels there are two possible causes: ACTH production from the contralateral pituitary or an ectopic source. The procedure then is of no diagnostic value. If, on the other hand, the ACTH concentration in the only central sample is significantly higher (as

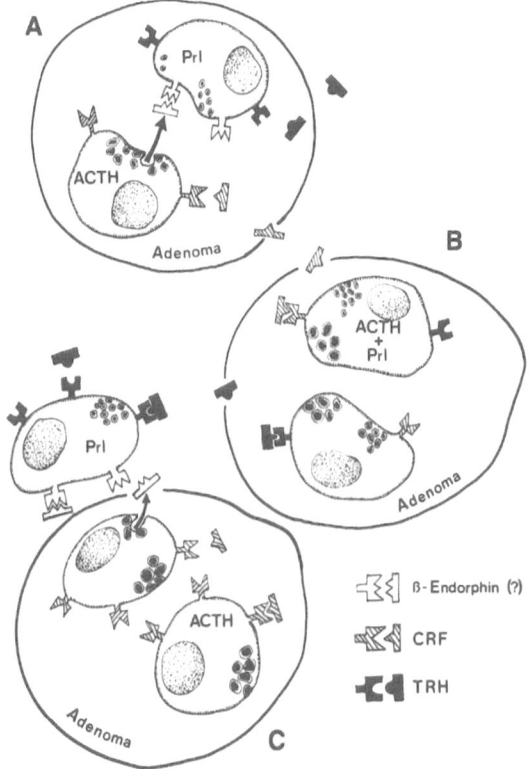

Figure 3.14. Three possible explanations of elevated prolactin levels (PRL) after CRF application. **A**: Two-cell-line tumor. **B**: Cosecretion of ACTH and prolactin from one cell line. **C**: Stimulation of normal lactotroph cells close to the adenoma.

mentioned above), this is diagnostic for central ACTH hypersecretion.

As hormonal assays have interassay variations (5 to 10%), small and borderline differences in hormonal concentrations are difficult to interpret. Thus, it seems reasonable to increase hormonal concentration gradients by stimulating pituitary hormonal secretion.

As already suggested in the literature (74,99) and recently demonstrated in detail (116), CRF further helps to discriminate the tumor side by stimulation of ACTH and/or prolactin in most patients with a pituitary microadenoma.

The observation that CRF stimulates prolactin and TRH may enhance ACTH levels in patients with a pituitary ACTH-producing adenoma is quite surprising. This stimulatory effect is not known to occur in healthy patients (as also demonstrated in our study). Peripheral hyper-prolactinemia is only rarely observed in patients with Cushing's disease. However, this may be a very constant feature of Cushing's disease, which was hidden until now by its very subtle expression in peripheral blood.

Three models can be proposed to explain this phenomenon of cosecretion (Fig. 3.13):

1. Secretion of prolactin and ACTH from two different cell lines, a hypothesis that is supported by a detailed immunohistochemical study (140).
2. Cosecretion of prolactin and ACTH from the same tumor cell, a proposition paralleling the findings from other pituitary adenomas (142–145).
3. Stimulation of prolactin by beta-endorphin which is secreted in stoichiometric amounts from any normal or tumoral adrenocorticotroph cell line (74,121,122,146).

The finding of pituitary hormone gradients other than ACTH may provide useful and confirmatory data to assist accurate lateralization of small microadenomas, which secrete ACTH plus other hormones. From the technical point of view, measurement of prolactin has some advantages when compared with ACTH: it can be measured by quite specific antibodies that exhibit no significant cross-reactivity to the chemically related growth hormone or placental lactogen. Like ACTH levels, prolactin concentration increases during periods of stress, but unlike ACTH, prolactin secretion does not seem to occur episodically. This improves discrimination of pathologic and normal levels, which are about 5 ng/ml in men and 8 ng/ml in women.

We also observed that TRH stimulated prolactin preferentially from the tumor side. In one patient with a pituitary microadenoma, in whom no lateralization of ACTH and prolactin was observed after CRF, TRH resulted in a pronounced increase of prolactin levels on the tumor side: the prolactin side-to-side ratio rose from 0.75 to 70.5. Thus, we suggest administering not only CRF for IPS sampling, but also TRH.

Besides being useful for lateralization of microadenomas, the described hormonal cosecretion may also enable better differentiation between central and ectopic ACTH-secreting tumors, since the latter do not secrete prolactin.

Conclusion

IPS sampling can be useful in selected patients with Cushing's syndrome; however, it has also been performed for non-ACTH secreting tumors (151). Eventhough from a theoretical point of view it seems to answer many diagnostic questions, it has problems of its own. The procedure requires bilaterally precise catheter placements, which is impossible due to anatomical variations in certain patients. This will be recognized only after angiographic demonstration of the anatomical situation. Ideal anatomical situations can be expected in only about half of the patients.

It cannot be overemphasized that unreliable results may be obtained

when sampling is done with less than ideal or
    even equivocal catheter placements, or
when the hemodynamic situation is altered.

The latter may be the case with large adenomas (which do not require IPS sampling for localization), and, unfortunately, after previous pituitary surgery. Thus lateralization of persisting or recurring secreting microadenomas after surgery cannot be reliably performed. In addition, even with correct catheter placement and normal hemodynamics, diagnostic problems may be observed. Therefore, IPS sampling may not be able to differentiate diffuse hyperplasia of adrenocorticotroph cells from a medially located microadenoma, even though this has not been reported to date (74,147,148,149).

Acknowledgment. The authors wish to thank Prof. U. Krause, Department of Endocrinology, for his support, assistance, and hormone determinations.

References

1. Liddle GW, Gibens JR, Nicholson WE, et al. The ectopic ACTH syndrome. *Cancer Res* 1965;25:1057–1061.
2. Schild H, Riedmiller H, Schweden F. Neben-

niere. In: Schild H, Schweden F, eds. *CT in der Urologie*. Stuttgart, New York: Georg Thieme Verlag; 1989.

3. Orth DN, Liddle GW. Results of treatment in 108 patients with Cushing's syndrome. *N Engl J Med* 1971;285:243–247.

4. Lüdecke D, Kautzky R, Saeger W, Schrader D. Selective removal of hypersecreting pituitary adenomas? *Acta Neurochir* 1976;35:27–42.

5. Tyrrell JB, Brooks RM, Fitzgerald PA, Cofoid PB, Forsham PH, Wilson CB. Selective transphenoidal resection of pituitary microadenomas. *N Engl J Med* 1978;298:753–758.

6. Soffer LJ, Iannaccone A, Gabrilove JL. Cushing's syndrome: a study of fifty patients. *Am J Med* 1961;30:129–146.

7. Crapo L. Cushing's syndromes: changing views of diagnosis and treatment. *Ann Intern Med* 1979;90:829–844.

8. Howlett TA, Drury PL, Perry L, Doniach I, Rees LH, Besser GM. Diagnosis and management of ACTH-dependent Cushing's syndrome: comparison of the features in ectopic and pituitary ACTH production. *Clin Endocrinol* 1986;24:699–713.

9. Orth DN. The old and the new in Cushing's syndrome. *N Engl J Med* 1984;310:649–651.

10. Murphy BEP. Some studies of the protein-binding of steroids and their application to the routine micro and ultramicro measurement of various steroids in body fluids by competitive protein-binding assay. *J Clin Endocrinol Metab* 1967;27:973–990.

11. Ruder HJ, Guy RL, Lipsett MB. A radioimmunoassay for cortisol in plasma and urine. *J Clin Endocrinol Metab* 1972;35:219–224.

12. Kabra PM, Tsai L, Marton LJ. Improved liquid-chromatography method for determination of serum cortisol. *Clin Chem* 1979;25:1293–1296.

13. Ballard PL, Carter JP, Graham BS, Baxter JO. A radioreceptor assay for evaluation of the plasma glucocorticoid activity of natural and synthetic steroids in man. *J Clin Endocrinol Metab* 1975;41:290–304.

14. Gore M, Cester E. Comparison of a fenorinetic and a competitive protein binding assay for determination of plasma hydrocycorticosteroids. *Ann Clin Biochem* 1975;12:160.

15. Millan MA, Abou Samra AB, Wynn PC, Catt KJ, Aguilera G. Receptors and actions of corticotropin-releasing hormone in the primate pituitary gland. *J Clin Endocrinol Metab* 1987;64:1036–1041.

16. Robin P, Predine J, Milgrom E. Assay of unbound cortisol in plasma. *J Clin Endocrinol Metab* 1977;46:277–283.

17. Evans PJ, Peters RJ, Dynas J, Walker RF, Riad-Fahnuy D, Hall R. Salivary cortisol levels in true and apparent hypercortisolism. *Clin Endocrinol* 1984;20:709–715.

18. Delacerda L, Kowarski A, Migeon CJ. Integrated concentration and diurnal variation of plasma cortisol. *J Clin Endocrinol Metab* 1973;36:227–283.

19. Crapo L. Cushing's syndrome: a review of diagnostic tests. *Metabolism* 1979;28:955–977.

20. Aron DC, Tyrrell JB, Fitzgerald PA, Findling JW, Forsham PH. Cushing syndrome: problems in diagnosis. *Medicine* 1981;60:25–35.

21. Liddle GW. Tests of pituitary adrenal suppressibility in the diagnosis of Cushing's syndrome. *J Clin Endocrinol Metab* 1960;20(2):1539–1560.

22. Tyrell JB, Findling JW, Aron DC, Fitzgerald PA, Forsham PH. An overnight high-dose dexamethasone suppression test for rapid differential diagnosis of Cushing's syndrome. *Ann Intern Med* 1986;104:180–186.

23. Lytras N, Grossman, Perry L. Corticotrophin relasing factor: responses in normal subjects and patients with disorders of the hypothalamus and pituitary. *Clin Endocrinol* 1984;20:71–84.

24. Boggan JE, Tyrell JB, Wilson CB. Transsphenoidal microsurgical management of Cushing's disease. *J Neurosurg* 1983;59(2):195–200.

25. MacErlean DP, Doyle DP. The pituitary fossa in Cushing's syndrome: a retrospective analysis of 93 patients. *Br J Radiol* 1976;49:820–826.

26. Turski PA, Newton Th, Horten BH. Sellar contour: anatomic-polytomographic correlation. *AJR* 1981;137:213–216.

27. Burrow GN, Wortzman G, Rewcastle HB, Holgate RC, Kovacs K. Microadenomas of the pituitary and abnormal sella tomograms in an unselected autopsy series. *N Engl J Med* 1981;304:156–158.

28. Taylor CR, Jaffe CC. Methodological problems in clinical radiology research: pituitary microadenoma detection as a paradigm. *Radiology* 1983;147:279–283.

29. Pojunas KW, Daniels DL, Williams AL, Thorsen MK, Haughton VM. Pituitary and adrenal CT of Cushing's syndrome. *AJR* 1986;146:1235–1238.

30. Teasdale E, Teasdale G, Mohsen F, MacPherson P. High-resolution computed tomography in pituitary microadenoma: is seeing believing? *Clin Radiol* 1986;37:227–232.

31. Saris SC, Patronas NJ, Doppman JL, et al. Cushing's syndrome: pituitary CT scanning. *Radiology* 1987;162:775–777.

32. Marcovitz S, Wee R, Chan S, Hardy J. Diagnostic accuracy of preoperative CT scanning of pituitary somatotroph adenomas. *AJNR* 1988;9:19–22.

33. Davis PC, Hoffman JC Jr, Spencer T, Tindall GT, Braun IF. MR Imaging of pituitary adenoma: CT, clinical, and surgical correlation. *AJR* 1987;148:797–802.

34. Irnberger Th. Die hochauflösende koronare Computertomographie bei endokrin aktiven Mikroadenomen der Hypophyse unter besonderer Berücksichtigung ihrer Kontrastmitteldynamik. *Fortschr Röntgenstr* 1985;143(3): 315–321.

35. Chambers EF, Turski PA, LaMasters D, Newton TH. Regions of low density in the contrast-enhanced pituitary gland: normal and pathologic processes. *Radiology* 1982;144:109–113.

36. Turski PA, Damm M. Role of computed tomography in the evaluation of pituitary disease. *Semin Ultrasound CT MR* 1985;6:276.

37. Peck WW, Dillon WP, Norman D, Newton TH, Wilson CB. High-resolution MR imaging of pituitary microadenomas at 1.5 T: experience with Cushing disease. *AJR* 1989;152:145–151.

38. Wichmann W, Schubiger O, Valavanis A, Kasdaglis K. Zur kernspintomographischen Diagnostik von Mikroadenomen der Hypophyse: Vergleich MRT, CT und OP. *Fortschr Röntgenstr* 1988;149;3:239–244.

39. Dwyer AJ, Frank JA, Doppman JL, et al. Pituitary adenomas in patients with Cushing disease: initial experience with Gd-DTPA-enhanced MR imaging. *Radiology* 1987;163: 421–426.

40. Kucharczyk W, Davis DO, Kelly WM, Sze G, Norman G, Newton TH. Pituitary adenomas: high-resolution MR imaging at 1.5 T1. *Radiology* 1986;161:761–765.

41. Doppman JL, Frank JA, Dwyer AJ, et al. Gadolinium DTPA enhanced MR imaging of ACTH-secreting microadenomas of the pituitary gland: correlation of MR appearance with surgical findings. *J Comput Assist Tomogr* 1988;12:728–735.

42. Scriba PC, Hacker R, Dieterle P, Kluge F, Hochheuser W, Schwarz K. ACTH-Bestimmungen im Plasma aus dem Bulbus cranialis venae jugularis. *Klin Wochenschr* 1966;24: 1393–1397.

43. Werder K v, Scriba PC. Jugular-vein sampling of ACTH (Letter to editor). *N Engl Med J* 1977;297:730.

44. Drury PL, Ratter S, Tomlin S, et al. Experience with selective venous sampling in diagnosis of ACTH-dependent Cushing's syndrome. *Br Med J* 1982;284:9–12.

45. Grant SJB, Stiel JN, Sorby WA, Henniker AJ. Venous ACTH sampling in Cushing's syndrome. *Med J Aust* 1983;1:336–337.

46. Yalow RS. Heterogenicity of peptide hormone. *Recent Prog Horm Res* 1976;32:33–79.

47. Liberman B, Wajchenberg BL, Tambascia MA, Mesquita CH. Periodic remission in Cushing's disease with paradoxical dexamethasone response: an expression of periodic hormonogenesis. *J Clin Endocrinol Metab* 1976;43:913–918.

48. Bailey RE. Periodic hormonogenesis—a new phenomenon: periodicity in function of a hormone-producing tumor in man. *J Clin Endocrinol Metab* 1971;32:317–327.

49. Blau N, Miller WE, Miller ER, Cervi-Steiner J. Spontaneous remission of Cushing's syndrome in a patient with an adrenal adenoma. *J Clin Endocrinol Metab* 1975;40:659–663.

50. Aron DC, Findling JW, Tyrrell JB, et al. Pituitary-ACTH dependency of nodular adrenal hyperplasia in Cushing's syndrome. *Am J Med* 1981;71:302–306.

51. Findling JW, Tyrrell B. Occult ectopic secretion of corticotropin. *Arch Intern Med* 1986; 146:929–933.

52. Parent AD, Begin J, Smith RR. Incidental pituitary adenomas. *J Neurosurg* 1981;54:228–231.

53. Salassa RM, Laws ER, Carpenter PC, Northcutt RC. Transsphenoidal removal of pituitary microadenoma in Cushing's disease. *Mayo Clin Proc* 1978;53:24–28.

54. Hardy J. Transsphenoidal microsurgery of the normal and pathological pituitary. *Clin Neurosurg* 1977;16:185.

55. Brown RD, van Loon GR, Orth ND, Liddle GW. Cushing's disease with periodic hormonogenesis: one explanation for paradoxixal response to dexamethasone. *J Clin Endocrinol Metab* 1973;36:445–451.

56. Carey RM. Suppression of ACTH by cortisol in dexamethasone-nonsuppressible Cushing's disease. *N Engl J Med* 1977;302:275–279.

57. Findling JW, Aron DC, Tyrrell JB. Selective venous sampling for ACTH in Cushing's syndrome: Differentiation between Cushing's disease and the ectopic ACTH syndrome. *Ann Intern Med* 1981;94:647–652.

58. Lamberts SWJ, de Jong FH, Birkenhäger JC. Evaluation of diagnostic and differential diagnostic tests in Cushing's syndrome. *Neth J Med* 1977;20:267–274.

59. Northrop G, Baldwin D, Faber LP, Schwartz TB. Dexamethasone suppression of urinary 17-hydroxycorticoids in a patient with an ACTH-producing bronchial adenoma. *Presbyterian-St.Luke's Medical Bulletin* 1970;9: 43–44.

60. Kley HK, Stolze T, Krüskemper HL. Letter to the editor. *N Engl J Med* 1977;297:731–732.

61. Corrigan DF, Schaaf M, Whaley RA, Czerwinski CL, Earll JM. Selective venous sampling to differentiate ectopic ACTH secretion from pituitary Cushing's syndrome. *N Engl J Med* 1977;296:861–862.

62. Boggan JE, Tyrrell JB, Wilson CB. Transsphenoidal microsurgical management of Cushing's disease. Report of 100 cases. *J Neurosurg* 1983;59:195–200.

63. Oldfield EH, Chrousos GP, Schulte HM. Preoperative lateralization of ACTH-secreting pituitary microadenomas by bilateral and simultaneous inferior petrosal venous sinus sampling. *N Engl J Med* 1985;312:100–103.

64. Xuereb GP, Prichard MML, Daniel PM. The arterial supply and venous drainage of the human hypophysis cerebri. *QJ Exp Physiol* 1954;39:199–218.

65. Green HT. The venous drainage of the human hypophysis cerebri. *Am J Anat* 1957;100:435–456.

66. Bergland RM, Ray BS, Torack RM. Anatomical variations in pituitary gland and adjacent structures in 225 human autopsy cases. *J Neurosurg* 1968;23:93–99.

67. Bergland RM, Page RB. Can the pituitary secrete directly to the brain? (affirmative anatomical evidence). *Endocrinology* 1978;102: 1325–1338.

68. Oliver C, Mical RS, Porter JC. Hypothalamic-pituitary vasculature. *Endocrinology* 1977;101: 598–604.

69. Page RB. Pituitary blood flow. *Am J Physiol* 1982;243:E427–E442.

70. Page RB. Directional pituitary blood flow: a microcinephotographic study. *Endocrinology* 1983;112:157–165.

71. Antunes JL, Muraszko K, Stark R, Chen R. Pituitary blood flow in primates: a Doppler study. *Neurosurgery* 1983;12:492–495.

72. Bonneville JF, Dietemann JL. *Radiology of the Sella Turcica.* Berlin-Heidelberg-New York: Springer; 1981.

73. Boskovic JF, Savic V, Josifov J. Über die Sinus petrosi und ihre Zuflüsse. *Gegenbaurs Morphol Verb* 1963;104:420.

74. Doppman JL, Oldfield E, Krudy AG. Petrosal sinus sampling for Cushing's syndrome: anatomical and technical considerations. *Radiology* 1984;150:99–103.

75. Gänshirt H. *Der Hirnkreislauf.* Stuttgart: Thieme; 1972.

76. Gejrot T, Lauren T. Retrograde venography of the internal jugular veins and transverse sinuses. *Acta Otolaryngol* 1964;57:177–179.

77. Hanafee WN. Orbital venography. *Radiol Clin North Am* 1982;10:63–65.

78. Hanafee WN, Rosen LM, Weidner W, Wilson GH. Venography of the cavernous sinus, orbital veins, and basal venous plexus. *Radiology* 1965;84:751–754.

79. Hanafee WN, Shiu PC, Dayton GO. Orbital venography. *Am J Roentgenol* 1968;104:29–35.

80. Harris FS, Rhoton AL. Anatomy of the cavernous sinus. *J Neurosurg* 1976;45:169–180.

81. Jacobs JB, Grivas NE. Interval cavernous sinography in the evaluation of intrasellar masses. *Am J Roentgenol* 1969;107:589–594.

82. Kaplan HA, Browder J, Krieger AJ. Intercavernous connections of the cavernous sinuses. *J Neurosurg* 1976;45:166–168.

83. Krayenbühl H, Yasargil MG. *Zerebrale Angiographie für Klinik und Praxis.* Stuttgart-New York: Thieme; 1979.

84. Krmpotic-Nemanic J, Draf W, Helms J. *Chirurgische Anatomie des Kopf-Hals-Bereiches.* Berlin-Heidelberg-New York-Tokyo: Springer; 1985.

85. Lang J. *Klinische Anatomie des Kopfes.* Berlin-Heidelberg-New York: Springer; 1981.

86. Lanz T von, Wachsmuth W. *Praktische Anatomie.* 1. Band, Teil 1 b. Berlin-Heidelberg-New York: Springer; 1979.

87. Lombardi G, Passerini A. Venography of the orbit: technique and anatomy. *Br J Radiol* 1968;41:282–286.

88. Nadjmi M, Mertens HG, Moissl G, Dommasch D. Jugularographie und Phlebogramm. *Radiologe* 1971;11:395–404.

89. Pernkopf E. *Topographische Anatomie des Menschen.* Band 4. München-Berlin-Wien: Urban & Schwarzenberg; 1960.

90. Piscol K. Die perkutane Katheterisierung der Vena frontalis zur Darstellung der orbitalen Venen und des Sinus cavernosus. *Fortschr Röntgenstr* 1970;112:56–60.

91. Renn WH, Rhoton AL. Microsurgical ana-
    tomy of the sella region. *J Neurosurg* 1975;
    43:288–298.
92. Shiu PC, Hanafee WN, Wilson GH, Rand
    RW. Cavernous sinus venography. *Am J
    Roentgenol* 1968;104:57–62.
93. Takahashi M, Tanaka M. Cavernosus sinus
    venography by transfemoral catheter tech-
    nique. *Neuroradiology* 1971;3:1.
94. Theron J, Moret J. *Spinal Phlebography.* Ber-
    lin, Heidelberg-New York: Springer; 1978.
95. Vignaud J, Clay C. Technique d'opacification
    par voie veineuse du plexus caverneux. *Ann
    Radiol* 1974;17:229–230.
96. Waga S, Kikuchi H, Handa J, Handa H.
    Cavernous sinus venography. *Am J Roentgenol*
    1970;109:130–137.
97. Weidner W, Rosen L, Hanafee W. Neuro-
    radiology of tumors of pituitary gland. *Am J
    Roentgenol* 1965;95:884–889.
98. Doppmann JL, Krudy AG, Girton ME, Old-
    field EH. Basilar venous plexus of the post-
    erior fossa: a potential source of error in
    petrosal sinus sampling. *Radiology* 1985;155:
    375–378.
98b. Wilson M. The anatomic foundation of
    neuroradiology of the brain. Little, Brown and
    Co., Boston, 1972.
99. Schild H, Strack T, Günther R, et al. Selek-
    tive Blutentnahme aus dem Sinus petrosus in-
    ferior mit digitaler Subtraktionsangiographie.
    Fortschr Röntgenstr 1986;144(6):627–635.
100. Brismar G, Brismar J, Cronquist S. Complica-
    tions of orbital and skull base phlebography.
    Acta Radiol Diagnosis 1976;17:274–280.
101. Oldfield EH, Girton ME, Doppman JL. Ab-
    sence of intercavernous mixing: evidence sup-
    porting lateralization of pituitary microadeno-
    mas by venous sampling. *J Clin Endocrinol
    Metab* 1985;61:644–647.
102. Krieger DT, Allen W. Relationship of bioas-
    sayable and immunoassayable plasma ACTH
    and cortisol concentrations in normal subjects
    and in patients with Cushing's disease. *J Clin
    Endocrinol Metab* 1975;40:675–687.
103. Vale W, Spiess J, Rivier C, Rivier J. Charac-
    terization of a 41-residue ovine hypothalamic
    peptide that stimulates secretion of corticotro-
    pin and β-endorphin. *Science* 1981;213:1394–
    1397.
104. Müller OA, Hartwimmer J, Hauer J.
    Corticotropin-releasing factor (CRF) stimula-
    tion in normal controls and in patients with
    Cushing's syndrome. *Psychoneuroendocrinol-
    ogy* 1986;11:49–60.
105. Pieters GF, Hermus AR, Smals AG. Respon-
    siveness of the hypophyseal-adrenal axis to
    corticotropin-releasing factor: in pituitary-
    dependent Cushing's disease. *J Clin Endocri-
    nol Metab* 1983;57:513–516.
106. Schuermeyer T, Averginos PC, Gold PW. Hu-
    man corticotropin releasing factor in man:
    pharmacokinetic properties and dose-response
    of plasma ACTH and cortisol secretion. *J Clin
    Endocrinol Metab* 1984;59:1103–1108.
107. Chrousos GA, Schulte HM, Oldfield EH,
    Gold PW, Cutler GB Jr, Lorianux DL. The
    corticotropin-releasing factor stimulation: an
    aid in the evaluation of patients with Cushing's
    syndrome. *N Engl J Med* 1984;310:622–626.
108. Cote J, Lefevre G, Labrie F, Barden N. Dis-
    tribution of corticotropin-releasing factor in
    ovine brain determined by radioimmunoassay.
    Regul Pept 1983;5:189–195.
109. Swanson LW, Sawchenko PE, Rivier J, Vale
    WW. Organization of ovine corticotropin-
    releasing factor immunoreactive cells and
    fibers in the rat brain: an immunohistochemi-
    cal study. *Neuroendocrinology* 1983;36:165–
    186.
110. Gibbs DM, Stewart RD, Lin JH, Vale W,
    Rivier J, Yen SSC. Effects of synthetic
    corticotropin-releasing factor and dopamine
    on the release of immunoreactive β-endorphin/
    β-lipotropin and α-melanocyte-stimulating
    hormone from human fetal pituitaries in-vitro.
    J Clin Endocrinol Metab 1982;55:1149–1152.
111. Furutani Y, Morimoto Y, Shibahara S. Clon-
    ing and sequence analysis of CDNA for ovine
    corticotropin-releasing factor precursor. *Na-
    ture* 1983;301:537–540.
112. Giguere V, Labrie F, Cote J, Coy DH,
    Sueiras-Diaz J, Schally AV. Stimulation of
    cyclic AMP accumulation and corticotropin re-
    lease by synthetic ovine corticotropin-releasing
    factor anterior pituitary cells: site of gluco-
    corticoid action. *Proc Natl Acad Sci USA*
    1982;79:3466–3469.
113. Peters JR, Foord SM, Diequez C, Scanlon
    MF, Hall R. Alpha1-adrenoreceptors on intact
    rat anterior pituitary cells. Correlation with
    adrenergic stimulation of thyrotropin secre-
    tion. *Endocrinology* 1983;113:133–140.
114. Johns MA, Azmitia EC, Krieger DT. Specific
    in-vitro uptake of serotonin by cells in the
    anterior pituitary of the rat. *Endocrinology*
    1982;110:754–760.
115. Grino M, Guillaume V, Boudouresque F, et
    al. Characterization of corticotropin-releasing
    hormone receptors on human pituitary corti-

cotroph adenomas and their correlation with endogenous glucocorticoids. *J Clin Endocrinol Metab* 1988;67:279–283.

116. Schulte HM, Allolio B, Günther RW, et al. Selective bilateral and simultaneous catheterization of the inferior petrosal sinus: CRF stimulates prolactin secretion from ACTH-producing microadenomas in Cushing's disease. *Clin Endocrinol* 1988;28:289–293.

117. Hyde JF, Ben-Jonathan N. The posterior pituitary contains a potent prolactin-releasing factor: in-vivo studies. *Endocrinology* 1989; 125:736–741.

118. Grossman A, Perry L, Schally AV. New hypothalamic hormone, corticotropin-releasing factor, specifically stimulates the release of adrenocorticotropic hormone and cortisol in man. *Lancet* 1982;1:921–925.

119. Orth DN, DeBold CR, DeCherney GS. Pituitary adenomas causing Cushing's disease respond to CRF. *J Clin Endocrinol Metab* 1982;55:1017–1019.

120. Hermus AR, Pieters GF, Pesman GJ. Responsivity of adrenocorticotropin to corticotropin-releasing hormone and lack of suppressibility by dexamethasone are related phenomena in Cushing's disease. *J Clin Endocrinol Metab* 1986;62:634–639.

121. Rivier C, Vale N, Cuig N, Brown M, Guillenni R. Stimulation in-vivo of the secretion of prolactin and growth hormone by β-endorphin. *Endocrinology* 1977;100:238–241.

122. Rivier C, Brownstein M, Spiess J, Rivier J, Vale W. In-vivo corticotropin-releasing factor-induced secretion of adrenocorticotropin beta-endorphin, and corticosternine. *Endocrinology* 1982;110:272–278.

123. Chrousos GP, Nieman L, Nisula B, et al. Corticotropin-releasing factor stimulation (Letter to the Editor). *N Engl J Med* 1984; 311:471–472.

124. Malchoff CD, Orth DN, Abboud C, Carney JA, Paivolero PC, Carey RM. Ectopic ACTH syndrome caused by a bronchial carcinoid tumor responsive to dexamethasone, metyrapone, and corticotropin-releasing factor. *Am J Med* 1988;12:728–735.

125. Manni A, Latshaw RF, Page JR, Santen RJ. Simultaneous bilateral venous sampling for adrenocorticotropin in pituitary-dependent Cushing's disease: evidence for lateralization of pituitary venous drainage. *J Clin Endocrinol Metab* 1983;57:1070.

126. Hauffa BP, Stolecke H, Schulte HM. Cushing disease: successful preoperative lateralization of an ACTH-producing pituitary microadenoma by simultaneous bilateral inferior petrosal venous sinus sampling with corticotropin releasing hormone stimulation. *Eur J Pediatr* 1986;145:559–562.

127. Doppman JL, Nieman L, Miller DL, et al. Ectopic Adrenocorticotropic Hormone Syndrome: Localization Studies in 28 Patients. *Radiology* 1989;172:115–124.

128. Alloh EN, Skelton MO. Increased adrenocortical activity associated with malignant disease. *Lancet* 1960;2:278–284.

129. Azzopardi JG, Williams ED. Pathology of "nonendocrine" tumors associated with Cushing's syndrome. *Cancer* 1968;22:274–286.

130. Imura H, Matsukura S, Yamamoto H. Studies on ectopic ACTH-producing tumors: Clinical and biochemical features of 30 cases. *Cancer* 1975;35:1430–1437.

131. Imura H. Ectopic hormone syndromes. *Clin Endocrinol Metab* 1980;9:235–249.

132. Mason AMS, Ratcliffe JG, Buckle RM, Mason AS. ACTH secretion by bronchial carcinoid tumors. *Clin Endocrinol* 1972;1:3–7.

133. O'Riordan JLH, Blanshard GP, Moxham A, Nabarro JDN. Corticotrophin-secreting carcinomas. *QJ Med* 1966;35:137–140.

134. Rees LH, Bloomfield GA, Gilkes JJH, Joffcoate J, Besser GM. ACTH as a tumor marker. *Ann NY Acad Sci* 1977;297:603.

135. Scriba PC, Werder K v, Richter J, Schwarz K. Ein Beitrag zur klinischen Diagnostik des ektopischen ACTH-Syndroms. *Klin Wochenschr* 1967;46:49–51.

136. Singer W, Kovacs K, Ryan N, Horvath E. Ectopic ACTH sndrome: clinicopathological correlations. *J Clin Pathol* 1978;31:591–598.

137. Strott CA, Nugent CA, Tyler FH. Cushing's syndrome caused by bronchial adenomas. *Am J Med* 1968;44:97–103.

138. Wahl TO, Kyner JL. Source of ACTH in Cushing's disease. *N Engl J Med* 1979;300:679.

139. Kahaly G, Strack T, Krause U, et al. A CRF-producing and -secreting tumor of the lung. In: Moody TW, ed. *Neural and Endocrine Peptides*. New York: Plenum; 1986:439.

140. Findling JW, Tyrrell JB. Occult ectopic secretion of corticotropin. *Arch Intern Med* 1986;146:929–933.

141. Sherry SH, Guay AT, Lee AK, et al. Concurrent production of adrenocorticotropin and prolactin from two distinct cell lines in a single pituitary adenoma: a detailed immunohistochemical analysis. *J Clin Endocrinol Metab* 1982;55:947–955.

142. Müller OA, Fink R, Werderk K v, Scriba PC. Hypersecretion of ACTH, growth hormone and prolactin in a patient with pituitary adenoma. *Acta Endocrinol* 1978;87(*Suppl* 215):4–5.

143. Heitz PU. Multihormonal pituitary adenomas. *Horm Res* 1979;10:1–13.

144. Bassetti M, Spada A, Arusio M, Vallar L, Brina M, Giannattasio G. Morphological studies on mixed growth-hormone (GH-) and prolactin (PRL-) secreting human pituitary adenomas. Co-existence of GM and PRL in the same secretory granule. *J Clin Endocrinol Metab* 1986;62:1093–1100.

145. Melmed S, Braunstein G, Chang RG, Becker DP. UCLA conference: pituitary tumors secreting growth hormone and prolactin. *Ann Intern Med* 1986;105:238–253.

146. Crock PA, Pestell RG, Calenti AJ, et al. Multiple pituitary hormone gradients from inferior petrosal sinus sampling in Cushing's disease. *Acta Endocrinol* 1988;119:75–80.

147. Lamberts SWJ, Stefanko SZ, de Lange SA, et al. Failure of clinical remission after transsphenoidal removal of microadenoma in a patient with Cushing's disease: multiple hyperplastic and adenomatous cell nests in surrounding pituitary tissue. *J Clin Endocrinol Metab* 1980;50:793–795.

148. Schnall AM, Kovacs K, Brodkey JS, Pearson OH. Pituitary Cushing's disease without adenoma. *Acta Endocrinol (Copenh)* 1980;94: 297–303.

149. Miller DL, Doppman JL, Nieman KL, et al. Petrosal sinus sampling: discordant lateralization of pituitary microadenomas before and after stimulation with corticotropin releasing hormone. *Radiology* 1990:176;429–431.

150. Miller DL, Doppman JL. Petrosal sinus sampling: technique and rationale. *Radiology* 1991;178:37–47.

151. Frank SJ, Gesundheit N, Doppman JL, et al. Preoperative lateralization of pituitary microadenomas by petrosal sinus sampling: utility in two patients with non-ACTH secreting tumors. *Am J Med* 1989;87:679.

4

Pancreatic Venous Sampling

—— *Renan Uflacker* ——

Introduction

Pancreatic islet cell tumors are often small lesions that are detected by the clinical syndromes they produce and not by their tumor mass. Localization, therefore, is difficult, yet important, as surgery is frequently curative (1).

Neuroendocrine cells from pancreatic islets release amines and polypeptides, which interfere with the physiologic processes of digestion and glucose metabolism. Excessive release of normal and abnormal hormones is encountered when pathologic dysplasias of the islets occur, overriding normal regulatory control. The action of the released hormones on target receptors will cause clinical syndromes reflecting the function of a single polypeptide, the secretion of multiple peptides, or the presence of abnormal peptides in function and structural characteristics. Clinical presentation, however, may be very subtle or not detectable at all and the diagnosis may be made only on family member screening or in retrospect (2).

Some of the endocrine tumors of the pancreas become manifest functionally only after special methods of study are used. Some of these tumors will remain below the threshold of detection by current techniques and are designated as nonfunctioning. Others release polypeptides that are biologically inactive and do not produce a recognizable clinical picture.

The observation of the ulcerogenic syndrome by Zollinger and Ellison caused a great increase in investigational activity regarding endocrine tumors of the pancreas which markedly expanded knowledge in that field. The most important developments were the formulation of the amine-precursor uptake and decarboxylation (APUD) concept, study of the pathogenetic types of endocrinopathies, improvement in diagnosis and localization of the lesions by biochemical and immunochemical identification of polypeptides, new imaging techniques, development of new therapeutic methods, and the recognition of clinical syndromes (3).

Functioning islet cell tumors are diagnosed by the hormones they elaborate and can be localized preoperatively with a combination of arteriography, selective venous sampling, bolus-dynamic computed tomography (CT), intraoperative ultrasound, and magnetic resonance imaging (MRI) (4). The accuracy of preoperative localization varies from a low of 15 to 70% (4,5) for gastrinomas to a high of 80 to 90% for insulinomas (4).

Regardless of the clinical presentation and the method of diagnosis the management of such lesions should include early detection of the islet cell tumor before nonreversible organic damage or metastases occur.

Population of Pancreatic Endocrine Cells

The islet of Langerhans represents the major locus of pancreatic endocrine cells; it is already established, however, that a small but variable proportion of similar endocrine cells are also present in noninsular locations along the pancreatic ductular epithelium and paraductular acinar elements. Both from a functional and ultrastructural standpoint, eight distinct cell types are currently recognized within the pancreatic islets (6). Not all cell types are normally present in all species, and some of these have only been identified in the developing embryo (6).

In early research, the production of the hormone insulin was detected to be derived from the beta cells (B cells) among a variety of islet cells. The islets were referred to as being composed of B cells and a group of nonbeta cells. Histochemical properties, reactivity to the varios impregnation procedure, and the discovery of glucagon, another pancreatic hormone, subsequently permitted the identification of the alpha (or A_2) cell. A third histochemically distinct islet cell type, the D cell, has been latterly identified, and without recognizable function until somatostatin was discovered.

The isolation of the vasoactive intestinal peptide (VIP) led to the discovery of the VIP cells present in small number (2 to 5%) in the islet cells and scattered along the acinar tissues.

Further studies in minor impurities in insulin preparation led to the discovery of the hormone human pancreatic polypeptide (hPP). Most of the pancreatic polypeptide immunoreactivity is confined to the posterior portion of the head and uncinate process, portions derived from the ventral pancreatic bud (6). PP cells are localized within the islet cells and also in occasional cells scattered within the ducts and acinar elements.

The presence of gastrin producing G cells in the gastroduodenal mucosa in humans and in a variety of species has been firmly established. The presence of similar cells in the pancreas, however, has not been convincingly demonstrated. The isolation of gastrin from islet cell tumors in patients with Zollinger-Ellison syndrome prompted a search for gastrin secreting cells (G cells) in normal pancreatic islets. Gastrin production was ascribed, initially, to the D cells. But D cells are now related to the production of somatostatin. Fetal and neonatal observations, as well as tissue cultures and the high incidence of pancreatic origin for the gastrinomas, strongly indicate that gastrin may indeed be secreted by an as-yet-unidentified cell that may be present in small numbers (6).

A number of other polypeptide hormones (secretin and substance P) and biogenic amines (serotonin and dopamine) are also associated with the pancreatic islets; however, no specific islet cell type has yet been identified. At the ultrastructural level, however, cellular secretory granules morphologically identical to those of the enterochromaffin cell of the gut have been identified and these cells have been designated as pancreatic EC cells and associated with serotonin (5-HT) (6).

Distribution of Hormone-Producing Islet Cells

Different islet cell hormone producing can be demonstrated by immunohistochemical methods (Fig. 4.1). For the demonstration of insulin, an indirect peroxidase technique employing guinea pig antiinsulin (1:1000 for 24 hours at 4°C) and peroxidase-conjugated rabbit anti-guinea pig IgG (1:50 for 30 minutes at 22°C) is used. Rabbit antivasoactive intestinal peptide serum is used for VIP cells.

The distribution pattern of the various cell types within the islet of Langerhans is related to the microcirculation. Immunohistochemical studies demonstrated that in humans the insulin-producing B cells occupy a central position within the islets, while the glucagon (A), somatostatin (D), pancreatic polypeptide (PP), and vasoactive intestinal peptide–producing cells are dispersed throughout with some preferential clustering of the A and D cells along the periphery of the islets (6) (Fig. 4.2). In humans the afferent vessels enter the islet at the periphery. The afferent blood has to pass the A and D cells before reaching the B cells, permit-

Figure 4.1. Demonstration of the normal distribution of islet of Langerhans in a normal human pancreas. Formalin-fixed paraffin-embedded tissue stained with immunoperoxidase technique for insulin-producing islet cells (× 40).

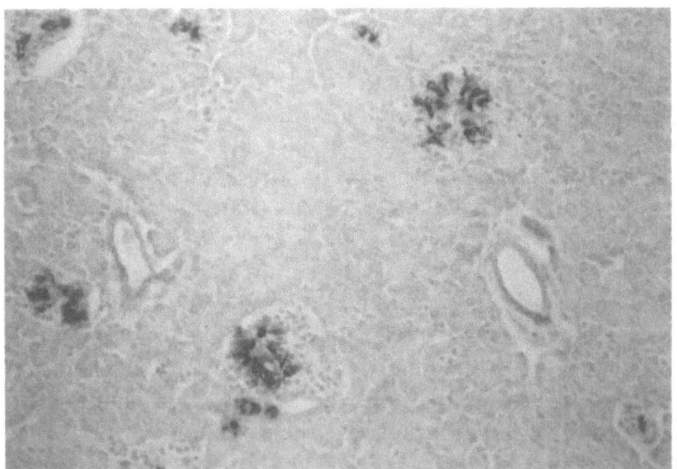

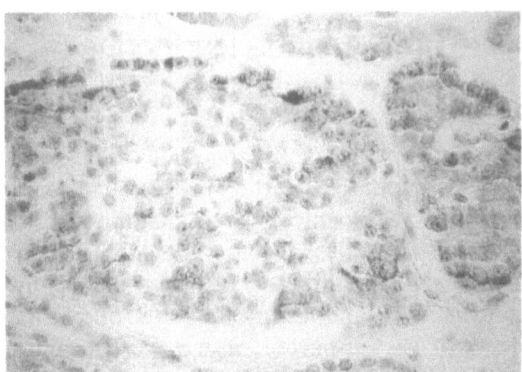

A

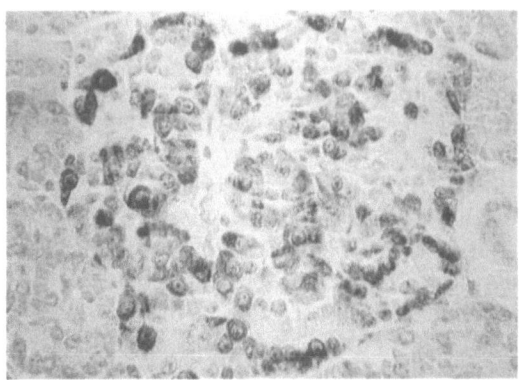

B

Figure 4.2. Immunocytochemical demonstration of the normal distribution of insulin and glucagon-producing cells in sections of normal pancreas. A: Insulin-producing islet cells (B cells) stained with the indirect immunoperoxidase technique with guinea pig antiinsulin at 1:1000 (× 400). B: Glucagon-producing islet cells (A cells) stained by the peroxidase-antiperoxidase technique using 1:500 antiglucagon (× 40).

ting glucagon and somatostatin to modulate the release of insulin from the B cells. The relative numbers of A, D, and B cells within the islet is relatively constant. The B cells accounts for 60 to 80% of the islet cells, A cells for 15 to 20%, and D cells for 5 to 15%. The PP cells are rare and irregularly dispersed within the pancreas representing about 0.5 to 1.0% of the islet cell population. The VIP cells represent about 2 to 5% of the islet cell population (6).

Based on data from 30 patients with normal peripheral levels of glucose Roche et al. (7) observed that the B-insulin producing cells are randomly distributed along the pancreas in a noncongruous way.

The APUD Concept

The development of the new cytologic techniques like cytochemistry, immunochemistry, and electron microscopy made it possible to identify a large population of neuroendocrine cells, particularly of the gastroenteropancreatic system. Highly specific functional morphology led to the observation that endocrine cells of the gastrointestinal tract have cytochemical characteristics in common with more centrally located cells and with neural-ganglion cells. A large part of the endocrine system and the autonomic nervous system could be cytologically encompassed, therefore, in a diffuse neuroendocrine system. The more pertinent common cytochemical characteristics include the cellular capability of the amine-precursor uptake and decarboxylation (APUD). The cells with such a common characteristic are called APUD cells and the tumors originated from these cells have been named APUD-omas (3).

The APUD concept integrates the neural and endocrine systems. Many of the polypeptides secreted by APUD cells have been identified in both the brain and the gut (2), strongly supporting the unifying concept of the APUD system. Because of the common properties of the different APUD cells synthesizing, storing, and secreting a variety of polypeptide hormones and biogenic amines, these cells were originally regarded as neural crest derivates (B). There is, however, recent evidence showing that the endocrine cells of the pancreas are derived from the neuroendocrine-programmed ectoblast (9). The endocrine cells of the pancreas, along with those of the gastroenteric axis, are now referred to as neuroendocrine in nature and are believed to have integrated endocrine, neuroendocrine, and paracrine functions orchestrating the normal digestive processes (6,10).

The relevance of the unifying concept is, however, illustrated by the clinical association of both neural tumors and endocrine tumors in type II multiple-endocrinopathy syndromes and in the presence of secretory-diarrhea syndrome produced by a tumor originating either in neural, islet, or other tissue, in which the prime hormone responsible is VIP, a neurotransmitter polypeptide (3).

The unifying concept is also important to understand entopic and ectopic release of islet cell tumor hormones. Tumors have been identified as arising from each of the five types of islet cells. The orthoendocrine tumors elaborate polypeptides that are native to the islets. This is an entopic release of hormone and includes glucagon from the A cells, insulin from the B cells, somatostatin from the D cells, human pancreatic polypeptides from the PP cells, and the amine serotonin from the enterochromaffin cells.

Other islet cell tumors release polypeptides ectopically, secreting polypeptides that are not normally native to the adult pancreas. These include the gastrinoma, vipoma, corticotropinoma, the parathyrinoma, and rarer entities. Gastrin-containing cells have been identified in the fetal pancreas but not in the normal adult pancreas. Ectopic hormone production may be multiple and mixed. The clinical presentation may be bizarre, or one clinical picture may predominate. Ectopically functioning tumors are, in general, potentially malignant. Endocrine tumors with ectopic function may be associated with APUD cell hyperplasia. An additional characteristic is that ectopic tumors may also elaborate large polypeptides (5).

Tumors of the Endocrine Pancreas

In February 1869, Paul Langerhans, a German medical student in Berlin, presented his dissertation on the microscopic anatomy of the pancreas without speculations on the physiologic function of the islets of the cells that now bear his name and, even though the endocrine function was suspected, it was not until the isolation of insulin in 1922 that the role of the pancreas as an endocrine organ was verified. Although the possible role of the pancreas in diabetes was mentioned in the first years of the 20th century, not before the splendid work by Banting was its role proved (11).

Insulin overdoses, subsequently, were documented as creating a hypoglycemic syndrome similar to that observed spontaneously in some rare patients. In 1927, Mayo found a pancreatic islet cell tumor with liver metastases in a patient with severe hypoglycemia. Graham and Whipple reported, separately, the cure of patients with attacks of hypoglycemia by surgical removal of functioning islet cell adenoma from the pancreas.

In 1955, Zollinger and Ellison described two patients with a syndrome of intractable, recurrent peptic ulcer disease needing total gastrectomy to prevent recurrency of ulcerations. Gregory found gastrin in a pancreatic tumor

Figure 4.3. Schematic representation of the macroscopic, microscopic, and electronic microscopy presentation of an endocrine pancreatic tumor. Note that the lesion is well delimited from the normal pancreatic parenchyma macroscopically and microscopically. The lesion is, however, covered by a pancreatic parenchyma layer. The lesion is surrounded by the pancreatic acini and the islet cell is disarranged with granular cells of the dominant type. Approximately × 900. Note the reticular fibers within the tumor and in the limits. Electronic microscopy shows the granular cells adjacent to one vessel releasing the granules with the hormone through the pores. Note that the Golgi complex is very prominent.

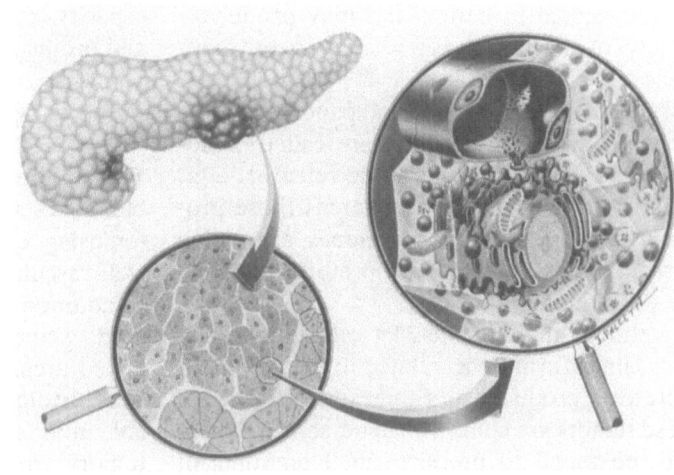

extracted from a patient with Zollinger-Ellison syndrome in 1964, giving rise to the concept of ectopic production of hormones. In 1966, McGravan described the glucagonoma syndrome related to a pancreatic adenoma-producing glucagon.

Islet cell neoplasms of the pancreas are relatively uncommon lesions accounting for 2 to 4% of all pancreatic tumors, but the exact incidence is not known. These tumors may arise anywhere in the pancreas with somewhat similar frequency. Dominant localization is still controversial, and some authors report higher frequency in the tail (10) and others in the head (12). Pancreatic adenomas may be single or multiple but are circumscribed lesions that contrast sharply with adjacent pancreatic parenchyma. Tumor size ranges from 0.5 to 5 cm, although tumors as large as 35 cm have been reported. Areas of tissue hyperplasia have also been found, producing large amounts of hormones causing clinical syndromes similar to islet cell tumors.

Macroscopic characteristics of the islet cell tumors may vary considerably due to differences in the amount of stroma, necrosis, hemorrhage, and cystic formation. Adjacent normal pancreatic tissues are frequently compressed, allowing the tumors to be "shelled out" during surgery. Areas of invasion, however, may be identified in benign and malignant islet cell tumors. The tumor cells are usually well differentiated and polygonal, with moderate eosinophilic or pale granular cytoplasm and small central nuclei (Fig. 4.3). Undifferentiated tumors are less organized and may show spindle cells and elongated nuclei with polyhedral cells and abundant granular cytoplasm. The only reliable criterion for malignancy in these tumors is the demonstration of metastases in lymph nodes, liver, or other sites.

Frequently islet cell tumors are shown to contain one or more polypeptide hormones within their cells and associated with well-defined syndromes, such as the multiple endocrine adenomatosis (MEA) type I syndrome.

Islet cell tumors are grouped on the basis of their predominant secretory product. Islet cell tumors producing large amounts of insulin are referred to as insulinomas, glucagon as glucagonomas, gastrin as gastrinomas, vasoactive intestinal peptide as VIP-omas, somatostatin as somatostatinomas, and pancreatic polypeptide as PP-omas. It should be kept in mind, however, that the majority of such tumors are multihormonal in nature and may produce a variety of hormones not related to the pancreas (6).

Tumors producing normal pancreatic hormones as the principal ones are called ortho-endocrine (or entopic hormone release), e.g., insulinoma, glucagonoma, whereas those producing "nonpancreatic" hormones are called paraendocrine (or ectopic hormone release), e.g., gastrinoma.

Although most of the islet cell tumors produce clinical symptoms related to the dominant secretory product, a significant number of these tumors are clinically silent; some of them may be found to' produce small amounts of polypeptide hormones, but the amounts are not sufficient to produce a clinical syndrome.

Insulinoma

Hypoglycemia is caused by pancreatic and extrapancreatic factors. Extrapancreatic factors causing hypoglycemia are nonendocrine lesions, such as mesodermal tumors, carcinoma of the adrenal gland, primary carcinoma of the liver, a few carcinomas of the GI tract, extensive liver disease, and hypofunction of the anterior pituitary and adrenal cortex. Insulinomas, however, are the most prominent cause of hypoglycemia syndrome (4).

Insulinomas are characterized by large production and secretion of insulin and proinsulin. These are the most common cause of entopic hormone release in the pancreas. Up to 90% of the insulinomas are single but may be multiple in a small proportion, especially in cases of MEA type I syndrome. Rarely, insulinomas may arise outside the pancreas.

Insulinomas are benign lesions in 90% or more of the cases. To date, the presence of distant metastases is the only reliable criterion for malignancy.

The clinical presentation of a functioning insulinoma is characterized by bizarre neurologic symptoms, severe fasting hypoglycemia reversed by glucose administration, and elevated levels of insulin and proinsulin in the blood. Most features of the insulinoma syndrome can be directly attributed to the decreased storage

capacity and uncontrolled release of insulin and proinsulin by the tumor cells (6).

Histologic and Architectural Data

The architecture of an insulinoma may resemble that of a giant distorted islet with thin anastomosing cords of tumor cells separated by well-vascularized connective tissue septa (6). In addition to the trabecular pattern, an organoid, acinar (glandular), diffuse (solid), or mixed architectural pattern may be observed. The histologic pattern of insulinomas is variable and similar to that of other islet cell tumors, making the distinction with other APUD-omas impossible. Amyloid substance is found in the connective tissue stroma in the proximity of the tumor cells, more often than in other types of islet cell tumors.

Histochemical stains employed for the specific demonstration of beta granules give positive reaction in up to 75% of insulinomas. Immunohistochemical staining with antiinsulin sera localizes insulin within the tumor cells in the majority of insulinomas, including those with histochemical stain negative for B granules. The staining density is variable among the B cells with positive insulin localization and the number of granules is smaller within the tumor cells (Fig. 4.4).

Insulinomas have been classified ultrastructurally into four categories based on the morphology of the secretory granules:

Type I: cells with typical B cell secretory granules
Type II: cells with typical and atypical granules
Type III: cells with atypical granules only
Type IV: cells with no identifiable granules.

The most common types of insulinomas are types I and II tumors with the highest insulin concentration. These tumors give positive histochemical and immunohistochemical staining reactions for insulin and can confidently be diagnosed as insulinomas. The diagnosis can only be suggested in type III tumors. The type IV tumors cannot be accurately diagnosed as insulinomas in the absence of corroborative

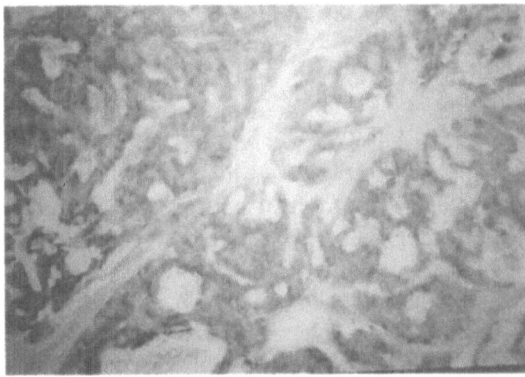
A

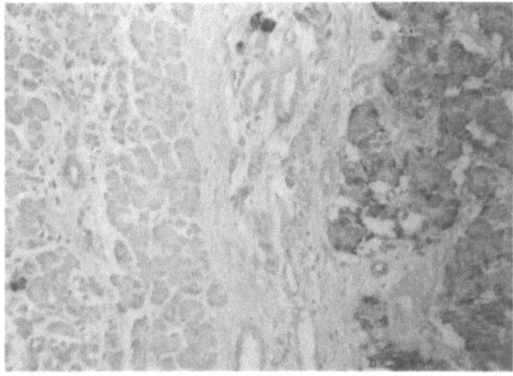
B

Figure 4.4. **A**: Pancreatic insulinoma showing positive staining for insulin in a majority of tumor cells. The staining is relatively faint in insulinomas due to the low granule content of the tumor cell. Formalin-fixed paraffin-embedded tissue stained by the indirect immunoperoxidase technique. Note the trabecular pattern of the tumor with the well-vascularized connective tissue septa within the tumor. **B**: Pancreatic nesidioblastosis showing positive staining for insulin in the hyperplastic cells (to the right) limited by the trabeculae made of connective tissue.

biochemical data regarding proinsulin levels in the tumor or blood, since they frequently give negative histochemical and immunohistochemical reactions for beta granules.

Islet cell hyperplasia producing insulin and hypoglycemic syndrome is very rare and may be diffuse in the newborn (nesidioblastosis) (Fig. 4.4) or restricted in adults. It may also be present as a companion to islet cell tumor. Islet cell hyperplasia is observed by counting the number of islet cells under low-power magnifications, and a semiquantitative estimate reveals that the islet frequency in the middle of the resected specimen exceeds the frequency of islets at the margins by a factor of 4 to 3.

Diagnostic Workup

The symptoms associated with hypoglycemia and hyperinsulinism occur in a fasting state. The symptoms of headache, blurred vision, incoherence, convulsions, and coma are due to the deleterious effect of hypoglycemia on brain function. Other symptoms such as sweating, weakness, hunger, palpitation, and trembling are homeostatic responses to hypoglycemia involving the secretion of catecholamines, demonstrating the interdependence of the neural

and humoral regulatory systems characteristic of the APUD cell system.

Prolonged fasting is the most useful diagnostic test. Fasting for 72 hours, with simultaneous blood glucose and immunoreactive insulin determination every 6 hours and during symptom occurrence is a reliable test. In normal patients during prolonged fast, blood glucose levels fall and immunoreactive insulin becomes undetectable. In patients with an autonomous secretion of insulin (insulinoma), insulin level is not suppressed during prolonged fast and a "normal" or slightly elevated concentration of immunoreactive insulin is detected.

A number of other laboratory diagnostic studies may be useful. In the diazoxide suppression test the administration of this compound results in an increase in blood glucose by depressing insulin secretion. If this happens in the presence of hypoglycemia, inappropriate secretion of insulin by a tumor is suggested. Tolbutamide tolerance test, leucine tolerance test, and oral glucose tolerance test may also be helpful. Intravenous injection of exogenous glucagon has also been used as a diagnostic (11) test for insulinoma. During diagnostic workup and the preoperative period, care should be exercised to avoid persistent severe hypoglycemia because of the risk of permanent brain damage.

The localization and surgical considerations in islet cell tumors is presented at the end of this section.

Glucagonoma

The glucagon-secreting tumor is an A-cell tumor of the pancreas and usually produces a definite clinical syndrome: diabetes-dermatitis syndrome. However, this syndrome is uncommon and recognition of the tumor is frequently late. The main reason for the delayed diagnosis is that mild diabetes, dermatitis, and anemia characteristic of the syndrome are nonspecific and common problems in adults. To the physician not commonly involved with endocrine problems, the clinical presentation of the syndrome does not readily suggest the possibility of an islet cell tumor (13).

Cutaneous rash, which has been characterized as a necrotizing, migratory erythema, is the most clinical diagnostic feature, when present. The syndrome reflects the catabolic glycogenolytic action of glucagon. Glucagon also has an inhibitory action on intestinal motility, causing ileus, constipation, and sometimes diarrhea. Additional problems include glossitis, angular stomatitis, and occasional blackout spells without hypoglycemia or electrolyte abnormalities. It has also been observed that patients with this syndrome present hypoaminoacidemia, mental depression, and a predeliction to develop infections, thromboses, and thromboembolic episodes (5,6).

The cutaneous rash involves the buttocks, intergluteal folds, perineum, groin, legs, feet, and circumoral areas. The lesions first appear as an erythematous rash, developing into bullae within 1 to 2 weeks. The excoriation of the bullae leads the exposed areas to become a necrosis with erythematous margins that gradually heals with crusts and hyperpigmentation, at the same time with development of new lesions at sites of pressure or friction.

Histologic and Architectural Data

Glucagonomas show architectural aspects common to all islet cell tumors with larger lesions presenting degeneration hemorrhage, and necrosis.

Amyloid deposition has not been observed in glucagonomas so far. Immunohistochemical localization of glucagon within the tumor cells and demonstration of high glucagon immunoreactivity in tumor extracts are the only reliable means for accurately establishing the diagnosis of these tumors. The improvement of the skin lesions and reversal of biochemical abnormalities following surgical removal of the pancreatic islet cell tumor is also an acceptable proof of the diagnosis of a glucagonoma (3,6).

On electronic microscopy, glucagonomas have relatively fewer granulated cells. The morphology of these cells is varied among tumors and between areas of the same tumor.

Three different types of secretory granules have been identified in glucagonomas (3): small (150 nm), medium (180 to 2,600 nm), and large granules (180 to 300 nm) identical to those of normal A-cell granules. Small granules are more immunoreactive to glucagon in functioning glucagonomas. Silent, small and multicentric tumors associated with Zollinger-Ellison syndrome, insulinomas, and MEA type I syndrome show the presence of the moderately large granules (6).

Diagnostic Workup

The diabetes-dermatitis syndrome is the indication for the diagnosis of a glucagonoma. The skin lesions described in the introduction, as coalescent adjacent lesions, responsible for the serpiginous configuration are characteristic of necrolytic migratory erythema. These lesions are invariably associated with an underlying pancreatic glucagon-producing tumor and since they may be the first to attract attention, glucagonomas are quite often diagnosed by dermatologists.

Glucagonomas may be located anywhere in the pancreas and may be solitary or multiple. Most of the solitary lesions reported in the literature have been over 5 cm in diameter and malignant with metastases in 68% of the cases (6). Hepatic metastases may be the first form of disease, due to the usually delayed diagnosis. A high clinical awareness and suspicion is necessary for the diagnosis of a glucagonoma tumor.

The diagnosis is readily confirmed by the finding of elevated plasma glucagon concentrations. An association of increased plasmatic insulin is characteristic and may account for the mildness of the diabetes. The intravenous tolbutamide test increases glucagon (paradoxically) but is superfluous in the majority of cases.

Localization of the tumor within the pancreas is a different story and several different imaging techniques are now available. Localization workup including pancreatic venous sampling will be described later in this chapter (14,15).

Somatostatinoma

A characteristic syndrome associated with somatostatinoma has not been clearly defined, and this tumor has often been described as a silent nonfunctioning islet cell tumor and found serendipitously at the time of cholecystectomy (16). The clinical picture, however, is full of nonspecific manifestations common in adults, such as diabetes mellitus, cholecystolithiasis, steatorrhea, diarrhea, indigestion, hypochlorhydria, weight loss, and occasionally anemia, and is sometimes called inhibitory syndrome or somatostatinoma syndrome (16,17). The clinical symptoms are related to the inhibitory actions of somatostatin on neighboring APUD cells that secrete a number of hormones such as insulin, glucagon, cholecystokinin, and gastrin. Somatostatin was originally designated as somatotropin-release–inhibiting factor due to the inhibitory action of pituitary release of growth hormone (18).

Histologic and Architectural Data

Somatostatin was established as a product of the pancreatic D cells and descriptions of delta-cell tumors soon followed in 1977.

Histologically, the tumors show the usual features common to islet cell tumors. Immunohistochemical staining with somatostatin antibodies is positive in the majority of tumor cells. Ultrastructural studies showed morphologic features similar to those of normal delta cells of human islets, including secretory granules of 250 to 400 mμ in size. The granules present a variable electron-dense core with somatostatin (6). Somatostatinomas also contain calcitonin, adrenocorticotropin, gastrin, and cortisol, consistent with the multihormonality of islet cell tumors. Somatostatin, on the other hand, also occurs as a minor component in about 20% of other pancreatic endocrine tumors (6).

Most of the somatostatinomas are malignant tumors presenting with liver metastases or lymphadenopathies by the time of diagnosis. Postoperative mortality is disproportionally high and long-term prognosis is still uncertain.

Diagnostic Workup

In addition to the elevated concentration of circulating somatostatin, the depressed plasma concentration of immunoreactive insulin and glucagon are diagnostic features. In contrast, patients with glucagonomas will present elevated levels of immunoreactive insulin and glucagon (3).

The inhibitory syndrome, however, has a very confusing clinical presentation with nonspecific symptoms rather common in elderly women, and preoperative detection has been reported in only a few instances. Most of the cases have been diagnosed during gallstone surgery.

Most of the tumors are single and malignant but very often may first be detected by hepatic and lymph nodes metastases through imaging methods. An abdominal mass may be the first finding, but the size ranges from 0.6 to 20 cm, according to the description of the few cases reported in the literature (6).

High clinical awareness and suspicion is necessary for the diagnosis of a somatostatinoma.

Localization of the small primary lesions within the pancreas follows the same guidelines for localization of other islet cell tumors and different imaging methods should be used to improve accuracy. Detailed localization workup will be discussed later, together with other kinds of pancreatic endocrine tumors. Localization of somatostatinomas is essential due to the high chance of most of the tumors becoming malignant.

Pancreatic Polypeptide Secreting Tumors (PP-omas)

The human pancreatic polypeptide (hPP) from the F (D_2 or PP) cells is probably the most recent polypeptide to be identified in the pancreas (16).

Patients are usually asymptomatic and detection of PP-omas are detected during prospective screening in families at risk for MEA I.

PP-omas are rare lesions and although several patients with tumors have been reported (6) no specific clinical syndrome has been described for pancreatic polypeptide excess. Sometimes patients with watery diarrhea syndrome with normal or minimally elevated VIP levels in the blood have very high levels of circulating hPP and a large amount of histologically demonstrable hPP immunoreactivity in the pancreatic tumor, demonstrating that at least in some patients the Verner-Morrison syndrome can be mediated by hPP excess (6).

PP-omas are usually single tumors, but when associated with the MEA Type I syndrome, multiple small tumors may be found (6). The F cells, also called PP or D_2 cells, are normally and preponderantly located in the posterior portion of the head of the pancreas; tumors producing hPP, however, have been found everywhere in the pancreas.

The biologic activity of hPP is not known; hPP, however, may have physiologic actions antithetical to those of cholecystokinin. hPP decreases gallbladder contractility, increases choledochal tone, inhibits pancreatic exocrine secretion, and inhibits pentagastrin-stimulated gastric acid secretions (3).

Histologic and Architectural Data

Immunohistochemically, the majority of tumor cells stain for hPP. Electronic microscopy shows the tumor cells with a large number of small secretory granules, morphologically indistinguishable from the normal pancreatic PP cells (F or D_2) (6).

Diagnostic Workup

The diagnosis is usually made during prospective screening in asymptomatic patients from families at risk for MEA I syndrome. Abnormal concentration of hPP in the plasma in basal fasting state and food-stimulated state are the most important features for the detection of the pancreatic component of MEA type I.

Elevated hPP concentrations, more than four times the level in age-matched controls, are indicative of tumor. On the other hand, a normal basal concentration with an increased response to a standard test meal appears to be associated with APUD cell hyperplasia, without tumor. Increased concentration of hPP in plasma and tumors are found in about half the patients with a variety of pancreatic endocrine tumors; the association, however, between abnormal hPP levels and genetic MEA type I syndrome is much more prominent.

The results of circulating plasma hPP in suspect patients must be interpreted in comparison with controls, because normal basal levels increase with age and there is a normal vagal and enteric response to food (3).

Localization of PP-omas is not so critical as in other pancreatic endocrine tumors, because they are rarely malignant and produce no significant recognizable syndrome. Angiography, percutaneous venous sampling, and other imaging methods are adequate for the localization diagnosis.

Gastrinoma (Ectopic Ulcerogenic Syndrome, Zollinger-Ellison Syndrome)

Gastrinoma is the second most common type of hormone-producing islet cell tumor. It was described by Zollinger and Ellison in 1955 as the association of a non-beta islet cell tumor of the pancreas with gastric acid hypersecretion and severe, recurrent peptic ulcer disease. It was thought at that time that hyperacidity and peptic ulcer disease were related to a gastric acid secretogogue overproduction. Within 5 years, Gregory, Tracy, and colleagues proved that the ulcerogenic tumor in the pancreas was producing a potent gastric secretogogue, identified as "gastrin-like." The tumoral-secreted gastrin is produced 35 to 45 times more than the normal gastric antrum, explaining the clinical findings of gastric acid hypersecretion, diarrhea, and steatorrhea (19).

Most of the gastrinomas arise in the pancreas (85 to 95%), although it is an ectopic endocrine tumor of the pancreas. Gastrinomas may also arise from the duodenum, stomach, bile ducts, and splenic hilum (20,21).

Pancreatic gastrinomas are usually small, multiple (70%), and malignant (60 to 70%) reinforcing the concept of ectopic hormone-producing tumor related to malignancy.

As discussed previously, gastrin-producing cells have not been demonstrated in normal human pancreatic islets and the histogenesis and the high incidence of pancreatic gastrinomas has not been explained satisfactorily (3).

Histologic and Architectural Data

The histologic pattern of gastrinomas is similar to that of other endocrine pancreatic tumors. Tumoral cells are arranged in trabeculae, sheets, nests, or mixed. Occasional amyloid deposits may be seen in the stroma.

The tumor cells are argyrophilic and stain positively with hematoxylin. The cells are usually well differentiated and even in malignant lesions may not show pleomorphism, atypicalities, or mitotic activity. Immunohistochemically, gastrin can be localized in the tumor cells with positive staining. At electronic microscopy gastrinomas are composed of a variable number of granular and agranular cells, and have been classified into four major categories: Type I, tumor with granular cells containing granules identical to those of antral G cells; Type II, cells containing typical G-cell granules and cells containing small round granules (up to 150 to 200 nm); Type III, cells containing small round granules (atypical) only; Type IV, cells containing granules characteristic of other endocrine cell types. Type II tumors are the most frequent (6).

The gastrinomas produce large amounts of gastrin, have a reduced capacity for its storage within the secretory granules, and give rise to hypergastrinemia and Zollinger-Ellison (Z-E) syndrome. However, gastrinomas should not be completely equated with the Z-E syndrome because not all gastrinomas produce enough gastrin to produce clinical symptoms and silent gastrinomas occur in the absence of the Z-E syndrome and the syndrome may occur in the absence of an identifiable tumor (6).

The syndrome associated with hyperplasia of the gastric antral G cells is called Z-E syndrome type I. Z-E syndrome type II is associated with a gastrinoma. Occasionally, a pancreatic islet cell tumor in a patient with Z-E syndrome does not show functional, histochemical, immunohistochemical or ultrastructural features of gastrinoma (6).

Diagnostic Workup

Clinical Features. Gastrin production is the cardinal feature of gastrinoma and most clinical features are related to its effect. Peptic ulceration is the predominant problem and is characterized by multiple ulcers of fulminant behavior, atypical sites, and recurrence. Currently, however, progressive awareness of the condition and detection of elevated gastrin levels by radioimmunoassay has enabled earlier diagnosis before the condition reaches such a florid state. Diarrhea occurs in 36 to 81% and may precede manifestations of ulceration. Aspiration of the gastric hypersecretion or total gastrectomy stops the diarrhea in most patients (22).

Diagnosis. Radioimmunoassay of plasmatic gastrin is critical in the diagnosis of gastrinoma, but values must be interpreted with care. Several other conditions, such as pernicious anemia, renal failure, and gastric outlet obstruction, may also elevate gastrin. Evidence of an elevated fasting gastrin level on two separate occasions is required for investigation of a diagnosis of gastrinoma, due to differences in laboratories and techniques.

Before the advent of reliable radioimmunoassay for plasma gastrin the diagnosis was often delayed. Gastrinomas were identified only after failed gastric operations for peptic ulcer and the advent of complications of the disease. There are a few clues that will lead to the suspected diagnosis of gastrinomas, such as ulcer recurrency after operation for peptic ulcer, which is the most common problem.

Bleeding, perforation, and reulceration are also common complications.

Ulcerations in the distal part of the duodenum and proximal jejunum are pathognomonic and uncommon.

Acid secretion studies have in the past been very helpful, but are not always correct, especially in previously operated patients. A basal acid output of more than 10 mmol per hour, a basal-acid output to maximal acid output ratio greater than 0.6, and a overnight 12-hour acid secretion of more than 100 mmol are all suggestive of the diagnosis. A high proportion of patients with basal acid hypersecretion have normal serum gastrin levels and no gastrin secreting tumor, whereas up to 50% of patients with a proved gastrinoma fail to meet the criteria for acid hypersecretion (11).

If serum gastrin levels are elevated to more than 10 times normal the probability of a diagnosis of gastrinoma is almost certain.

Due to the earlier diagnosis of gastrinoma in less advanced forms of the disease, the serum gastrin levels may not be so elevated and provocative tests have been developed. Calcium and secretin infusion are the most commonly used (11,23,24).

Localization techniques have been developed using imaging techniques, including arteriography, computed tomography, and ultrasound. Selective pancreatic venous sampling, performed in conjunction with provocation tests, can provide very accurate delineation of tumor sites. Endoscopy is of limited use but will demonstrate the peptic ulcerations and the rare gastrinomas of the stomach or duodenal wall (25).

VIP-oma of the Pancreas
(Watery Diarrhea, Hypokalemia, Achlorhydria (WDHR) Syndrome, Verner-Morrison Syndrome, Pancreatic Cholera Syndrome)

The clinical presentation of Verner-Morrison syndrome is profuse, explosive, tea-colored watery diarrhea, associated with hypokalemia and hypochlorhydria. Dehydration and weakness are common complications. The most probable cause of the diarrhea is the vasoactive intestinal polypeptide (VIP) (25). All the clinical features of the syndrome can be attributed to the physiologic actions of VIP. The specific action accounts for the massive secretion of water and electrolytes from the small bowel and pancreas, overwhelming the absorptive capacity of the colon (15). Hyperglycemia, fluctuating hypercalcemia, hypotension, and episodic flushing may also be present. The WDHA syndrome occurs most commonly in late adult life in both sexes.

Most of the patients have solitary pancreatic tumors (VIP-omas) but those are malignant in over 60% of the cases; the rest are adenomas. A diffuse pancreatic islet hyperplasia has been observed with the syndrome (6).

Histologic and Architectural Data

The usual histologic features of islet cell tumors are encountered. The tumor cells are nonargentaffin and are argyrophilic only when stained by the Grimelius technique. Immunohistochemical procedures using VIP antisera stain the tumor cells in variable numbers not correlating with the number of argyrophil cells. VIP-omas are frequently found to be multihormonal and hPP is found in a fair number of tumor cells.

Electron-microscopy shows that these tumors are composed of a large population of agranular or paucigranular cells, and the granules measure up to 150 nm with osmiophilic cores, identical to those seen in normal D cells of human islets. Secretory granules of tumor cells of some VIP-omas are identical to those of VIP-producing D_1 cells, also morphologically indistinguishable from the atypical granules of insulinomas, glucagonomas, and gastrinomas (16).

Diagnostic Workup

The clinical features of the Verner-Morrison syndrome are nonspecific but very suggestive of the disease. Hormone assay is diagnostic in most patients. Imaging of the pancreas and liver may show the primary lesion, usually single, anywhere in the pancreas and hepatic metastases in a large number of patients. Recurrence of symptoms after surgical treatment with enucleation of the tumor or pancreatectomy, is often related to liver metastatic disease, which is readily demonstrated by ultrasound, CT, and angiography (26,27).

Nesidioblastosis

Nesidioblastosis occurs most commonly in infants and children under the age of 2 years (11). It may represent a pretumor situation with diffuse hyperplasia and even microadenomatous transformation of the endocrine cells of the pancreas.

At least four cell types, A, B, D, and D_2, are involved in abnormal clusters of islet cells. Insulin secretion is the dominant feature and the other hormones produced are silent. Hypoglycemia is the main clinical finding which may be associated with neurologic and mental problems, early diagnosis being necessary to prevent permanent sequelae (11).

Diagnosis is more difficult than in adults and many patients have well-established neurologic damage caused by repeated hypoglycemic attacks (28). Operation may be mandatory if drug therapy fails. Subtotal pancreatectomy of 80 to 90% of the distal pancreas may cure most of the children. Total pancreatectomy might be necessary if the first partial resection fails (29,30), and occasionally treatment with diazoxide may be required after surgery (11).

There is no crucial need for lesion localization, although sometimes a larger number of clusters of hyperplastic cells are localized in particular areas of the pancreas. Angiography is negative, as are CT and ultrasound (US). Percutaneous selective pancreatic venous sampling may aid in the diagnosis, showing generalized and diffuse insulin elevation or localized sites of hormone production (31,32).

Other Pancreatic Abnormalities and Pancreatic Endocrine Tumors

The identification of a widely dispersed group of cells of common origin and biochemical characteristics, the APUD cells, has allowed a better understanding of the endocrine tumors of the pancreas. It has also helped to establish the relationships between the endocrine tumors of the multiple endocrine neoplasia type I syndrome. Any of the APUD polypeptides may be produced ectopically from islet cells tumors (33). Hormones such as antidiuretic hormone (vasopressin), cholecystokinin, pancreatic corticotropinoma (ectopic-ACTH syndrome), pancreatic parathyrinoma (ectopic-hypercalcemia syndrome), and 5-hydroxytryptamine (carcinoid-like syndrome) have been reported in the literature (3,11,34).

The pluripotential capacity of the pancreatic islet cells to produce a number of polypeptides combined with the certain existence of many unidentified peptides suggests the likelihood of other undescribed pancreatic endocrine tumors (11).

A large proportion of the islet cell tumors are multihormonal and the presence of a number of different hormones within them is to be expected; however, one of the hormones dominates, giving the clinical syndrome.

Hyperplasia of pancreatic islet cells in the nontumoral areas of the pancreas may be found in more than half of the islet cell tumors where a hyperplasia involving all endocrine cell types occur (6).

Multiple endocrine adenopathy (MEA) warrants additional discussion. MEA is a set of syndromes of inherited endocrine hyperfunction disorders. There are three distinct types (33): MEA-I, MEA-II, and MEA-IIB. The MEA-I, or Werner's syndrome, is manifest as hyperparathyroidism (HPT), pancreatic islet cell tumor (gastrinoma or insulinoma), and pituitary adenoma. The MEA-II, or Sipple's syndrome, presents HPT, medullary carcinoma of the thyroid gland (MCT), and pheochromocytoma (PCC). The MEA-IIB is characterized by MCT and PCC without hyperparathyroidism but associated to neuromas (33).

In MEA-I, syndrome pancreatic islet cell tumors occur in 50% of the patients and gastrinomas are more frequent than insulinomas. Clinical manifestations include renal lithiasis, osteoporosis, psychosis, and abdominal pain from an ulcer or pancreatitis. Acromegaly, galactorrhea, amenorrhea, or Cushing's disease may also be found, depending on the cell type of the pituitary gland tumor. If the islet

Table 4.1. Algorithmic approach for diagnosis and localization of pancreatic insulinoma.

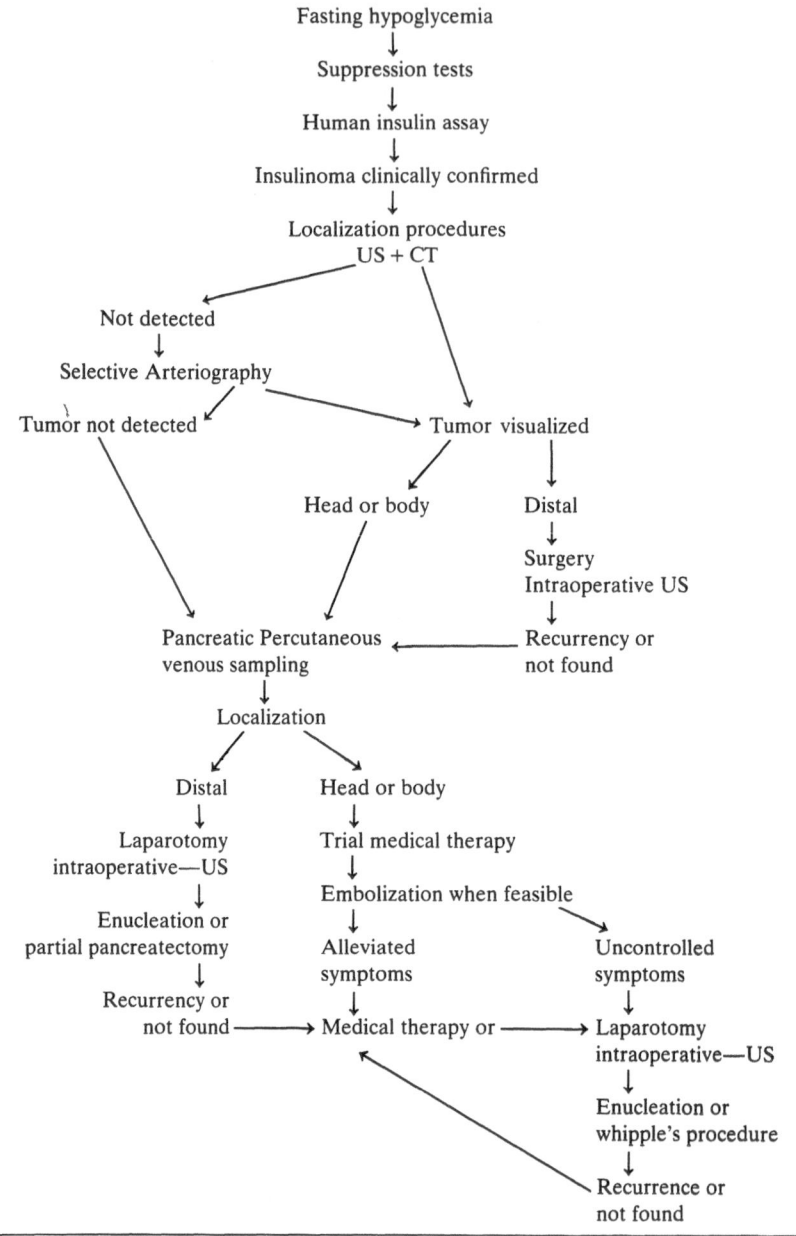

cell is an insulinoma the effects of hypo-glycemia will be the prominent ones (33).

Localization of Islet Cell Tumors

The diagnosis of islet cell tumors is clinically made and confirmed by laboratory tests.

The confirmation of the existing pancreatic hormone producing tumor is currently performed using radioimmunoassays of the peripheral blood.

The association of the clinical characteristic syndrome and elevated polypeptide concentration, with or without using the suppression tests, will seal the clinical diagnosis of the disease in most cases (3). Clinical diagnosis of multihormonal tumors without a dominant

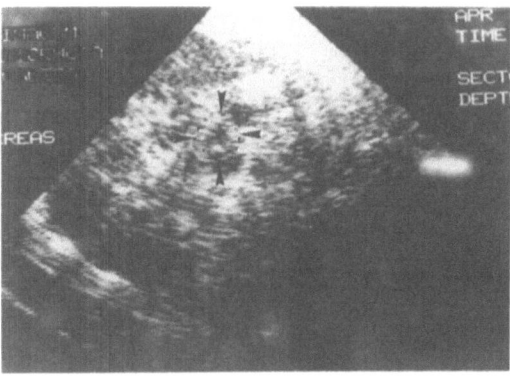
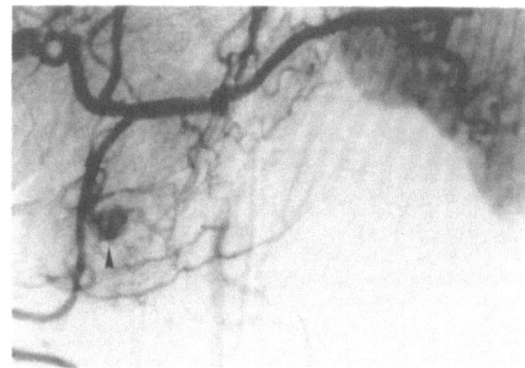

A   B

Figure 4.5. Pancreatic insulinoma in a 50-year-old woman with recurrent episodes of headache, convulsions, coma, and changes in behavior. The patient was in psychiatric treatment for 2 years. **A**: Ultrasonography showing a small hypoacoustic nodule in the head of the pancreas (arrowheads). **B**: The ultrasonographic finding was confirmed by angiography of the celiac artery. Note the hypervascular tumor in the pancreas head close to the gastroduodenal artery (arrowhead). Patient was operated on and single insulinoma was proved.

polypeptide or with mixed symptoms may be very difficult (35). The silent APUD-omas, although producing a variety of hormones, even some still undetected by current immunoassay techniques, may be identified by incidental US, CT, angiographic examinations or by symptoms related to growth (36).

Imaging for pancreatic islet cell tumor localization turned out to be the keystone for adequate treatment and a lot of developments have been introduced in that technology lately (4).

The current imaging armamentarium for islet cell tumor localization includes ultrasound, computed tomography, pancreatic arteriography, pancreatic venous sampling, and intraoperative ultrasound, in addition to surgical inspection and palpation (Table 4.1). Some authors, however, suggest that the diagnostic workup can be limited (37).

Ultrasound

Ultrasound examination of the pancreas for islet cell tumor localization has relatively low sensitivity and low specificity (1). However, pancreatic adenomas larger than 0.7 cm in diameter may be detected in favorable situations. Sonographically, pancreatic islet cell tumors are characteristically round or oval, well de-

marcated, and less echogenic than the surrounding pancreatic tissue (Fig. 4.5). Islet cell tumors of the pancreas are more easily detected on transverse than on longitudinal scans. The search for smaller lesions by sonography is unrealistic within the limitations of the currently available technology. Ultrasound, however, is generally more flexible than CT, independent of contrast material, and provides several different planes for evaluation. Limitations of the technique are overlying bowel gas and insufficient transducer resolution.

Previous reports in the literature (1) yielded a low sensitivity for US in the detection of islet cell tumors of only 25% (1). A recent report, however, presented a much better result of 50% localization of insulinomas in previously unknown lesions and up to 71% in lesions previously known by other techniques (38). Another series shows a sensitivity of 61% in lesions not known previous to the examination (39).

To be reliable, however, sonographic demonstration of a pancreatic endocrine tumor must be shown in at least two planes. Differential diagnosis of small pancreatic adenomas includes peripancreatic lymph nodes and lymphatic metastases, which are usually seen as hypoechoic and well circumscribed as APUD tumors (38).

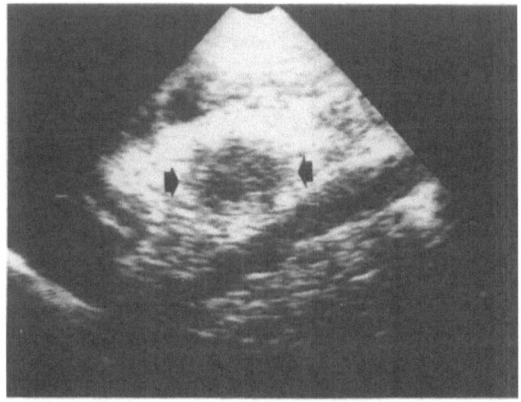

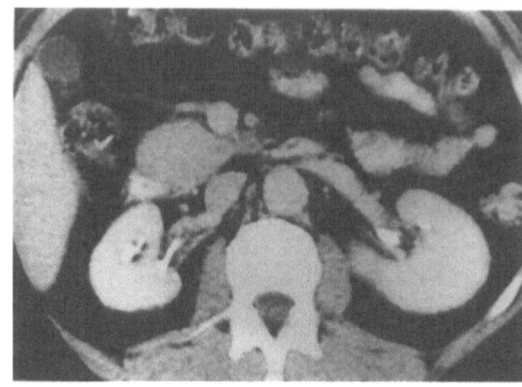

A

B

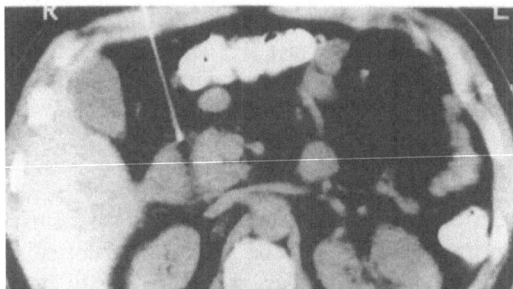

Figure 4.6. Nonfunctioning pancreatic islet cell tumor in the head of the pancreas. **A**: Ultrasonography, showing a relatively large hypoechogenic mass in the head of the pancreas (arrows). **B**: CT demonstrates the tumor in the head of the pancreas. Note that there is no contrast impregnation during the infusion. **C**: CT was also used for biopsy of the lesion, which let to the diagnosis of APUD-oma. No specific hormone was detected at the immunohistochemistry examination.

C

Larger islet cell tumors are readily localized by ultrasonography and CT and are amenable to percutaneous biopsy, either using ultrasound or CT orientation (Fig. 4.6). Larger lesions, however, are most probably nonfunctioning tumors or a glucagonoma and very unlikely to be a insulinoma or gastrinoma.

Ultrasonography is also very sensitive for hepatic metastatic disease identification. All the known islet cell tumors may be malignant in a small percentage of the cases, except glucagonomas and somatostatinomas which are malignant in 68% or more of the patients (6). Hepatic metastases may be the first findings in such patients.

Computed Tomography (CT)

Computed tomography is a noninvasive procedure that is used preoperatively for islet cell tumor localizations. To CT was granted a rel-atively low sensitivity and low specificity in the detection of pancreatic endocrine tumors. A recent large series shows sensitivity as low as 30% (39). Another study yields better results, reaching 42.1% (1). An additional one shows 25% for previously unknown lesions and 62.5% for previously known lesions (38). A more recent study however showed identification of 78% of the tumors and a specifity of 100% (40).

Size and location of gastrinomas are not independent concerning CT detection; 21 of 22 pancreatic gastrinomas were greater than 1 cm in diameter, whereas 6 of 17 extrapancreatic gastrinomas were less than 1 cm. Seventy-seven percent of pancreatic gastrinomas were correctly located with CT, but only 35% of extrapancreatic gastrinomas were correctly detected (40).

It is commonly agreed that CT of small islet cell tumors requires a bolus injection of contrast material and rapid sequential scanning, since transient increases in contrast enhancement (tumor blush) are characteristic of these tumors, which generally cannot be differentiated from the surrounding pancreatic tissue on the precontrast scan (Figs. 4.7 and 4.8). Increased tumor density without administration of contrast medium was reported in an early report from 1978 (41) but was not subsequently confirmed.

Protrusion of the lesion from the pancreatic contour by itself is nonspecific but may be useful information in some cases (Fig. 4.7) particularly with contrast enhancement.

Calcification of islet cell tumor was a reliable sign related with malignancy in 7 of 10 cases in a report from 1977 (42) and another one from 1984 (32). The only lesion with calcification in our series proved to be benign (Fig. 4.8). Calcifications are characteristically discrete and nodular, and distinguishable from the calcifications of pancreatitis (43).

Large lesions are readily identified by CT of the pancreas, but the differential diagnosis with pancreatic carcinoma is not easy and may require preoperative biopsy (Fig. 4.6).

Respiratory movements during dynamic scanning may obscure details. The splenic vein and artery must not be mistaken for tumors; neither must intestinal loops and lymph nodes.

The size limit for CT detection of pancreatic islet cell tumors appears to be 1.5 cm according to one report (43). Improved spatial resolution and faster scan time may increase sensitivity for tumor detection within a smaller size range. A normal CT, however, does not satisfactorily exclude either liver metastasis or pancreatic islet cell tumor. Other imaging methods seem warranted in patients with a normal CT scan.

Arteriography

Since Olsson's (44) angiographic description of an insulinoma in 1963, arteriography became a popular method for diagnosis and localization of the islet cell tumors of the pancreas and a large number of reports are available in the literature (4,45–53).

Pancreatic angiography has been very successful in detecting islet cell tumors in several reports and very unsuccessful in another group of reports. Successful results vary from 20% (46) to 88% (45). In one of the largest series a correct diagnosis was obtained in 63 of 82 patients (77%) with insulinoma. In a recent series, 62% of the single insulinomas were seen on arteriography, but only 29% are typically hypervascular and only 13% of the gastrinomas were correctly localized (7). The low success rate for localizing gastrinomas was corroborated by another series where only 15% of the lesions were identified. The success rate of angiography in the diagnosis of other islet cell tumors has been higher (1).

Angiography showed a specificity of 100% and a sensitivity of 86% for gastrinomas in the liver. For extrahepatic gastrinomas, angiography showed a specificity of 94% and a lower sensitivity of 68% (53). For lesions outside the liver, CT scanning detected 57%, angiography 70%, and the combination 73% of tumors with a false-positive rate of 7% (53). The overall success rate may be around 50 to 60% for all islet cell tumors.

The angiographic abnormalities vary with the size of the tumor. In small lesions, the dominant finding is a well-circumscribed, rounded area of increased contrast accumulation in the capillary and venous phase (47) (Fig. 4.9). No tumor vessels, or very few, are seen within small tumors. As the adenomas become larger, more tumor vessels appear and the arteries supplying the lesion dilate. The degree of vascularization may vary considerably. Some tumors contain dilated sinusoids, some have a rich network of capillaries between tumor cells arranged in a trabecular or rosette-like fashion. In others with prominent degeneration, fibrosis, or hyalinization, the vascularization is poor (47). Lesions as small as 0.5 cm may be detected satisfactorily by arteriography when hypervascular. Islet cell hyperplasia is not detected by any imaging method, except percutaneous venous sampling and hormone assay.

Regardless of the hormone they produce, pancreatic islet cell tumors have similar angiographic appearances. There is a tendency, however, for nonfunctioning adenomas to be larger before they are discovered, because they produce very few symptoms or none at all. For

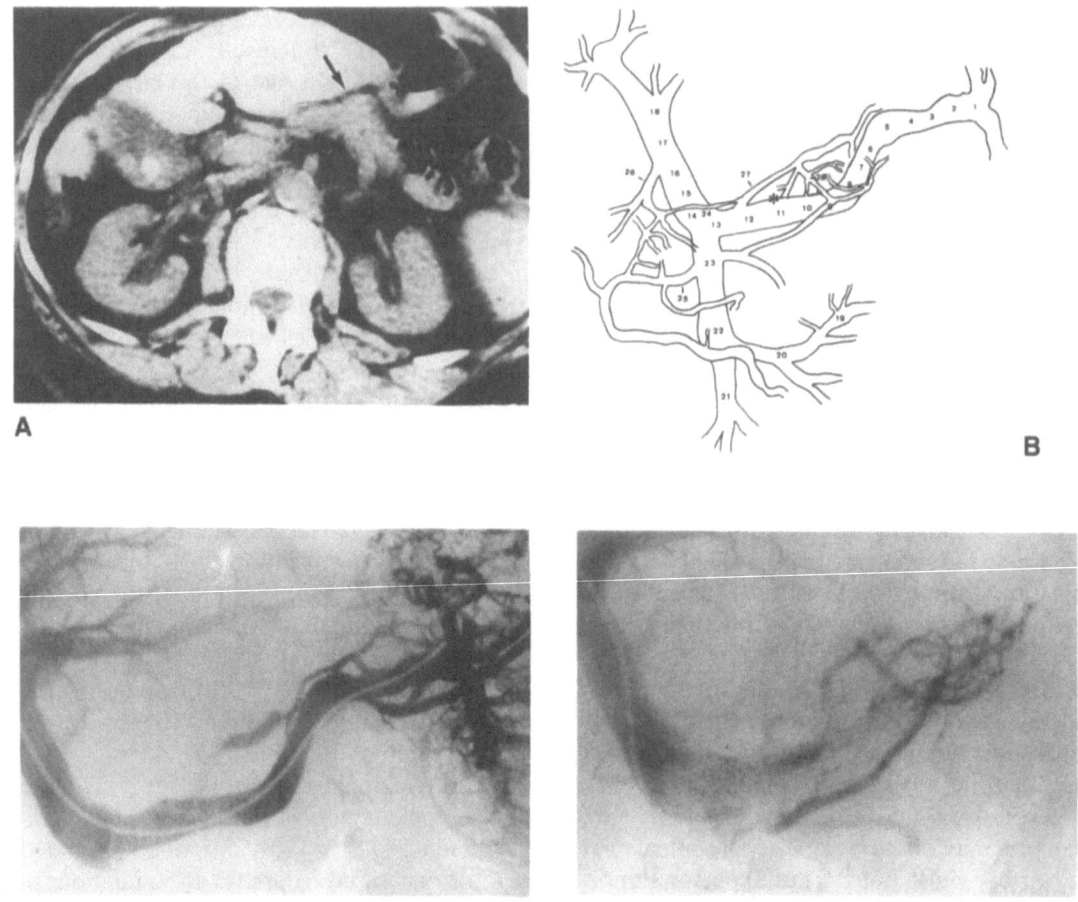

Figure 4.7. Pancreatic insulinoma in a 79-year-old woman characterized by severe hypoglycemia and neurologic symptoms. **A**: CT showing one bulging area in the pancreatic contour, anteriorly. Note that there is no contrast impregnation (arrow). Angiography was negative. To confirm the finding a percutaneous pancreatic venous sampling was performed. **B**: Schematic drawing with the venous sampling map. The following values were obtained for insulin:

1. 107 μU/ml	11. 133 μU/ml	21. 89 μU/ml
2. 111 μU/ml	12. 104 μU/ml	22. 90 μU/ml
3. 146 μU/ml	13. 89 μU/ml	23. 95 μU/ml
4. 151 μU/ml	14. 178 μU/ml	24. 127 μU/ml
5. 107 μU/ml	15. 85 μU/ml	25. 67 μU/ml
6. 109 μU/ml	16. 84 μU/ml	26. 175 μU/ml
7. 143 μU/ml	17. 92 μU/ml	27. 1,730 μU/ml
8. 148 μU/ml	18. 92 μU/ml	28. 121 μU/ml
9. 142 μU/ml	19. 76 μU/ml	Peripheral: 15 μU/ml
10. 139 μU/ml	20. 85 μU/ml	

Note that the lesion is located in the body of the pancreas in the ventral aspect and the highest hormone level is in sample 27, from the left gastric vein. **C** and **D**: Venography of the splenic vein and transverse pancreatic vein showing the connection of the left gastric vein with the pancreatic body venous drainage.

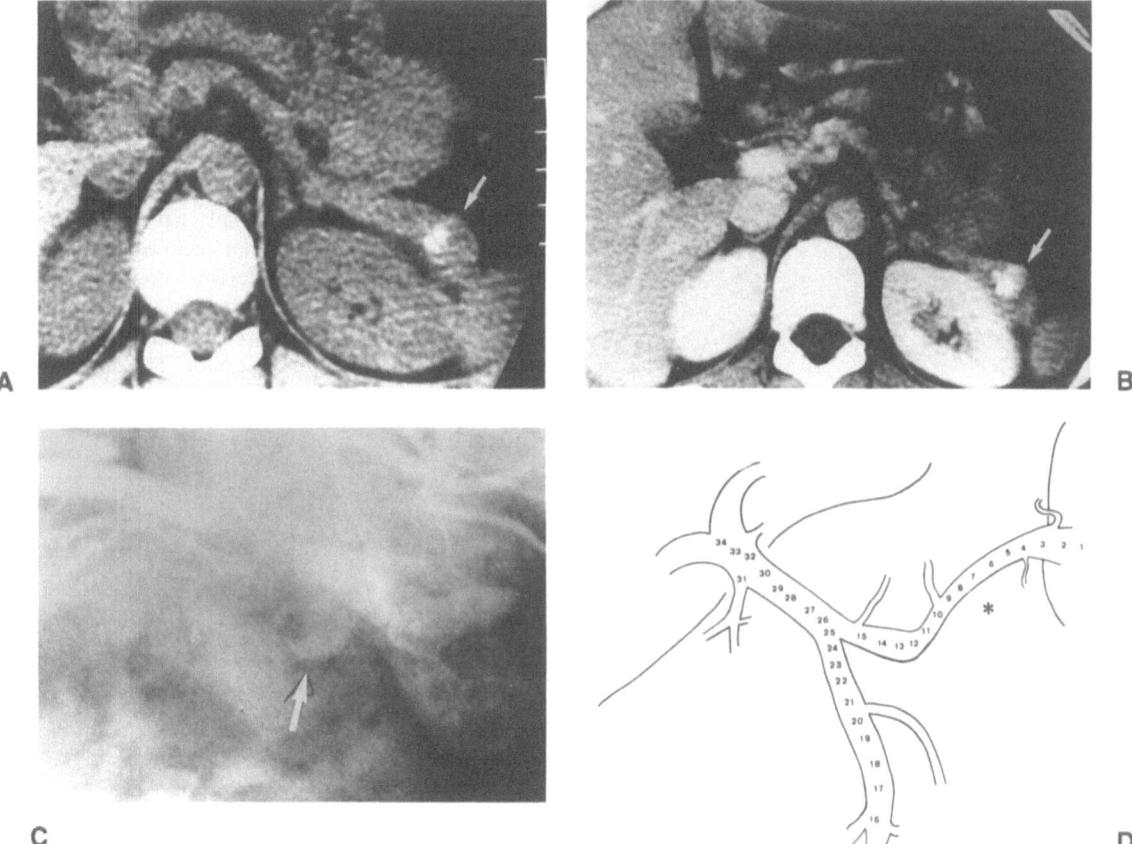

Figure 4.8. Benign pancreatic insulinoma with calcification. **A**: CT showing a bulging area at the pancreatic tail with nodular calcification (arrow). **B**: After the contrast infusion there is impregnation of the tumor (arrow). **C**: Angiography showed a small hypervascular adenoma at the tail of the pancreas (arrow). **D**: Pancreatic venous blood sampling was performed and the following values were obtained for insulin (only main vein samples were obtained, not selective):

1. 45 μU/ml
2. 38 μU/ml
3. 50 μU/ml
4. 48 μU/ml
5. 50 μU/ml
6. 45 μU/ml
7. 45 μU/ml
8. 620 μU/ml
9. 82 μU/ml
10. 82 μU/ml
11. 180 μU/ml
12. 78 μU/ml
13. 57 μU/ml
14. 45 μU/ml
15. 42 μU/ml
16. 39 μU/ml
17. 45 μU/ml
18. 42 μU/ml
19. 35 μU/ml
20. 42 μU/ml
21. 38 μU/ml
22. 41 μU/ml
23. 45 μU/ml
24. 41 μU/ml
25. 41 μU/ml
26. 40 μU/ml
27. 140 μU/ml
28. 86 μU/ml
29. 48 μU/ml
30. 50 μU/ml
31. 54 μU/ml
32. 62 μU/ml
33. 76 μU/ml
34. 70 μU/ml

Note that sample number 8 shows the highest value of insulin, consistent with insulinoma in the tail of the pancreas.

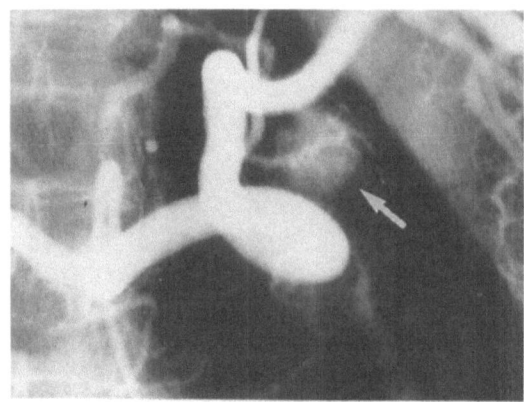

A

Figure 4.9. Insulinoma in the tail of the pancreas.
A: Note the hypervascular tumor, with well-defined
limits and one feeding vessel (arrow) branch of the
splenic artery. **B**: The tumor was enucleated. The
pathologic specimen shows well-vascularized connective tissue septa within the tumor. The diameter
was 15 mm.

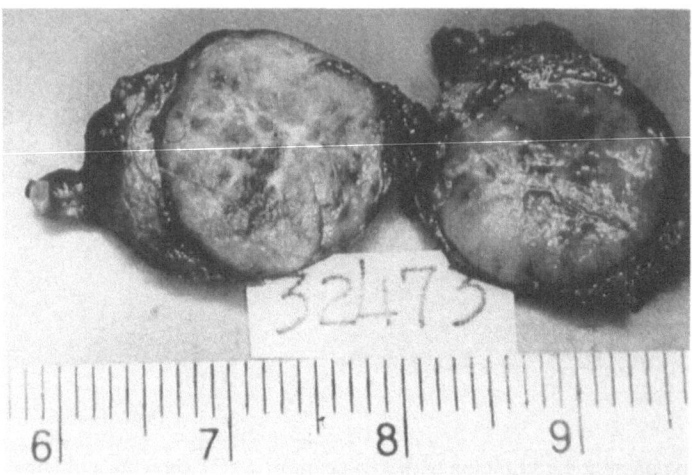

B

the same reason they have a higher incidence
of liver metastases than functioning pancreatic
adenomas (49).

Hepatic metastases are generally hypervascular and show dense blush in the late arterial phase and venous phase. Very small and
tiny hepatic metastases may be observed easily
in the liver against the normal stain of liver
parenchyma (Fig. 4.10). Larger and diffuse
metastatic lesions on the liver are readily
visualized (Fig. 4.11) on angiography.

The most important pitfall in the arteriographic diagnosis and localization of pancreatic
islet cell tumors is the unpredictable behavior
of such lesions concerning contrast impregnation (50).

The angiographic findings can be very subtle
and the use of a digital angiography apparatus

may improve the visualization of the lesion
(Fig. 4.5). Superselective techniques may also
aid in the diagnosis. Selective injections in
the gastroduodenal artery, dorsal pancreatic
artery, and splenic artery should be part of the
protocol for pancreatic adenomas localization
in addition to celiac artery and superior mesenteric artery angiography.

Although the poorly vascularized adenomas
may be missed, there is a risk of a false-positive
diagnosis in some patients with areas of increased contrast accumulation at the distal
third of the pancreas, related to the area supplied by the dorsal pancreatic or pancreatica
magna arteries. Other causes of false-positive
diagnosis are accessory spleens and hypervascular metastases to lymph nodes (Fig. 4.12)
(50).

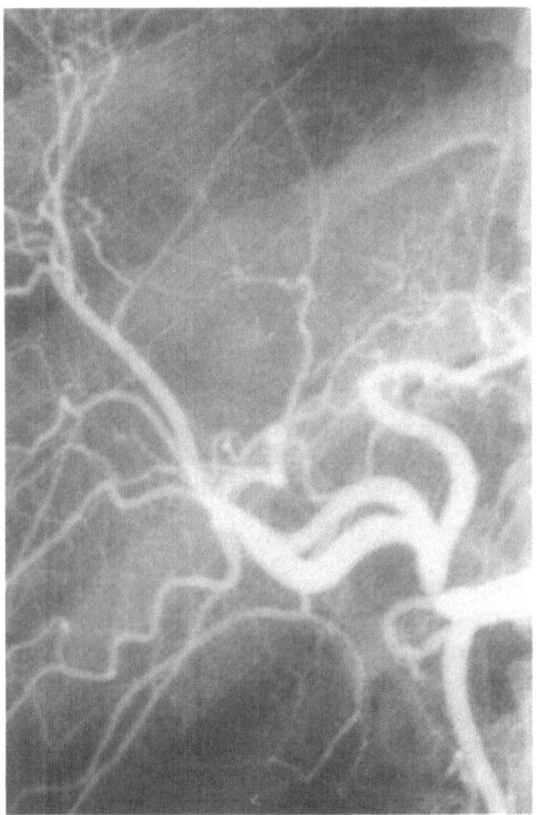 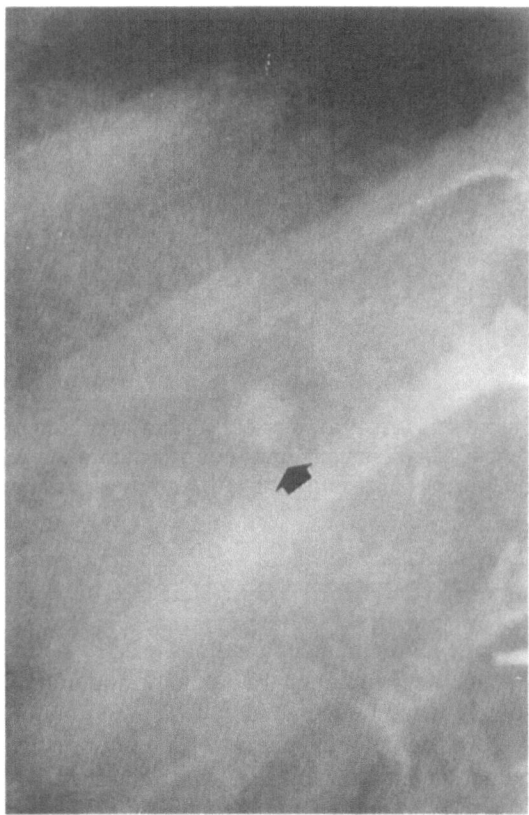

A   B

Figure 4.10. **A**: Liver metastatic disease of malignant insulinoma. Note the nodular lesion already starting with tumor blush at the early arterial phase. **B**: Late arterial phase showing the well-defined hypervascular lesion against the liver background (arrow).

Figure 4.11. Diffuse metastatic disease in the liver due to a pancreatic insulinoma. Note the hypervascular nodules throughout the liver with different sizes.

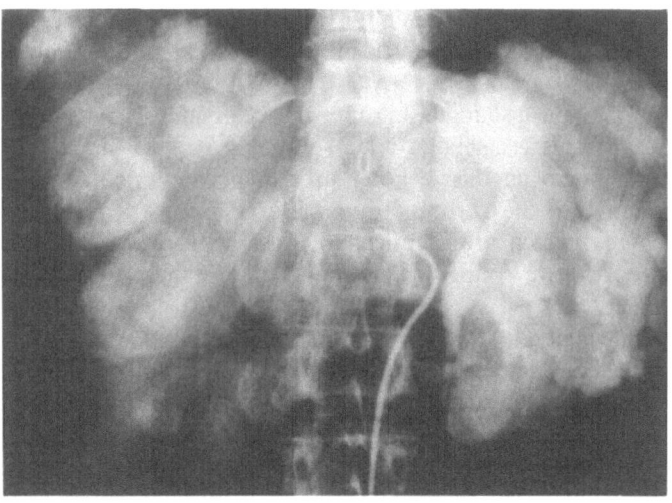

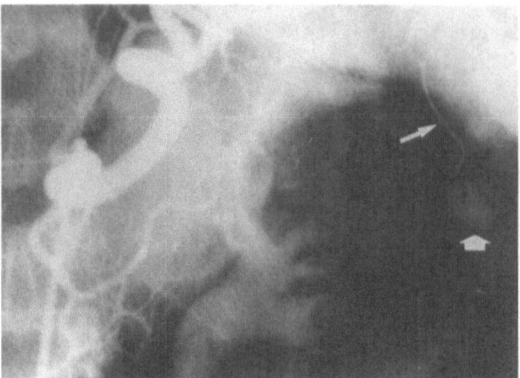 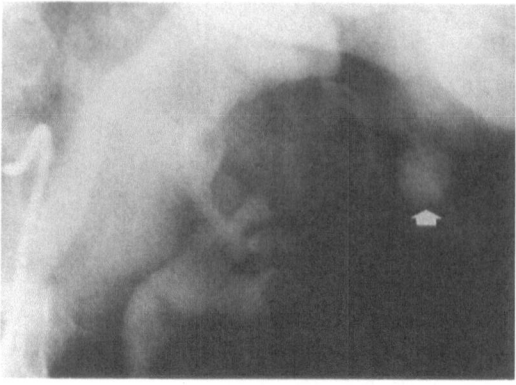

A   **B**

Figure 4.12. **A**: A 29-year-old woman with insulinoma localized in the tail of the pancreas by pancreatic venous blood sampling (not shown), with simultaneous ectopic spleen (short arrow) fed by a single artery (long arrow) at arteriography. **B**: The late arterial phase shows the splenic tissue blush (short arrow).

Intraoperative Ultrasound

Despite all the imaging methods used to localize islet cell tumors, a careful intraoperative search for a previously identified lesion or for an occult lesion is mandatory, either using palpation and dissection or, more recently, intraoperative ultrasound scanning (39,54–56). It is necessary to use a high-resolution, real-time scanner with a 7.5- or 10-mHz transducer. The transducers are covered with a sheath containing sterile gel and placed within the fluid-filled peritoneal cavity about 1 cm above the pancreas. The lesion may or may not be known to the radiologist during the examination, which takes about 10 minutes to perform. The whole procedure, however, may take as long as 60 minutes.

The typical sonographic appearance of an insulinoma is as a small, round, solid mass with a fine homogeneous echotexture, hypoechoic relative to the surrounding pancreatic parenchyma, which are identical to those seen on preoperative sonogram except for the higher clarity (39).

Intraoperative ultrasound used in a blind way showed a sensitivity of 84% for detection of insulinomas and when combined with surgical palpation, the sensitivity for localization of solitary insulinomas was 100% in one series of 25 patients (39). In another report, sensitivity for insulinomas using palpation was 71% and intraoperative ultrasound was 86% and the sensitivity for gastrinomas using palpation was 94% and intraoperative ultrasound was 83%, showing no significant overall difference between palpation and ultrasound to localize intraoperatively pancreatic islet cell tumors. However, it demonstrated that in 11% of patients ultrasound provides additional information not obtained by palpation alone (55). For localizing extrapancreatic tumors, however, palpation is significantly better than ultrasound. In fact, up to 50% of the gastrinomas may be extrapancreatic, suggesting that ultrasound used intraoperatively may be more useful for insulinomas localization than gastrinomas (56).

The pancreatic tail is more difficult to scan with ultrasound during surgery, requiring pancreatic tail and splenic mobilization for adequate examination, increasing the risk of organ injury.

False-positive lesions may be identified within the pancreas appearing as sonolucent mass lesions similar to islet cell tumors. Again, normal lymph nodes may be detected as lesions (55).

Lesions with indistinct borders may suggest pancreatic invasion and malignancy, requiring resection rather than enucleation (55).

The high sensitivity of palpation and intraoperative ultrasound lead some authors to suggest that preoperative localization procedures

Figure 4.13. Schematic drawing showing the percutaneous trans-hepatic access for portography and selective pancreatic venous sampling. Note the relationship of the liver, portal vein, and the rib cage.

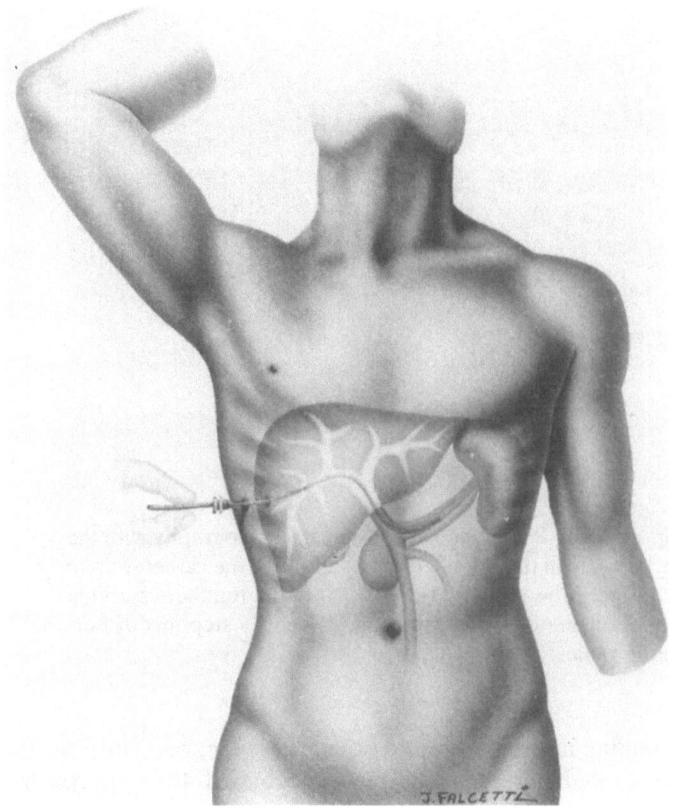

are not necessary in patients with clinical and biochemical evidence of insulinoma (39). This suggestion, however, is not valid for gastrinomas, and this series may have a falsely elevated sensitivity due to inherent referral bias (56).

Intraoperative ultrasound, however, is a great improvement in pancreatic islet cell localization and will be universally used in the near future.

Venous Sampling

Technique of Catheterization and Blood Sampling

The technique of transhepatic puncture and catheterization of the portal vein and its tributaries is performed according to the technique introduced by Wiechel (57) in 1971 and developed by Göthlin et al. (58) in 1974 and Hoevels et al. (59) in 1978. Since that time, a large number of reports appeared in the litera-

ture (60–71) on the diagnosis and localization of a variety of pancreatic endocrine tumors.

The puncture of the portal system is performed in the right midaxillary line, midway between the diaphragm and lower margin of the liver, toward the hilum of the liver. The puncture is oriented by fluoroscopy and a biplane system may be occasionally useful.

A 25-cm–long sheathed needle with a 5F polyethylene catheter is used for portal access. After puncture the needle is withdrawn and the catheter is slowly pulled back until brisk blood flow is obtained. A small, nonforceful, injection of contrast medium is made to confirm the catheter position in a portal vein branch and a J-tipped guide wire is manipulated into the portal vein and advanced into the splenic or the superior mesenteric vein. The catheter is then pushed over the guide wire to the desired site (Fig. 4.13).

The catheter needle sheath may be used for blood sampling in the large veins. Selective

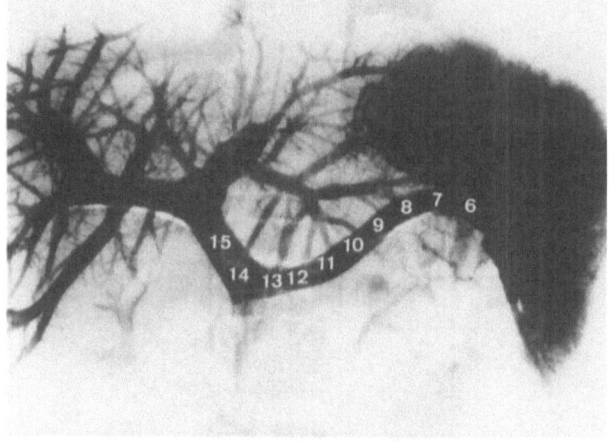

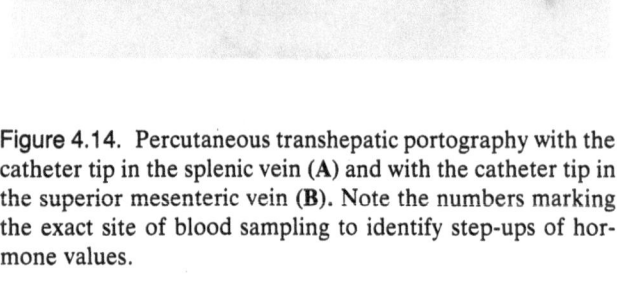

A

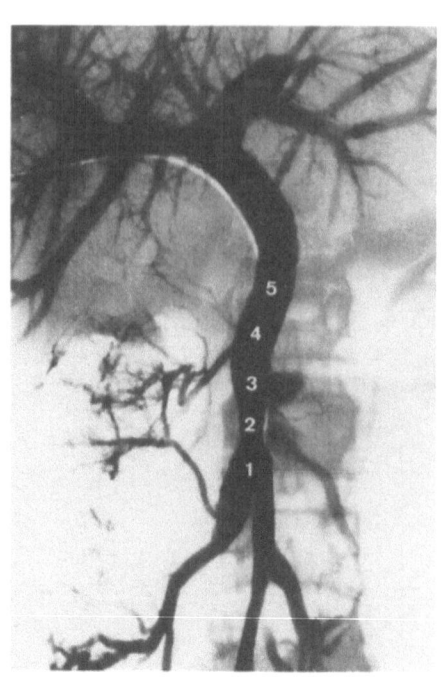

Figure 4.14. Percutaneous transhepatic portography with the catheter tip in the splenic vein (**A**) and with the catheter tip in the superior mesenteric vein (**B**). Note the numbers marking the exact site of blood sampling to identify step-ups of hormone values.

B

sampling in the pancreatic veins, however, requires catheter exchange for a preshaped 40-cm–long catheter with a side hole near the tip to facilitate blood aspiration.

The percutaneous puncture should not be made in a cranial direction, to avoid a sharp intrahepatic angle of the catheter which would make catheter manipulation and catheter exchange much more difficult. A slightly caudally oriented puncture or a right-angle puncture in relation to the spine is preferable.

Portography covering the splenic vein and the superior mesenteric vein is the initial angiographic procedure. A series of 12 films, 2 films/sec for 3 sec followed by 1 film/sec for 6 sec is obtained after the injection of 25 to 40 ml of contrast medium at a rate of 8 ml/sec, with the tip of the catheter near the splenic hilus and subsequently with the catheter tip deep into the superior mesenteric vein (Fig. 4.14). After obtaining the whole map of the portal system the blood sampling may be performed (60). Blood samples are obtained from the splenic, superior mesenteric, and portal veins. The splenic and mesenteric portograms are labeled with serial numbers at about 1.0 cm intervals, and samples are obtained at sites correspond-

ing to the serial numbers. This systematic approach is essential for identification of the sampling sites and interpretation of hormone data.

Following splenic, portal, and mesenteric sampling, selective catheterization of the pancreatic veins is undertaken. For selective catheterization and pancreatic venous sampling, a 1-cm curved-tip catheter should be used. The posterior superior pancreaticoduodenal (PSPD), anterior superior pancreaticoduodenal (ASPD), dorsal pancreatic (DP), transverse pancreatic (TP), and caudal pancreatic (CP) veins are catheterized selectively, using a torque-control guide wire (Fig. 4.15). After successful manipulation of the guide wire into the pancreatic vein the catheter is pushed over it. Catheterization with the catheter alone should be carefully avoided because it could result in damage to the vein wall and extravasation of contrast medium, and blood sampling consequently would be impaired. The guide wire tip should go beyond the catheter tip during positioning.

When selective and safe catheterization of the pancreatic vein is achieved, under fluoroscopic surveillance, a small amount of contrast

Figure 4.15. Anatomy of the pancreatic venous drainage. PV, portal vein; SV, splenic vein, SMV, superior mesenteric vein; IMV, inferior mesenteric vein; DP, dorsal pancreatic vein; GT, gastrocolic trunk; TP, transverse pancreatic vein; CPV, pancreatic veins; JV, jejunal vein; LGV, left gastric vein; PSPD, posterior superior pancreaticoduodenal vein; ASPD, anterior superior pancreaticoduodenal vein; PIPD, posterior inferior pancreaticoduodenal vein; AIPD, anterior inferior pancreaticoduodenal vein.

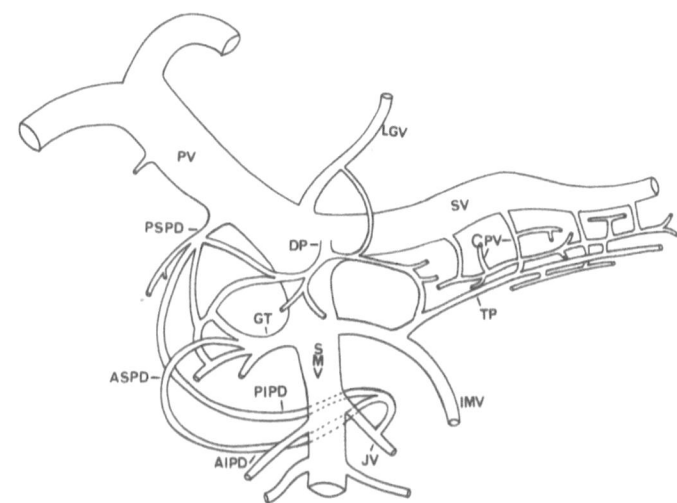

medium is injected to assure correct positioning of the catheter. This injection should be very gentle to avoid venous damage and inversion of the venous blood flow. After aspiration of the contrast medium out of the catheter a blood sample may be obtained. Phlebography is performed after sampling to document the correct place of the blood sampling and to map the venous system and the anatomy of the anastomoses. Phlebography into the ASPD and PSPD of normal caliber requires a hand injection of 6 to 8 ml of contrast medium. A series of six to eight films are exposed at a rate of two films/sec.

The easiest pancreatic vein to be catheterized is usually the ASPD vein, but it requires a circular shape of the tip of the guide wire with a radius of about 2 cm. The PSPD vein should be searched for at the caudal wall of the portal vein and a simple 90° or 80° curve at the tip of the guide wire is sufficient. The TP vein is searched for at the left lateral wall of the superior mesenteric vein near the confluence or at the lateral wall of the inferior mesenteric vein. The guide wire tip shape should be of a double reverse curve. The TP vein is usually visualized when one of the pancreatic body veins draining to the splenic vein are injected, facilitating identification and catheterization. The DP vein is not always present or possible to catheterize, but should be searched for at the anterior wall at the confluence. The veins

of the pancreatic tail are searched for at the ventrocaudal aspect of the splenic vein using a 1-cm–long curve with 90° at the tip of the guide wire. The positioning of the catheter may be a little more difficult at the pancreatic caudal veins because the guide wire slips out of the vein when the catheter is pushed over it. A curved-tip catheter helps to minimize this problem. A side hole close to the catheter tip helps in blood sampling. Hand injection of contrast medium for phlebography at the body and pancreas tail veins should be limited to 2 to 7 ml due to the smaller size of these veins.

Sampling Technique

The patient fasts for 8 hours. Transhepatic portal vein catheterization is performed under local anesthesia and sedation in adults and under general anesthesia in children. Celiac artery and hepatic vein catheterization may also be performed, especially when hepatic metastatic disease is suspected. A peripheral venous blood sampling should be obtained at the beginning and end of the examination (61).

At the superior mesenteric and splenic veins blood samples should be obtained at every 1 cm from the periphery to the confluence and at the portal vein samples are obtained from the confluence to the bifurcation. Selective catheterization of the pancreatic veins, as described above, should be attempted in the largest number of veins possible. The number of pancreatic veins one can catheterize per procedure increases with training and with familiarity with the anatomy of the pancreatic veins. Pancreatic venous blood samples in general should not be vigorously aspirated, to avoid blood flow reversion in adjacent venous territories. In fact, most of the blood sampling from pancreatic veins can only be collected by dripping, which more accurately represents venous flow and actual specific territory drainage. Selective pancreatic venous blood sampling should comprise four to six veins.

The blood samples must be handled appropriately. When gastrin and insulin are sampled for radioimmunoassay the samples may be stored for up to 2 hours in ice-chilled laboratory tubes before centrifugation, and the serum must be stored at $-20°C$ until assayed, whereas glucagon, pancreatic polypeptide (PP), vasoactive intestinal polypeptide (VIP), and somatostatin must be collected in ice-chilled tubes containing Trasylol and heparin, and immediately centrifuged at $+4°C$. The plasma is stored at $-20°C$ until assayed as well. Blood sampling is the most time-consuming part of the procedure and may take from 2 to 4 hours. From each vein 8 to 10 ml of blood should be obtained to allow repeated assays if necessary.

Blood samples are centrifuged and the serum stored at $-20°C$, until radioimmunologic determination of the hormone is performed. Radioimmunoassay of insulin in the serum is performed using ^{125}I-labeled pig insulin and guinea pig antipig insulin. Insulin standard and unknown samples and antisera are pipetted into a small glass tube, mixed and incubated for 20 hours at 4°C. ^{125}I-labeled insulin is added, mixed, and incubated for 4 hours at 4°C. Thereafter, 96% alcohol is added, and the solution is centrifuged for 20 minutes at 2,000 times gravity. The supernatant is pipetted into a plastic tube that is stoppered and radioactivity is counted. After plotting the standard curve of counts per minute versus the insulin concentration, the unknown insulin concentration is read (32).

All samples from the same patient should be assayed in the same run and all in triplicate.

Anatomy of the Pancreatic Veins

The anatomy of the pancreatic veins corresponds roughly to the distribution of the pancreatic arteries (Fig. 4.15) (61,72).

The head of the pancreas has the venous drainage related to the main stem of the portal vein and to the superior mesenteric vein (72). The venous drainage of the head of the pancreas is constituted by four main veins, forming two arcades, one posterior and one anterior. The posterior aspect of the pancreas head is drained by one or several posterior superior pancreaticoduodenal (PSPD) veins directly connected to the dorsal aspect of the portal vein, usually about 2 cm from the point of confluence of the splenic, the superior mesenteric, and the portal veins (Fig. 4.16A). The posterior arcade also empties into the first jejunal vein or directly into the superior mesenteric veins via the posterior inferior pancreaticoduodenal vein (PIPD). This arcade runs posteriorly to the pancreatic head in the pancreaticoduodenal sulcus, receiving tributaries from the pancreas and the duodenum. The anterior aspect of the pancreas head is drained by the anterior superior pancreaticoduodenal vein (ASPD) (Fig. 4.16B) emptying directly into the gastrocolic trunk (GT) beside several smaller veins. The GT receives the right gastroepiploic (RGE) vein (Fig 4.16C) and the middle colic vein (MCV) and empties itself into the right aspect of the superior mesenteric vein (SMV), from 1 to 3 cm from the junction of the superior mesenteric, splenic (SV), and portal (PV) veins.

The lower ventral aspect of the head of the pancreas is drained by the anterior inferior pancreaticoduodenal vein (AIPD) which drains into the first jejunal vein or, in some cases, into the SMV. The AIPD is usually joined by the PIPD vein in the last few centimeters before emptying into the first jejunal artery.

The ventral aspect of the pancreas head may be occasionally drained by a vein emptying in the ventral surface of the PV, near the confluence or up to 3 or 4 cm from that point.

The larger pancreatic veins draining the pancreas head run on the surface of the organ and not within the parenchyma itself.

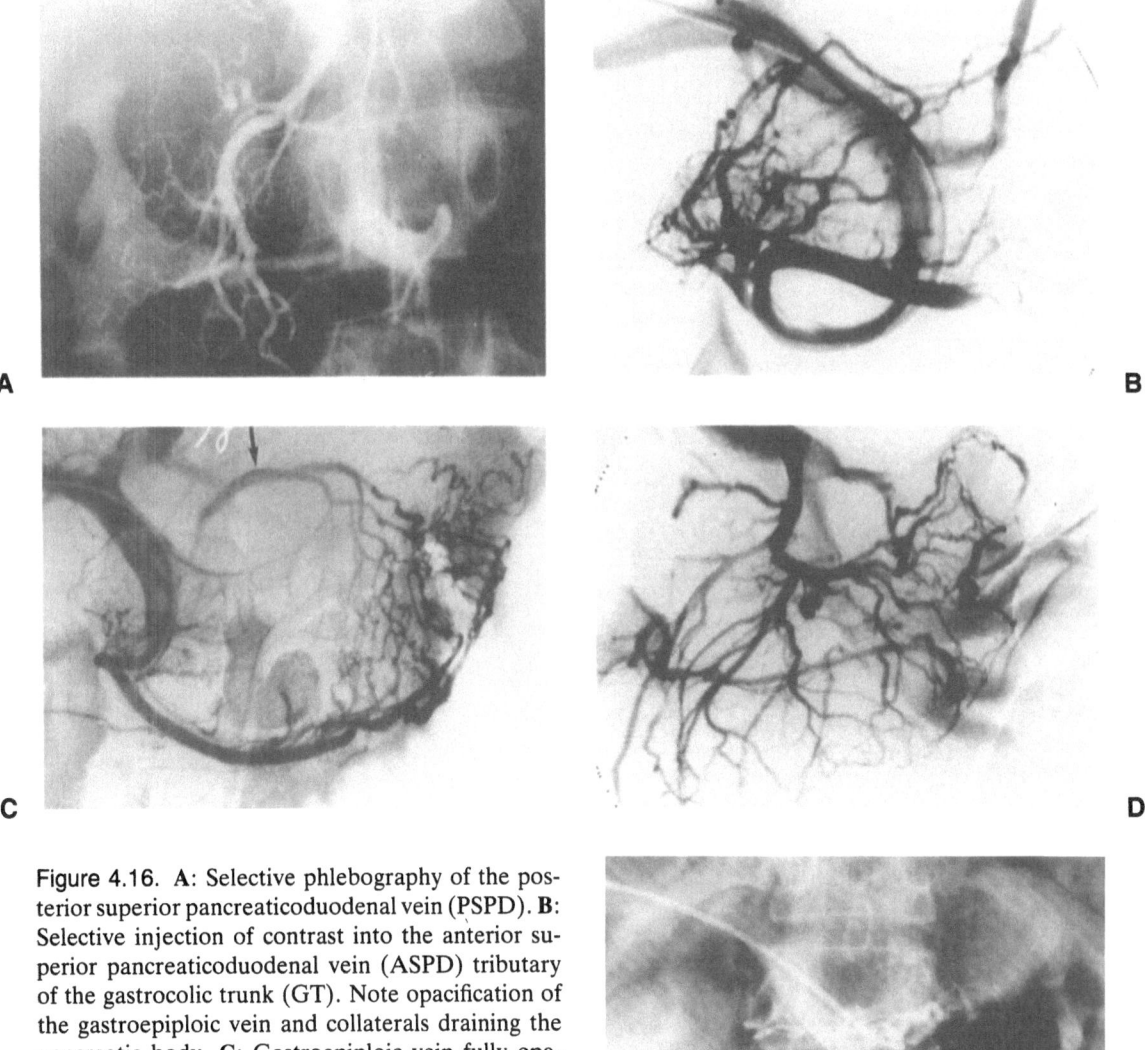

Figure 4.16. A: Selective phlebography of the posterior superior pancreaticoduodenal vein (PSPD). B: Selective injection of contrast into the anterior superior pancreaticoduodenal vein (ASPD) tributary of the gastrocolic trunk (GT). Note opacification of the gastroepiploic vein and collaterals draining the pancreatic body. C: Gastroepiploic vein fully opacified by injection at the GT. Note opacification over collaterals of the left gastric vein (LGV) (arrow). D: Injection of contrast into the dorsal pancreatic vein (DP), which is a dominant vein. Note the anastomosis with the pancreatic veins in the body and proximal tail. E: Small DP vein.

The venous drainage of the pancreas head is usually connected through collaterals to the dorsal pancreatic vein (DP) which drains part of the mediodorsal part of the head and empties in the dorsal aspect of the portal confluence wall (Fig. 4.16D,E).

The body of the pancreas is drained by the transverse pancreatic (TP) vein, which empties either into the inferior mesenteric vein, SMV, or SV (Fig. 4.17A). The TP vein runs along the inferior border of the pancreatic body, parallel to the SV and receives a large number of small branches from the pancreas body and may be connected to the left gastric vein (LGV) (Fig. 4.17B). Several of the smaller veins draining the body of the pancreas empty into the PSPD, the LGV, or directly into the large venous trunks near the confluence (Fig. 4.17B,C).

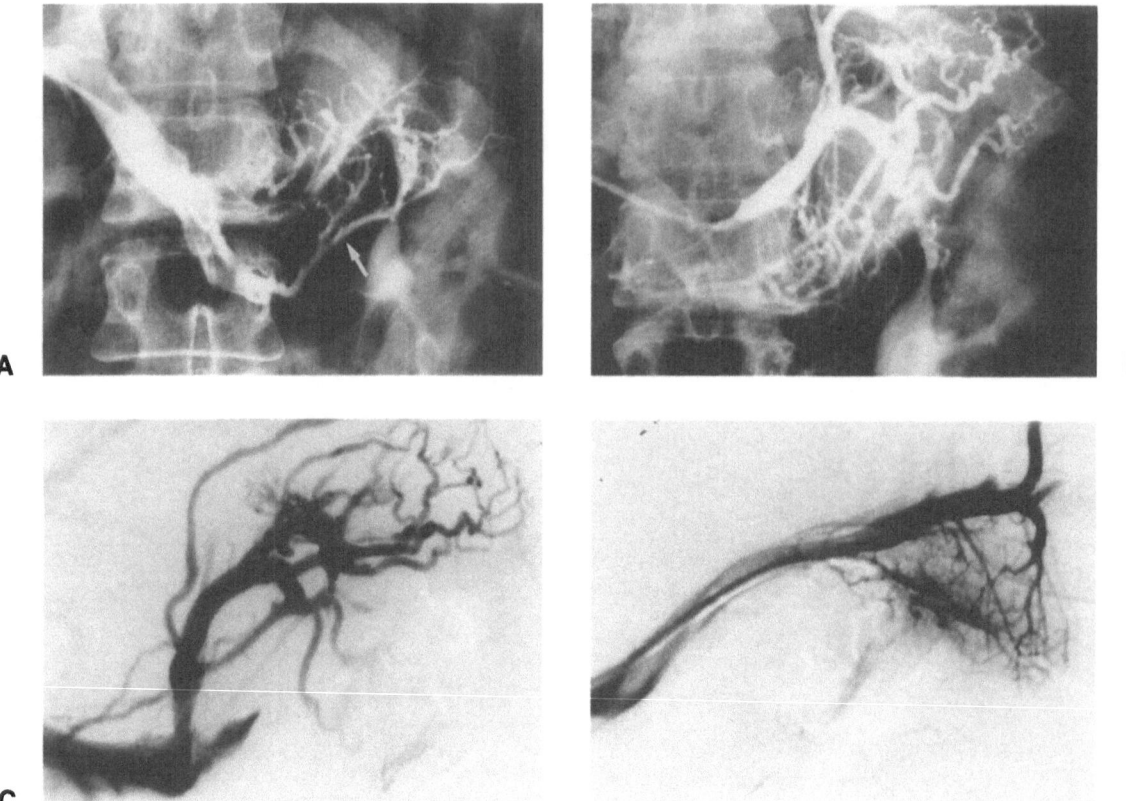

Figure 4.17. **A**: Selective injection into the transverse pancreatic vein (TP) (arrow). Note the collateral anastomosis of the TP with the pancreatic veins (CPV) in the tail of the pancreas. **B**: Injection into the left gastric vein (LGV). Note the collateral anastomosis with the CPV and TP vein. **C**: Selective injection into the LGV without collateral anastomosis to the CPV. **D**: Injection into one of the main CPV$_s$ in the tail of the pancreas.

The tail of the pancreas is drained by a large number of small and short veins that are usually connected to the caudal aspect of the splenic vein (Fig. 4.17D). These are mainly intrapancreatic veins that are part of a rich anastomotic venous bed connecting the TP vein and the splenic vein. Some of the lower polar veins of the spleen may also participate in the distal caudal pancreatic venous drainage.

The angiographer must be aware of the presence of the rich venous anastomoses in and around the pancreas because high hormone levels may be sampled in veins remote from the tumor site. Venous sampling in veins not directly related to the pancreatic venous drainage, such as the LGV, may present high hormone values due to secondary drainage of the

tumor site through small venous anastomoses (Fig. 4.17).

Interpretation of Hormone Data

Localized elevation of hormone concentration in the peripancreatic veins with abnormally high portal venous-arterial gradients may be found in the pancreatic venous effluent corresponding to the tumor site in the large majority of the patients (Fig. 4.18) (60,61).

Step-ups of hormone concentration in the SMV and PV are caused by tumors in the head of the pancreas. Tumors in the neck of the pancreas cause abnormal hormone elevation in the SV near the confluence. The tumors in the

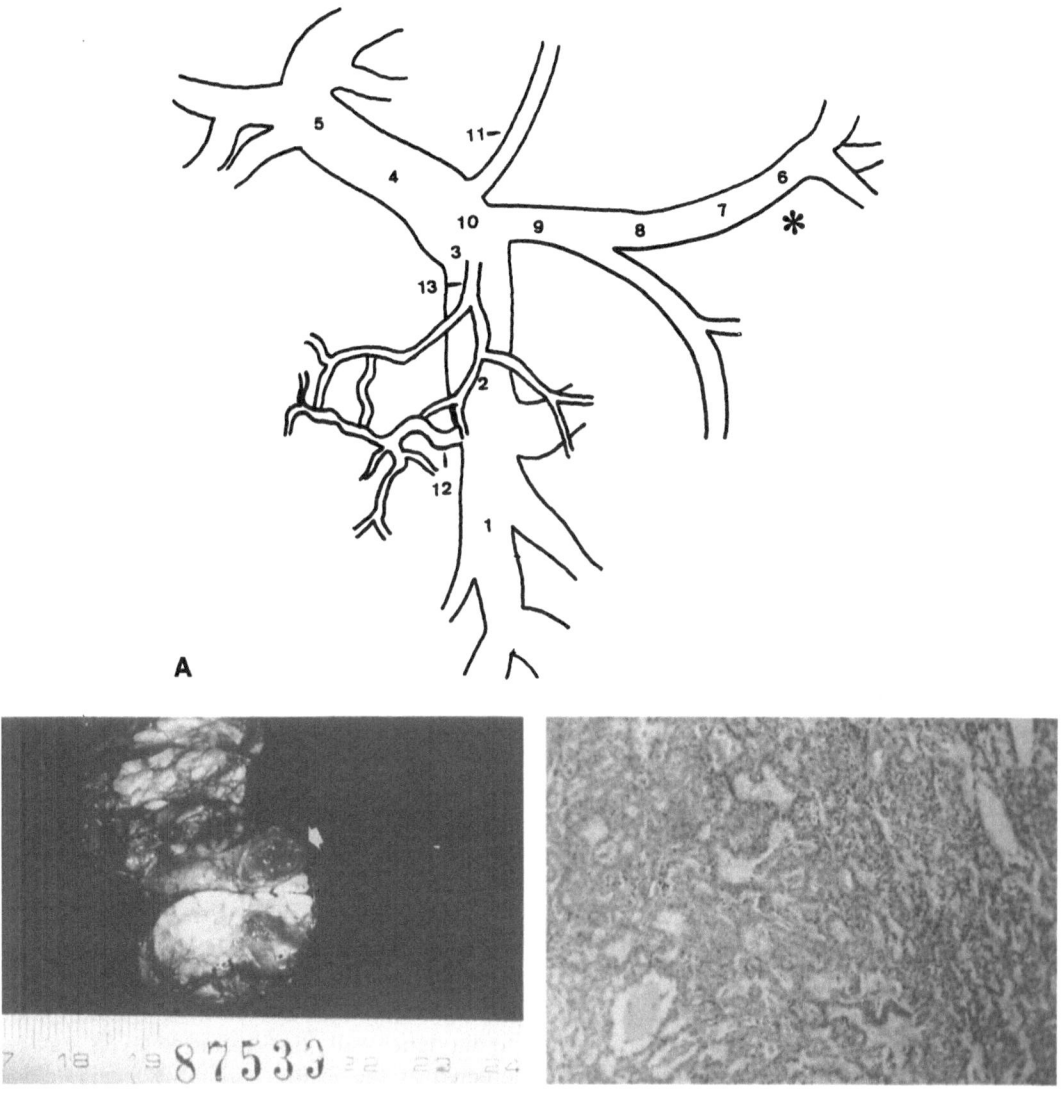

Figure 4.18. **A**: Insulin concentration in the mainstream of the splenic vein, superior mesenteric vein, and various portal tributaries and pancreatic veins in a 9-year-old girl with insulinoma of the tail of the pancreas. Highest insulin level in sample number 6. The patient had had two negative arteriographies and one negative CT previous to the pancreatic venous sampling:

1. 11 μU/ml
2. 17 μUlml
3. 15 μU/ml
4. 25 μU/ml
5. 40 μU/ml

6. *90* μU/ml
7. 28 μU/ml
8. 65 μU/ml
9. 45 μU/ml
10. 55 μU/ml

11. 35 μU/ml
12. 18 μU/ml
13. 16 μU/ml

B: Surgical specimen showing the insulinoma at the pancreas tail (arrow). **C**: Microscopy of the insulinoma (H-E) ($\times$ 400).

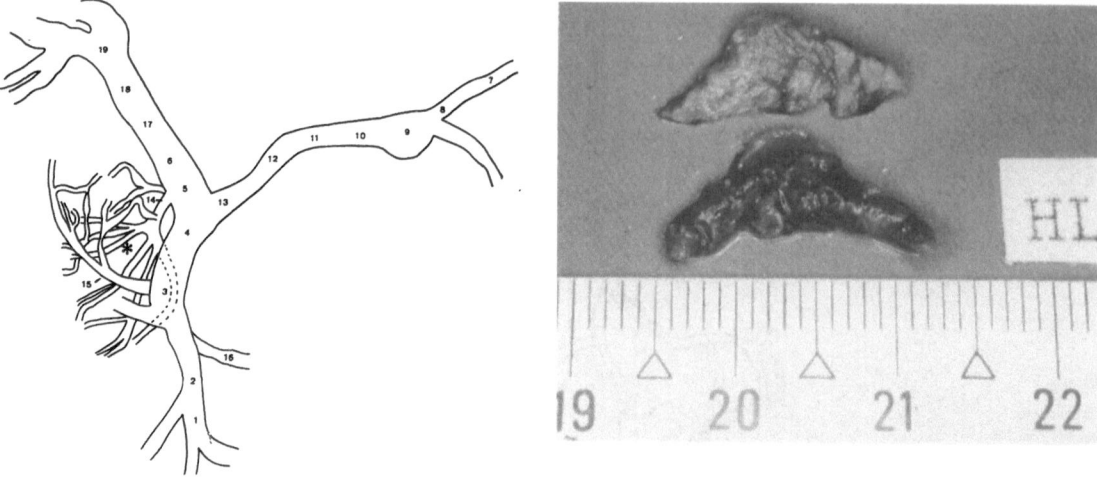

Figure 4.19. **A**: Insulin concentration in the mainstream of the splenic vein, superior mesenteric vein, portal vein, and various pancreatic tributaries in a 31-year-old man with an insulinoma in the posterior aspect of the head of the pancreas, mainly drained by the posterior superior pancreaticoduodenal vein (PSPD), sample 14. Arteriography and ultrasound were negative.

1. 35 μU/ml	8. 50 μU/ml	15. 51 μU/ml
2. 27 μU/ml	9. 49 μU/ml	16. 50 μU/ml
3. <5 μU/ml	10. 20 μU/ml	17. 29 μU/ml
4. 25 μU/ml	11. 40 μU/ml	18. 120 μU/ml
5. 40 μU/ml	12. 76 μU/ml	19. 160 μU/ml
6. 95 μU/ml	13. 70 μU/ml	Peripheral: 82 μU/ml
7. 31 μU/ml	14. >400 μU/ml	

B: The lesion was enucleated and pathological analysis showed insulin-producing adenoma.

body and tail of the pancreas cause increased hormone levels in the SV (Fig. 4.8).

Compared with sampling in the large peripancreatic veins, selective pancreatic vein catheterization and venous sampling for hormone assay increases the sensitivity of the test from 65% to 85 to 90% (6).

High hormone concentration in the PSPD will indicate a lesion in the posterior-superior aspect of the head of the pancreas (Figs. 4.19 and 4.20). Hormone elevation in the ASPD will be consistent with a lesion in the anterior-superior part of the pancreas head. High hormone values observed in samples obtained from the GT may indicate either a lesion in the anterior aspect of the pancreas head or in the tail of the pancreas because the gastroepiploic vein connects the veins from the splenic hilus to the GT. It is important, therefore, to sample selectively the ASPD in addition to the GT itself (Fig. 4.16B,C).

Special care should be taken regarding lesions (gastrinoma) located at the duodenal, gastric, or jejunal wall. When the lesion is at the duodenal wall, high hormone levels may be detected at the PSPD and ASPD veins (Fig. 4.21). Gastric lesions will be drained by the LG or gastroepiploic veins (Fig. 4.16C). The lesions at the jejunal wall are usually near the ligament of Treitz and increased hormone levels may be found at the first jejunal vein. It should be remembered that all those alternative sites for tumor localization are drained ultimately by pancreatic or peripancreatic veins and the positive predictive value of the finding may be reduced.

Lesions in the posterior and anterior-inferior segment of the pancreas head will produce high hormone concentration in the draining vein, usually at the first jejunal vein. The PIPD and AIPD veins may, however, drain directly to the SMV or inferior mesenteric veins.

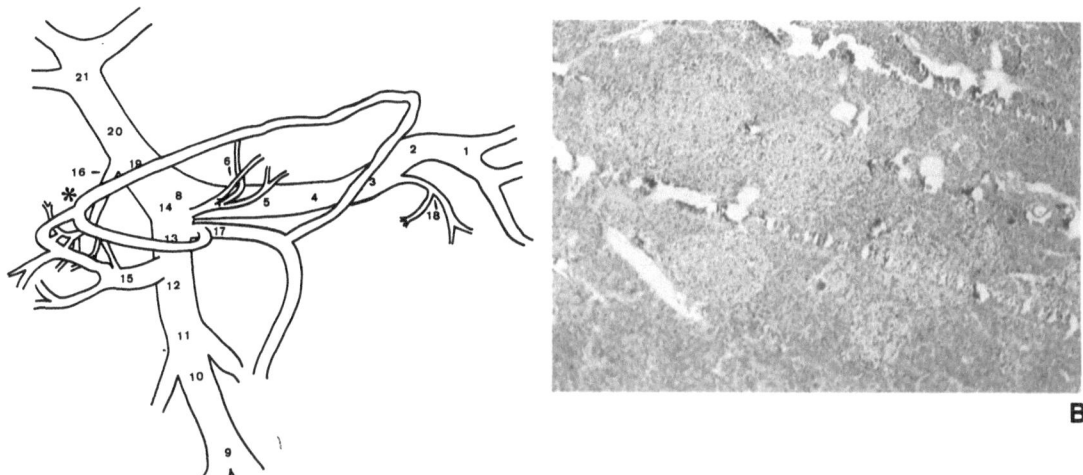

Figure 4.20. **A**: A 12-year-old boy with hypoglycemia had previous arteriography negative for pancreatic adenoma. Percutaneous pancreatic venous sampling showed elevated concentration of insulin into the posterior superior pancreaticoduodenal vein, sample number 16.

1. 52 μU/ml	9. 66 μU/ml	17. 55 μU/ml
2. 53 μU/ml	10. 66 μU/ml	18. 71 μU/ml
3. 62 μU/ml	11. 57 μU/ml	19. 62 μU/ml
4. 53 μU/ml	12. 55 μU/ml	20. 135 μU/ml
5. 53 μU/ml	13. 60 μU/ml	21. 23 μU/ml
6. 65 μU/ml	14. 58 μU/ml	Peripheral:
7. 71 μU/ml	15. 55 μU/ml	22. 73 μU/ml
8. 50 μU/ml	16. *410* μU/ml	

B: Surgical inspection and palpation showed no tumor. Partial resection of the head of the pancreas showed islet cell hyperplasia in the posterior aspect of the head of the pancreas. There are a lot of artifacts in the slide but islet cell hyperplasia is clearly seen (× 100).

Tumors in the mediodorsal part of the pancreas head and neck will be detected by high hormone levels at the DP vein. One must be aware, however, that the DP vein is largely connected through venous collaterals to the LG, TP, PSPD, and ASPD veins and energetic aspiration of the blood sample at the DP vein may get samples from different regions not normally drained by the DP vein (Fig. 4.16D).

Samples with high hormone concentration in the TP and LG veins (Fig. 4.7) will usually indicate a lesion in the body of the pancreas. The LG vein is not a usual pancreatic venous drainage; however, it is frequently part of the rich anastomotic bed that drains the body of the pancreas (Fig. 4.17B,C).

The tail of the pancreas is directly drained by the small CPV to the SV, and the sequential sampling of the SV is usually very efficient to demonstrate the gradient of hormone concentration if a tumor exists in the tail of the pancreas. Selective catheterization, however, obtains very selective blood samples, giving a very precise idea of the hormone production in that territory (Fig. 4.17D). It must be remembered, however, that the small veins at the tail may be connected to the TP vein and sampling from the TP with high hormone levels may also translate to a lesion in the tail of the pancreas. The distal part of the pancreatic tail may also be drained by some of the inferior polar splenic veins and those may be connected to the GT by the gastroepiploic vein.

Patients with nesidioblastosis show abnormal hormone levels at several sites in the SV, SMV, and PV (Fig. 4.22). Several pancreatic adenomas may also present with a diffuse increase in hormone level.

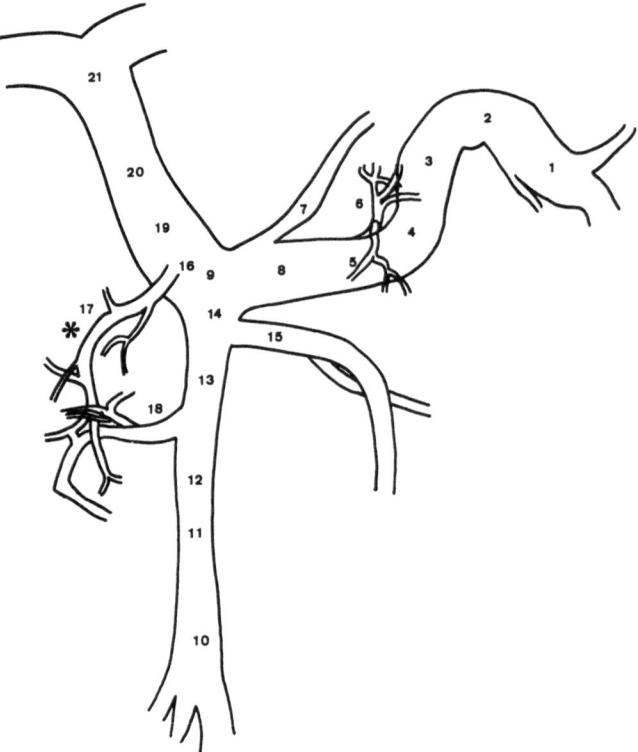

Figure 4.21. Patient with Zollinger-Ellison syndrome, multiple duodenal ulcerations, and GI bleeding. Angiography and ultrasound were negative. Percutaneous portal and pancreatic venous sampling for gastrin assay showed one lesion in the posterior aspect of the head of the pancreas, with increased level of gastrin on sample 17, posterior superior pancreaticoduodenal vein.

1. 212 pg/ml
2. 217 pg/ml
3. 129 pg/ml
4. 141 pg/ml
5. 159 pg/ml
6. 223 pg/ml
7. 186 pg/ml

8. 174 pg/ml
9. 190 pg/ml
10. 141 pg/ml
11. 130 pg/ml
12. 185 pg/ml
13. 177 pg/ml
14. 153 pg/ml

15. 264 pg/ml
16. 191 pg/ml
17. *680* pg/ml
18. 149 pg/ml
19. 210 pg/ml
20. 143 pg/ml
21. 241 pg/ml

Peripheral:
22. 154 pg/ml Ca stimulation 5 mg/kg/h p/3h
Peripheral:

23.   0 min 90 pg/ml
24. 30 min 162 pg/ml

25. 60 min 131 pg/ml
26. 120 min 203 pg/ml

27. 180 min 213 pg/ml
28. 180 min 226 pg/ml

Surgery was negative and no pancreatic lesion was found. The recovering of the patient was stormy but he did well for a few weeks and then started to deteriorate and eventually died of sepsis and GI bleeding. A small duodenal wall lesion was found at necropsy, consistent with gastrin-producing adenoma.

The presence of rich venous anastomoses in and around the pancreas may cause step-ups in hormone concentration in pancreatic veins remote from tumor site. Such findings may lead to the false diagnosis of multiple adenomas or nesidioblastosis. Other factors that may cause false elevated hormone concentration may include compression and occlusion of the pancreatic veins by tumors, previous surgery, and vigorous aspiration of the catheter wedged in the pancreatic veins.

The lower accuracy of the technique

Figure 4.22. A 2-month-old boy with hypoglycemia since birth and with clinical diagnosis of nesidioblastosis. Percutaneous portal venous sampling for insulin assay showed diffusely increased insulin levels.
1. 11.0 μU/ml
2. 13.5 μU/ml
3. 14.5 μU/ml
4. 10.0 μU/ml
5. 15.0 μU/ml
Ninety-five percent of the pancreas was removed surgically and insulin and glucose levels returned to normal levels.

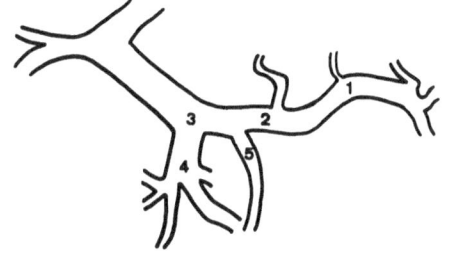

observed in some cases where samples were obtained only from the large peripancreatic veins (62) is explained by the portal blood flow that follows a lamellar pattern that generates a variability of hormone levels in large venous trunks. This explains the differences registered between two samples made at the same level but in different points of the vessel, leading to the conclusion that those nonselective pancreatic samplings are not good enough for accurate tumor localization (7). On the other hand selective pancreatic vein sampling generates extremely accurate and reproducible data, as demonstrated by Roche et al (7).

Intraarterial injection close to the tumor site may dump hormone production. So it is wise not to follow selective or superselective arteriography by venous sampling, to avoid reduction in tumoral hormone production. Contamination of blood samples by contrast medium disturbs hormone radioimmunoassay. Thus, blood sampling by wedge catheterization must be performed before contrast medium injection or after a thorough drainage of the vein (7).

Provocative tests using the secretin test for gastrin and the calcium test for insulin, although propugnated to improve tumor diagnosis and localization (23,39), were found to be worthless in Roche et al.'s (7) experience when performing selective pancreatic venous blood sampling.

Because of the variable venous anatomy of the pancreas and because of all these factors explained above that may mislead the interpretation of the hormone data, it is important for surgeons and angiographers to review together the venous anatomy and correspond-

ing hormone levels in individual cases. It is also essential that the pancreas be entirely explored and mobilized to avoid missing a second adenoma that might have an affluent vein draining into a vein near a preidentified tumor (66). The foreknowledge of tumor localization is very helpful for the surgical inspection, since small intrapancreatic adenomas may not be palpated and islet cell hyperplasia is not detected at all during surgical inspection.

Complications of the Procedure

Complications are infrequent following transhepatic catheterization of the portal vein and its tributaries for pancreatic venous sampling. The complications of the procedure are mainly related to mechanical injury to the liver tissue, the blood vessels, bile ducts, and gallbladder. Complications reported following transhepatic puncture and catheterization of the portal vein have been intraperitoneal hemorrhage, perforation of visceral veins, bleeding from the intercostal artery, perforation of the right flexure of the colon, pleural effusion (ascitic or hemorrhagic), tear in the inferior vena cava, and perforation of the duodenum. Minor lesions include intrahepatic hematoma, subintimal injections, and intraperitoneal bleeding during the procedure followed by pain and fever (73).

Most of the reported complications were observed in severely ill patients, such as those with cirrhosis of the liver, coagulopathy, and extrahepatic cholestasis (73). The patients with pancreatic adenoma are usually in better clinical shape and the complications are minimal. Reichardt et al. (63) reported pain and fever following inadvertent gallbladder puncture and an intrahepatic hematoma without the need for specific treatment. In our own series only one complication has arisen so far. Due to the long-lasting catheterization of the superior mesenteric artery following diagnostic arteriography performed before percutaneous pancreatic venous sampling, a small clot developed and ischemic infarction of a short ileal segment required surgical treatment. The pancreatic adenoma was found by venous sampling and resected at a later surgery.

Intraperitoneal hemorrhage is currently prevented by Gelfoam embolization of the percutaneous transhepatic puncture tract.

Clinical and Surgical Considerations

Localization and surgical treatment of insulinomas, gastrinomas, and the other various types of islet cell tumors pose different problems and alternate solutions, because of the varying clinical outcomes, number of lesions, variety of locations, and malignant potential that may be very different among the different tumor types.

Just to mention insulinomas and gastrinomas, which are the most common islet cell tumors, several distinct points should be emphasized regarding outcome and surgical treatment.

Zollinger-Ellison Syndrome

In general the gastrinomas producing the Zollinger-Ellison syndrome carry a reasonable prognosis, and even patients with known liver metastases have a 10-year survival of over 40% (74). Currently, it is possible to control the effects of acid hypersecretion effectively by pharmacological means using the H_2-receptor antagonists, reducing, therefore, the need for total gastrectomy.

Laparotomy is performed today in the hope that a single isolated gastrinoma will be discovered and lead to cure by resection. Solitary tumors of the pancreas, however, are relatively rare and the main hope lies in finding a lesion in the vicinity of the duodenal wall, which is found in about half the alleged 13% of patients with a duodenal wall tumor (74).

Confusion may arise about whether exploration is seen as an additional diagnostic procedure, an operation directed against the tumor, an attempt to control acid secretion regardless of tumor status, or all the above. Since in most cases the disease is malignant, the ideal treatment would be a safe type of chemotherapy that would suppress endocrine function and halt the spread of the tumor. But although some gastrinomas may respond to streptozocin (75), 5-fluorouracil, or tubercidin, no currently used chemotherapy has predictable efficacy (76). It is, therefore, important to examine what surgery can offer.

Due to late diagnosis, patients in early studies had more advanced disease than the populations being studied today. Early diagnosis, however, has not been shown to improve the prognosis or alter the distribution of tumors or the potential for long-term clinical deterioration. The earlier data provide still pertinent information.

About 60% of gastrinomas are malignant and around 50% have liver metastatic disease at the time of diagnosis. The syndrome recurs in more than 50% of the patients thought to have had all tumors correctly resected. A number of patients show no tumor at the surgical procedure either because of the small size or nonpancreatic location, or because there is no tumor at all (76).

Pancreatic islet cell hyperplasia accompanies gastrinoma quite frequently and if found alone, there is no proof that it may cause the syndrome, being most probably a consequence rather than the cause of elevated hormone secretion (76). It is most unlikely that antral G-cell hyperplasia causes Zollinger-Ellison syndrome. Rather, it is a nonspecific diagnosis that may occur in association with a variety of diseases including peptic-ulcer disease, pernicious anemia, acromegaly, hyperparathyroidism, uremia, and after ulcer therapy (76).

The head/body/tail ratio is 4:1:4 for gastrinomas in the pancreas. In a large series previously published, the patients with tumors in the head and body of the pancreas treated by pancreatectomy or pancreaticoduodenectomy generally fared very poorly because of multiple lesions, recurrence, and high perioperative mortality. Even single lesions in the tail, apparently well-suited for surgery, rarely resulted in cure (76). Many of the gastrinomas are slow growing, although some tumors may progress very rapidly. True cure from excision of tumors appears to be an exception and is theoretically impossible in over 80% of the patients (76). Noncurative excision, however, might benefit the management of the case and prolong life, but it has not been proved so far.

Since cimetidine therapy, H_2-receptor blocker, is available, it has been easier to treat recurrences after surgery. Attempts to find and remove the tumor surgically is advisable in some cases where the preoperative investigation has been negative, but in most cases such attempts appear doomed to failure. Total gastrectomy or excision of the tumor, therefore, will probably not prevent, but may delay, death from malignant disease (76). Mortality and morbidity are very high for total gastrectomy. Mortality ranges from 5 to 27% (76). Gastric resection should be avoided as stomal ulceration is probably far more dangerous and difficult to manage than recurrent ulceration in the duodenum. For these reason, pharmacologic control of acid secretion is the preferred treatment. For the past 15 years, cimetidine has been the main form of this therapy. There are, however, a variety of newer H_2-receptor–blocking antihistamines, prostaglandin analogues, anticholinergic agents, and beta-adrenergic agonists (76). Cimetidine by itself suppresses acid secretion, relieves symptoms, and allows ulcers to heal in more than 80% of the patients.

Although H_2-receptor blockers are extremely effective in controlling the acid hypersecretion and its effects, they do require long-term treatment with careful attention to dosage and compliance. Vagotomy and pyloroplasty may improve the response to the H_2-receptor blocker, carrying with it a life-long commitment to taking cimetidine (74).

Hypoglycemic Syndrome

The clinical diagnosis of insulinomas rests on the demonstration of Whipple's triad: symptoms of hypoglycemia, low circulating glucose, and prompt relief of symptoms after glucose administration (77). Insulinomas occur twice as often in women as in men and are uncommon before the age of 20. The average duration of symptoms before diagnosis was 19 months in a recent study (78), but the duration is probably decreasing in recent years due to increased awareness of the disease and more appropriate diagnostic means. About 80% of the patients have confusion or abnormal behavior, 50% being amnesic during the episode of hypoglycemia or in a frank coma (78).

Insulinomas are evenly distributed throughout the pancreas in most series among the head, body, and tail (23:27:31) (78) and about 11% of the patients have multiple tumors. Ectopic insulinomas are very rare. Some reports, however, show increased frequency of location of insulinomas in the pancreatic head (50%:25%) compared with the tail (79).

Prior to treatment the clinical diagnosis must be confirmed and the tumor localized adequately. Although the hypoglycemic syndrome may be successfully controlled in selected patients by embolization of the feeding artery, surgery is still the time-honored treatment for insulinomas.

Surgical treatment requires several hours of fasting, and except for a few patients who cannot tolerate it, intravenous glucose is not used. Glucose solutions are not used during the procedure itself.

An epigastric transverse incision is normally necessary for complete access to the pancreas. Before addressing the pancreas, a detailed search for neoplastic spread is performed. It must be noted that most adenomas are not visible by inspection, because they are covered by a thin layer of normal pancreatic parenchyma. The pancreas must be carefully palpated to feel slight differences in consistency (78). The procedures performed for adenoma extraction may be enucleation, partial pancreatectomy, Whipple's procedure, and total pancreatectomy. The extent of the pancreatectomy in multiple and malignant disease is dictated by the extent of the disease. The defect in the pancreas surface should be closed meticulously with permanent interrupted sutures followed by drainage with an aspiration system.

Blind pancreatic resections for suspected insulinoma warrants further discussion, even though the procedure is not advisable anymore, except in exceptional cases.

The origin of distal blind pancreatic resection was based on a large review performed in the late 1950s when many of the patients would not fit the present criteria for diagnosis and localization of the insulinomas (79). The clinical and laboratorial diagnosis, as well as the localization methods, are much more accurate; as a result many patients with hypoglycemia who might previously have been treated by laparotomy and blind distal resection can now be accurately assessed and spared a fruitless operation.

The rationale for blind distal pancreatectomy in suspected insulinoma arose from the mistaken belief that the majority of insulinomas occur in the tail of the pancreas. It should be kept in mind, however, that the distribution of pancreatic insulinomas is even, or slightly predominant in the head of the pancreas. It has been also suggested that when the adenoma cannot be felt at palpation it is more likely to be buried in the head than in the thinner and more accessible body and tail (79). There is also a suggestion for blind resection of the proximal pancreas as more appropriate than blind resection of the body and tail (79). It must be recalled that about 12% of patients with distal blind resection then have a total pancreatectomy, associated with increased morbidity and mortality. It seems likely that the more patients subjected to blind distal pancreatectomy, the greater will be the number of patients requiring total pancreatectomy.

It should be emphasized that the blind distal pancreatectomy will find only one of three tumors in the tail, whereas the formidable blind pancreaticoduodenectomy still would leave behind one of four occult tumors. These considerations emphasize the need for discretion in the use of blind pancreatectomy, and precise tumor localization is necessary before and during surgical treatment (71). The correct procedure is still disputed, however, because in patients with severe symptoms the danger of blind resection may be less than those of nonresection, and in those with mild symptoms nonresection may be more appropriate. A second-look procedure in 1 or 2 years may be safer.

Immediate first-operative complications have been reported to be about 15%, including fever, pancreatic pseudocyst, intraperitoneal abscess, peritonitis, pancreatitis, intestinal obstruction, biliary fistula, and gastrointestinal bleeding (78). Mortality may be as high as 6% (79).

Analysis of long-term results reveals a cure rate of 91.7% with only an 8.3% recurrence rate (78). Recurrence due to a malignant lesion is more likely to occur but still the prognosis is not so bad as in ordinary pancreatic cancer.

Persistent hypoglycemia usually can be controlled by the use of diazoxide, which has no antitumor effect but inhibits the release of insulin, thus reducing the level of plasma insulin to a lower concentration. Streptozotocin may be used in combination to treat malignant disease (78).

Infants with nesidioblastosis are usually treated by 85% pancreatectomy and splenectomy to control hypoglycemia at the neonatal period. The prognosis has not been very satisfactory due to postsplenectomy sepsis, recurrent hypoglycemia, permanent brain damage, and high mortality. More recently, removal of at least 95% of the pancreas has been proposed, preserving the blood supply to the spleen as well as the duodenum, permitting satisfactory control of the hypoglycemia and avoiding long-term septic complications (30).

Islet Cell Tumor Embolization

Therapeutic intraarterial embolization is a well-known palliative treatment for neoplastic lesions in a variety of organs, acting by decreasing blood flow and starting an ischemic

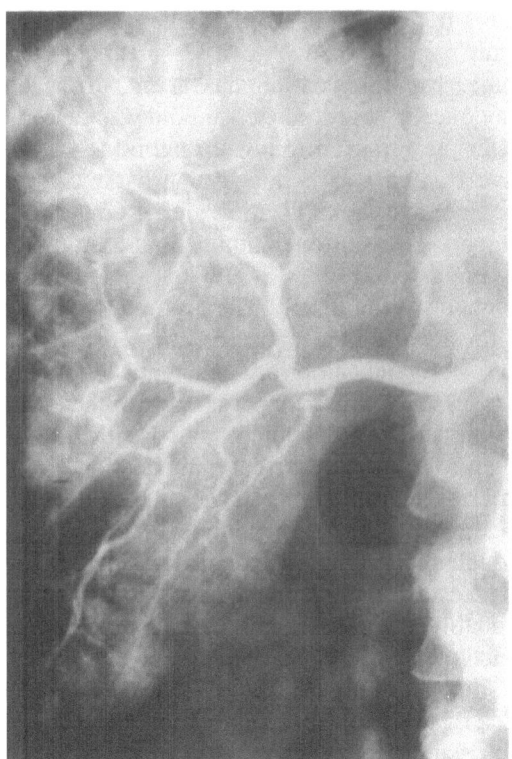

A

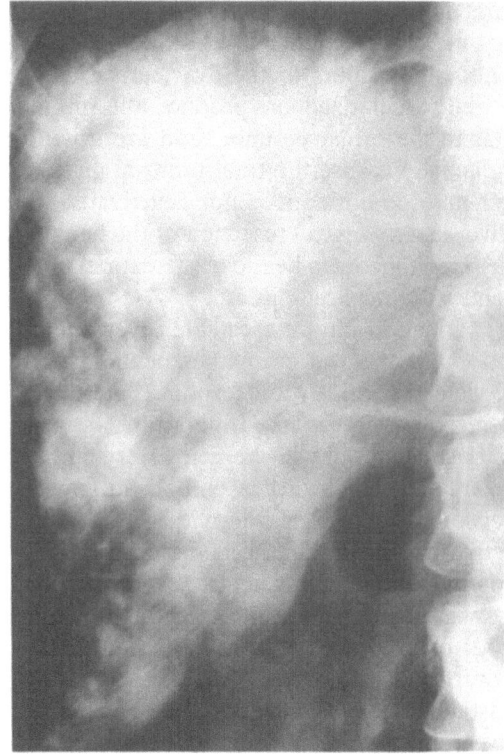

B

Figure 4.23. A 48-years-old woman with a VIP-oma massively metastatic to the liver producing the Verner-Morrison syndrome [watery diarrhea, hypokalemia and achlorhydria (WDHR)] with untreatable diarrhea. **A** and **B**: Note the diffuse metastatic disease to the liver with multiple hypervascular nodules. **C**: Embolization with Gelfoam particles was performed and the hepatic arterial circulation was totally occluded. Diarrhea was controlled for $2\frac{1}{2}$ years. Diarrhea recurred, new angiography demonstrated recurrence of the metastatic disease (not shown), and embolization was again performed, successfully controlling the symptoms for 2 additional years when the patient eventually died due to diffuse metastatic disease.

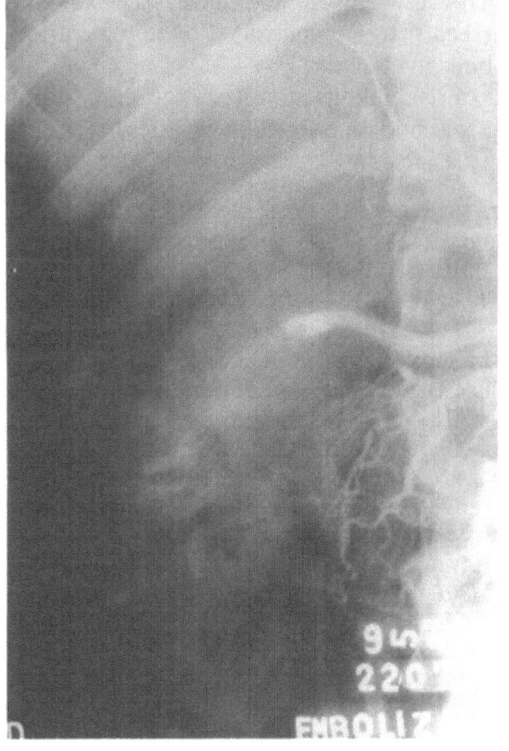

C

process that may lead to necrosis in the total or partial mass of the tumor. Metastatic pancreatic endocrine tumors to the liver, are usually very well vascularized and produce a hormone similar to the primary tumor, and are usually more active because the total tumoral mass is bigger and the hormone is not deactivated by the liver itself. Surgical resection of the hepatic metastases appears to be the best treatment for patients with localized disease.

In patients with unresectable liver metastases, interferon and chemotherapeutic agents have yielded relatively low response rates. The best responses in carcinoid metastatic disease have been achieved with hepatic artery embolization (80). Hepatic artery embolization with nonabsorbable particles provides the most effective treatment for the hepatic metastatic endocrine tumors, and when repeated periodically will maintain clinical remissions for long periods of time due to the suppression of the tumoral endocrine function. Besides carcinoid metastatic disease we have had the opportunity to treat by liver embolization patients with extensive metastatic disease from VIP-oma, which caused severe and untreatable aqueous diarrhea that was controlled by hepatic artery embolization alone (Fig. 4.23).

Arterial embolization has also been used to control endocrine function in a few secretory tumors including parathyroid adenomas (81)

and adrenal lesions. Treatment of hypoglycemic syndrome, due to a pancreatic insulinoma, by embolization has been performed only once, to our knowledge, and was successful in the reported follow-up period (82). We have treated two hypoglycemic patients with insulinoma by embolization alone. One of the patients did well for 6 months and then hypoglycemia recurred. A follow-up angiogram is planned for the future. The lesion was located in the head of the pancreas and fed by both posterior and anterior pancreaticoduodenal arcades. Embolization was performed with Ivalon particles (150 micra) and great care was taken to avoid inadvertent embolization of the superior mesenteric artery branches through the inferior pancreaticoduodenal artery. Although the lesion was totally embolized, the main arteries remained patent, and this was probably the reason for recurrent endocrine function.

The other patient had an insulinoma in the neck of the pancreas, totally fed by the dorsal pancreatic artery which was a branch of the superior mesenteric artery. The dorsal pancreatic artery was selectively catheterized and embolized with Ivalon particles (150 micra) and Gelfoam. After embolization the patient became hyperglycemic for almost 1 week due to normal pancreas suppression and gradually returned to normal glucose and insulin levels, which have

▷

Figure 4.24. A 49-year-old man with severe hypoglycemia, several coma episodes, and car accidents in the last 2 years. CT and ultrasound were negative. A and D: Angiography showed a 2-cm pancreatic adenoma in the body of the pancreas vascularized by terminal branches of the dorsal pancreatic artery (DPA). Late arterial phase (B) shows dense tumoral blush. Note that the DPA arises as a branch of the superior mesenteric artery. C: Embolization with Ivalon particles (150 micra) was performed and the tumoral vessels were completely occluded. D: Late arterial phase shows pancreatic parenchyma impregnation without tumoral blush. The follow-up of this patient showed hyperglycemia for 1 week which gradually tapered to normal glucose levels, remaining stable for more than two years. E: Percutaneous pancreatic venous blood sampling was also consistent with a single lesion and in the body of the pancreas. Samples number 2, 3, 4, 5, 7, 12, and 19 were the highest ones for insulin assay.

1. 360 (peripheral) μU/ml

2. *177 μU/ml*	10. 97 μU/ml	18. 40 μU/ml
3. *133 μU/ml*	11. 78 μU/ml	19. *141 μU/ml*
4. *140 μU/ml*	12. *128 μU/ml*	20. 34 μU/ml
5. *130 μU/ml*	13. 55 μU/ml	21. 26 μU/ml
6. 113 μU/ml	14. 52 μU/ml	22. 30 μU/ml
7. *130 μU/ml*	15. 51 μU/ml	23. 30 μU/ml
8. 109 μU/ml	16. 54 μU/ml	24. 25 μU/ml
9. 159 μU/ml	17. 47 μU/ml	

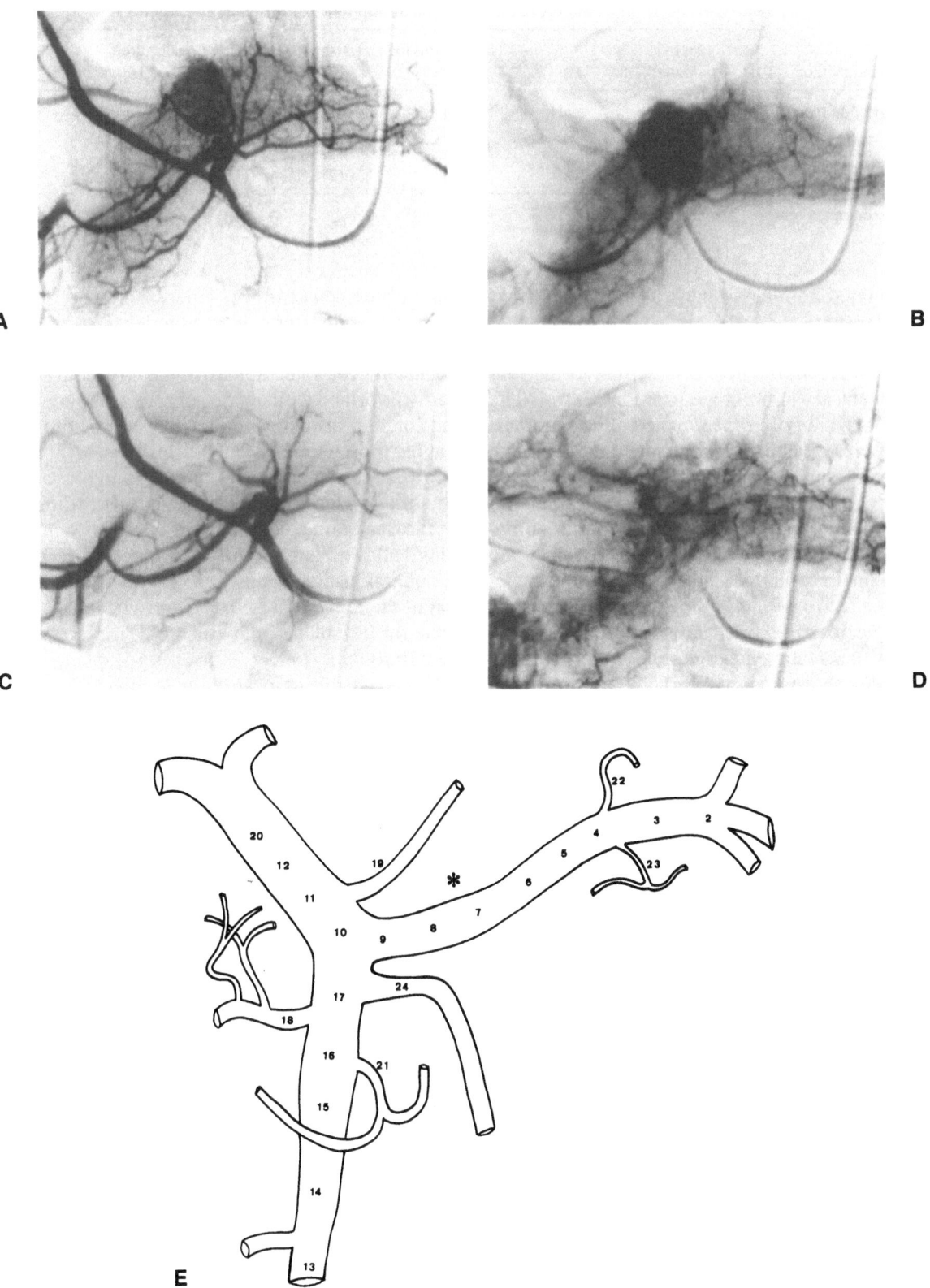

Table 4.2. Preoperative localization of pancreatic lesions causing hyperinsulinism in 26 patients.

Imaging method	No. of patients	Total lesions localized (total no. studies) Localization				
		Head	Body	Tail	Diffuse	Hepatic METS
Arteriography	25	4(11)	1(4)	5(10)	0(1)	3(3)
CT	9	1(3)	1(4)	1(3)	–	1(1)
US	6	0(2)	0(3)	0(1)	–	–
Venous sampling	16	7(7)	4(4)	7(7)	1(1)	–

CT, computed tomography; US, ultrasound.

remained normal for more than 2 years (Fig. 4.24).

Islet cell tumor embolization has a definite role in metastatic liver disease due to the reliable efficacy in hormone function control. The embolization of primary pancreatic adenomas, however, is still experimental and although effective in some patients, it should be reserved for carefully selected patients. The main indication for pancreatic endocrine tumor embolization is tumors with single feeder vessel and terminal circulation. In those cases the ischemic effect is maximized by total occlusion and the necrosis is extensive. It is important to note that pancreatic endocrine tumors that are not readily shown by arteriography are not candidates for embolization.

Author's Experience in Hyperinsulinism

Twenty-six patients with hyperinsulinism were studied. All patients presented fast hypoglycemia and elevated plasmatic levels of insulin. The ages ranged from 7 months to 79 years. Nine of the patients were male and 17 female. Eighteen patients underwent surgical treatment, two were treated by embolization alone, three were treated clinically because of metastatic disease, and the remaining three patients refused treatment.

Pancreatic high-resolution CT was performed in nine patients, using rapid infusion of the contrast material. Preoperative US was performed in six patients.

Arteriography was performed in 25 of the patients for tumor localization and liver evaluation. Arteriography included a complete study of the celiac artery, superior mesenteric artery, splenic artery, gastroduodenal artery, dorsal pancreatic and pancreatica magna when technically feasible. Some of the procedures were performed with digital subtraction system and some in the conventional way with photographic subtraction.

In 16 patients, pancreatic venous sampling of insulin and glucose was performed, according to the technique described in Venous Sampling, above, and in the literature (57–71). Peripheral insulin values were considered normal in the range of 5 to 20 μU/ml. The normal value for the splenic vein was considered to be 28 ± 10 μU/ml.

It was possible to localize the lesion in 23 patients. In two patients only hepatic metastases were identified. In 19 patients only one lesion was responsible for the hypoglycemia. In two patients multiple insulinomas were seen. One patient had islet cell hyperplasia, another patient had nesidioblastosis (Table 4.2). In 10 patients the lesion was found in the head of the pancreas, in 4 patients in the body, in ten in the pancreatic tail, and in the remaining patient with nesidioblastosis the lesion was diffuse.

Fifteen patients were treated by surgery. In two patients superselective embolization was the treatment, and three patients have had negative surgical exploration and no pancreatic tissue or tumor was resected.

Ultrasonography was used in six patients and showed only one lesion, which was confirmed by angiography. The diagnosis and localization procedures of the additional patients were pancreatic venous sampling, arteriography, and CT.

CT was performed in nine patients and showed the lesion in only two cases and the hepatic metastases in a third patient. The negative patients were examined by pancreatic venous sampling in five cases, and/or arteriography in three cases. In one case CT demonstrated the lesion in the pancreas body, which was not seen at the arteriography and was confirmed by pancreatic venous sampling.

Arteriography was performed in 25 patients and localized the lesion in 10 cases and hepatic metastases in 3 patients. Five of these patients underwent surgery without further diagnosis. In one of these patients no lesion was found (false positive).

Pancreatic venous blood sampling was performed in 16 patients, confirming lesions already localized by arteriography or CT in 3 cases. In one patient arteriography and CT have already localized one lesion, whereas blood sampling allowed the localization of two additional adenomas.

In 12 patients pancreatic venous blood sampling was the only successful method for insulinoma localization.

Thirteen patients underwent surgical treatment. Three enucleations and eight partial pancreatectomies confirmed all the lesions previously localized. In two patients where palpation was negative, no resection was performed.

Two patients underwent intraarterial embolization as the single treatment.

The most recent patient has been not operated so far.

Sensitivity of CT, in our series, for the detection of pancreatic insulinomas was 22%, whereas in the literature it varies from 30 to 62% (39,40). Arteriography showed a sensitivity of 35% with only one false positive compared to 20 to 90% in the literature (45,46). Pancreatic venous sampling was 100% effective in insulinoma localization in our series, confirming the findings in the literature (60–71).

References

1. Dunnick NR, Long JA, Krudy A, et al. Localizing insulinomas with combined radiographic methods. *AJR* 1980;135:747–752.
2. Gould VE, Memoli V, Chejfec G, Johannessen JV. The APUD cell system and its neoplasms. *Surg Clin North Am* 1979;59:93–108.
3. Friesen SR. Tumors of the endocrine pancreas. *N Engl J Med* 1982;306:580–590.
4. Freeny PC. Radiology of the pancreas: two decades of progress in imaging and intervention. *AJR* 1988;150:975–981.
5. Norton JA, Doppman JL, Collen MJ, et al. Prospective study of gastrinoma localization and resection in patients with Zollinger-Ellison syndrome. *Ann Surg* 1986;204:468–479.
6. Dayal Y, O'Brian DS. The pathology of the pancreatic endocrine cells. In: DeLellis RA, ed. *Diagnostic immunohistochemistry*, 1st ed. New York: Masson; 1981;111–135.
7. Roche A, Raisonnier A, Gillon-Savouret MC. Pancreatic venous sampling and arteriography in localizing insulinomas and gastrinomas: procedure and results in 55 cases. *Radiology* 1982; 145:621–627.
8. Turner RC, Morris PJ, Lee ECG, Harris EA. Localization of insulinomas. *Lancet* 1978;515–518.
9. Andrew A, Kramer B, Rawdon BB. Gut and pancreatic amine precursor uptake and decarboxylation cells are not neural crest derivates. *Gastroenterology* 1983;84:429–431.
10. Pearse AG. The diffuse endocrine system and the implications of the APUD concept. *Int Surg* 1979;64:5–7.
11. Modlin IM. Endocrine tumors of the pancreas. *Surg Gynecol Obstet* 1979;149:751–769.
12. Ingemansson S, Lunderquist A, Lundquist I, et al. Portal and pancreatic vein catheterization with radioimmunologic determination of insulin. *Surg Gynecol Obstet* 1975;141:705–711.
13. Higgins GA. Pancreatic islet cell tumors: insulinoma, gastrinoma, and glucagonoma. *Surg Clin North Am* 1979;59:131–141.
14. Ingemansson S, Lunderquist A, Holst J. Selective catheterization of the pancreatic vein for radioimmunoassay in glucagon-secreting carcinoma of the pancreas. *Radiology* 1976;119:555–556.
15. Ingemansson S, Holst J, Larsson LI, Lunderquist A. Localization of glucagonomas by catheterization of the pancreatic veins and with glucagon assay. *Surg Gynecol Obstet* 1977;145:509–516.
16. Visser PA, Friesen SR. Uncommon tumors of the APUD system. *Surg Clin North Am* 1979;59:143–158.
17. Sakazaki S, Umeyama K, Nakagawa H, Hashimoto H, et al. Pancreatic somatostatinoma. *Am J Surg* 1983;146:674–679.
18. Kelly TR. Pancreatic somatostatinoma. *Am J Surg* 1983;146:671–673.
19. Jensen RT, Gardner JD, Reufman JP, et al.

Zollinger-Ellison syndrome: current concepts and management. *Ann Intern Med* 1983;98:59–75.

20. Wolfe MM, Jensen RT. Zollinger-Ellison syndrome: current concepts in diagnosis and management. *N Engl J Med* 1987;317:1200–1209.

21. Wolfe MM, Alexander RW, McGuigan JE. Extrapancreatic, extraintestinal gastrinoma. *N Engl J Med* 1982;306:1533–1536.

22. Deveney CW, Deveney KE, Stark D, et al. Resection of gastrinomas. *Ann Surg* 1983;198:546–553.

23. Imamura M, Takahashi K, Adachi H, et al. Usefulness of selective arterial secretin injection test for localization of gastrinoma in the Zollinger-Ellison syndrome. *Ann Surg* 1987;205:230–239.

24. Modlin IM, Jaffe BM, Sank A, Albert D. The early diagnosis of gastrinoma. *Ann Surg* 1982;196:512–517.

25. Ingemansson S, Larsson LI, Lunderquist A, Stadil F. Pancreatic vein catheterization with gastrin assay in normal patients and in patients with the Zollinger-Ellison syndrome. *Am J Surg* 1977;134:558–563.

26. Lea Thomas M, Lamb GHR, Barra Clough MA. Angiographic demonstration of a pancreatic "VIP-oma" in the WDHA syndrome. *AJR* 1976;127:2037–1039.

27. Long RG, Bryant MG, Yuille PM, et al. Mixed pancreatic apudoma with symptoms of excess vasoactive intestinal polypeptide and insulin: improvement of diarrhoea with metoclopramide. *GT* 1981;22:505–511.

28. Keller A, Stone AM, Valderrama E, Kolodny H. Pancreatic nesidioblastosis in adults. Report of a patient with hyperinsulinemic hypoglycemia. *Am J Surg* 1983;145:413–416.

29. Telander RL, Wolf SA, Simmons P, et al. Endocrine disorders of the pancreas and adrenal cortex in pediatric patients. *Mayo Clin Proc* 1986;61:459–466.

30. Martin LW, Ryckman FC, Sheldon CA. Experience with 95% pancreatectomy and splenic salvage for neonatal nesidioblastosis. *Ann Surg* 1984;200:355–362.

31. Ingemansson S, Kühl C, Larsson LI, et al. Islet cell hyperplasia localized by pancreatic vein catheterization and insulin radioimmunoassay. *Am J Surg* 1977;133:643–645.

32. Ingemansson S, Kühl C, Larsson LI, et al. Localization of insulinomas and islet cell hyperplasias by pancreatic vein catheterization and insulin assay. *Surg Gynecol Obstet* 1978;146:725–734.

33. Greene BM, Golladay ES, Mollitt DL. Multiple endocrine adenopathy. *Surg Gynecol Obstet* 1983;156:665–678.

34. Irvine GB, Murphy RF. Multiple forms of gastroenteropancreatic hormones. *GT* 1981;22:1048–1069.

35. Feurle GE, Helmstaedter V, Tischbirek K, et al. A multihormonal tumor of the pancreas producing neurotensin. *Dig Dis Sci* 1981;26:1125–1133.

36. Stewart R, Sirinek KR, Levine BA. The asymptomatic pancreatic islet cell tumor: a novel presentation. *Surgery* 1986;100:108–112.

37. Case Records of the Massachusetts General Hospital. *N Engl J Med* 1988;318:1523–1532.

38. Günther RW, Klose KJ, Rückert K, et al. Islet-cell tumors: detection of small lesions with computed tomography and ultrasound. *Radiology* 1983;148:485–488.

39. Galiber AK, Reading CC, Charboneau JW, et al. Localization of pancreatic insulinomas: comparison of pre- and intraoperative US with CT and angiography. *Radiology* 1988;166:405–408.

40. Wank SA, Doppman JL, Miller DL. Prospective study of the ability of computed axial tomography to localize gastrinomas in patients with Zollinger-Ellison syndrome. *Gastroenterology* 1987;92:905–912.

41. Fricke M, Zick R, Mitzkat HJ. Das Insulinom im Computer-Tomogramm. *Radiologe* 1978;18:252–254.

42. Imhof H, Frank P. Pancreatic calcifications in malignant islet cell tumors. *Radiology* 1977;122:333–337.

43. Stark DD, Moss AA, Goldberg HI, Deveney CW. CT of pancreatic islet cell tumors. *Radiology* 1984;150:491–494.

44. Olsson O. Angiographic diagnosis of an islet-cell tumor of the pancreas. *Acta Chir Scand* 1963;126:346–351.

45. Boijsen E. Selective pancreatic angiography. *Br J Radiol* 1966;39:481–487.

46. Bookstein JJ, Obernan HA. Appraisal of selective angiography in localizing islet-cell tumors of the pancreas. *Radiology* 1966;86:682–685.

47. Gray RK, Rösch J, Grollman JH. Arteriography in the diagnosis of islet-cell tumors. *Radiology* 1970;97:39–44.

48. Alfidi RJ, Bhyun DS, Crile G. Arteriography and hypoglycemia. *Surg Gynecol Obstet* 1971;133:447–452.

49. Baghery S, Alfidi RJ, Zeich MG. Angiography of nonfunctioning islet cell tumors of the pancreas. *Radiology* 1976;120:57–59.

50. Korobkin MT, Palubinskas AJ, Glickman MG.

Pitfalls in arteriography of islet-cell tumors of the pancreas. *Radiology* 1978;100:319–328.

51. Roche A. Méthodes radiologiques de localisation des tumeurs endocrines du pancreas. Acta *Gastroenterol Belg* 1982;45:328–339.

52. Roche A, Capeau J, Halimi P. Méthodes radiologiques de localisation des tumeurs endocrines du pancreas. *Gastroenterol Clin Biol* 1983;7:49–58.

53. Maton PN, Miller DL, Doppman JL, et al. Role of selective angiography in the management of patients with Zollinger-Ellison syndrome. *Gastroenterology* 1987;92:913–918.

54. Gorman B, Charboneau JW, James EM, et al. Benign pancreatic insulinoma: preoperative and intraoperative sonografic localization. *AJR* 1986;147:929–934.

55. Norton JA, Cromack DT, Shawker TH, et al. Intraoperative ultrasonographic localization of islet cell tumors. A prospective comparison to palpation. *Ann Surg* 1988;207:160–168.

56. Shawker TH, Doppman JL. Intraoperative US. *Radiology* 1988;166:568–569.

57. Wiechel KL. Tekniken vid perkutan transhepatisk portapunktion (PTP). *Nord Med* 1971;86:912–914.

58. Göthlin J, Lunderquist A, Tylen U. Selective phlebography of the pancreas. *Acta Radiol (Diag)* 1974;15:474–480.

59. Hoevels J, Lunderquist A, Tylen V. Percutaneous transhepatic portography. *Acta Radiol (Diag)* 1978;19:643–648.

60. Lunderquist A, Eriksson M, Ingemansson S, et al. Selective pancreatic vein catheterization for hormone assay in endocrine tumors. *Cardiovasc Radiol* 1978;1:117–124.

61. Lunderquist A, Owman T, Reichardt W. Pancreatic venography. In: Abrams HL, ed. *Abrams Angiography*, 3rd ed. Boston: Little, Brown; 1983;1467–1477.

62. Passariello R. Localization of pancreatic functioning tumors with transhepatic venous sampling: results of an italian cooperative study on 54 cases. Presented at the 6th Annual Course on Diagnostic and Therapeutic Angiography and Interventional Radiology 1981; 16–19 March, Society of Cardiovascular Radiology, Orlando, Florida.

63. Reichardt W, Ingemansson S, Lunderquist A, Nobin A. Selective mesenteric phlebography in patients with carcinoid tumors. *Gastrointest Radiol* 1979;4:179–189.

64. Doppman JL, Brennan MF, Dunnick NR, et al. The role of pancreatic venous sampling in the localization of occult insulinomas. *Radiology* 1981;138:557–582.

65. Reichardt W. Selective phlebography in pancreatic and peripancreatic disease. *Acta Radiol (Diag)* 1980;21:513–522.

66. Cho KJ, Vinik AI, Thompson NW, et al. Localization of the source of hyperinsulinism: percutaneous transhepatic portal and pancreatic vein catheterization with hormone assay. *AJR* 1982;139:237–245.

67. Glowniak JV, Shapiro B, Vinik AI, et al. Percutaneous transhepatic venous sampling of gastrin. Value in sporadic and familial islet-cell tumors and G-cell hyperfunction. *N Engl J Med* 1982;307:293–297.

68. Burcharth F, Stage JG, Stadil F, et al. Localization of gastrinomas by transhepatic portal catheterization and gastrin assay. *Gastroenterology* 1979;77:444–450.

69. Kallio H, Suoranta H. Localization of occult insulin secreting tumors of the pancreas. *Ann Surg* 1979;189:49–52.

70. Pedrazzoli S, Feltrin G, Dodi G, et al. Usefulness of transhepatic portal catheterization in the treatment of insulinomas. *Br J Surg* 1980;67:557–561.

71. Uflacker R, Feldman CJ, Golbert M, Geiger AM. Diagnóstico de insulinoma oculto por colheita de amostras para dosagem de insulina no sistema porta. *Rev AMRIGS* 1983;27:48–53.

72. Reichardt W, Cameron R. Anatomy of the pancreatic veins. A post mortem and clinical phlebographic investigation. *Acta Radiol (Diag)* 1980;21:33–41.

73. Hoevels J, Lunderquist A, Owman T. Complications of percutaneous transhepatic catheterization of the portal vein and its tributaries. *Acta Radiol (Diag)* 1980;21:593–601.

74. Mee AS, Bornman PC, Marks IN. Conservative surgery in the Zollinger-Ellison syndrome. *Br J Surg* 1984;71:423–424.

75. Stadil F, Stage G, Rehfeld JF, et al. Treatment of Zollinger-Ellison syndrome with streptozotocin. *N Engl J Med* 1976;294:1440–1442.

76. McCarthy DM. The place of surgery in the Zollinger-Ellison syndrome. *N Engl J Med* 1980;302:1244–1347.

77. Stefanini P, Carboni M, Patrassi N, Basoli A. Beta-islet cell tumors of the pancreas: results of a study on 1,067 cases. *Surgery* 1974;75:597–609.

78. van Heerden JA, Edis AJ, Service FJ. The surgical aspects of insulinomas. *Ann Surg* 1979;189:677–682.

79. Mengoli L, Le Quesne LP. Blind pancreatic resection for suspected insulinoma: a review of

the problem. *Br J Surg* 1967;54:749–756.

80. Carrasco CH, Charnsangavej C, Ajani J, et al.
    The carcinoid syndrome: palliation by hepatic
    artery embolization. *AJR* 1986;147:149–154.

81. Doppman JL, Marx SJ, Spiegel AM, et al.
    Treatment of hyperparathyroidism by percu-

taneous embolization of a mediastinal adenoma. *Radiology* 1975;115:37–42.

82. Moore TJ, Peterson LM, Harrington DP, Smith
    RJ. Successful arterial embolization of an insuli-
    noma. *JAMA* 1982;248:1353–1355.

5

Pathophysiology and Detection of Renovascular Hypertension – Combination of Renal Vein Renin Sampling and Digital Subtraction Angiography

—— Thomas A. Sos ——

Introduction

The rapid improvements and recent changes in the biochemical and radiological detection of renovascular hypertension leave many physicians confused and perhaps make a report on the topic obsolete before it is published. Nevertheless, if the general physiologic principles of renovascular hypertension are understood, further changes in methodology can be placed in proper perspective. Knowledge of the mechanism of the release, action, and interaction of the renin-angiotensin-aldosterone system is fundamental to the understanding of renovascular hypertension (1).

Normal Renin Metabolism

Renin is produced by and stored in the cells of the juxtaglomerular apparatus located in the angle between the afferent and efferent arterioles in the glomerulus. It is released in response to a decrease in the renal perfusion pressure, plasma sodium concentration, or both. Renin acts to maintain the blood pressure (or hypertension in pathological states) by mediating the conversion of renin substrate produced in the liver to angiotensin I, a weak pressor agent. Angiotensin I, a decapeptide, is changed to the active octapeptide angiotensin II during a single pass through the lungs by a converting enzyme. Angiotensin II has multiple actions. It is the most powerful vasoconstrictor agent known and it also acts on the zona glomerulosa of the adrenal cortex to release aldosterone, which mediates sodium retention and potassium excretion in the kidney.

Selective sampling of renal vein, systemic arterial, and low inferior vena cava renin in patients with essential hypertension and, more recently, in a series of normotensive individuals has shown that a steady-state systemic plasma renin level is maintained by an equal contribution from each kidney. Each kidney secretes an increment of renin to produce a 25% increase in plasma renin level in the renal vein (V) compared to the renin level in the renal artery (A), which is equal to the aortic and infrarenal inferior vena cava renin levels.

$$\frac{V - A}{A} \simeq 0.25 \ (25\%)$$

Collectively, the two kidneys contribute a 0.5 (50%) renin increment in normotensives and in patients with essential or renovascular hypertension to maintain a steady state.

$$\frac{V_{\text{left}} - A_{\text{left}}}{A_{\text{left}}} + \frac{V_{\text{right}} - A_{\text{right}}}{A_{\text{right}}} \simeq 0.5 \ (50\%)$$

Peripheral plasma renin level is closely influenced by the state of the patient's hydration and sodium balance (Fig. 5.1). There is thus a large range of renin levels in normals with an

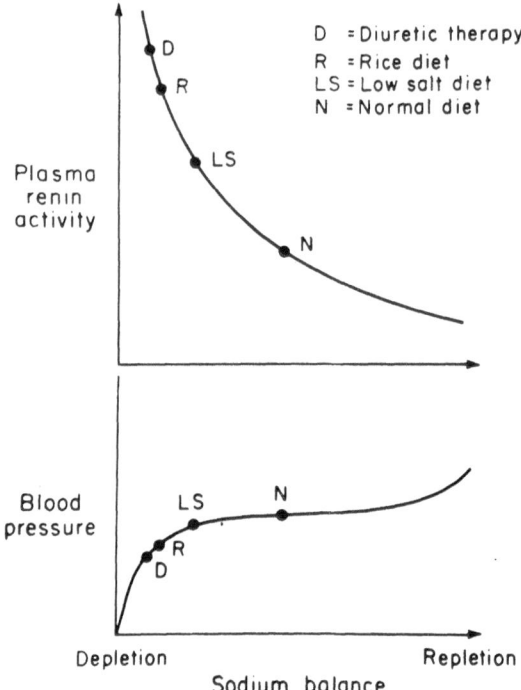

D = Diuretic therapy
R = Rice diet
LS = Low salt diet
N = Normal diet

Figure 5.1. Hypothetical relationship among body sodium balance, blood pressure, and renin.

overlap between normal and pathologic values. Therefore, any given peripheral plasma renin level must be indexed against the 24-hour urinary sodium concentration, which is a good indicator of hydration and sodium balance.

Renin in Pathologic States

Renal parenchymal ischemia, whether due to decreased arterial perfusion pressure or to parenchymal disease, stimulates renin release. Such hyperreninemia, or that due to renin-secreting tumor, produces hypertension. In humans if only one kidney is involved and the contralateral kidney is normal, the sodium retained due to the secondary hyperaldosteronemic state is excreted by the normal kidney, and the hypertension remains mediated by the hyperreninemic state. On the other hand, if the contralateral kidney is also abnormal due to parenchymal disease or renal artery stenosis, then neither kidney can excrete the retained sodium and therefore fluid retention, another

cause of hypertension, is produced and renin secretion is decreased by a negative feedback mechanism. The hypertension is thus soon converted from renin dependence to volume dependence and the renin levels may become normal. In patients with hemodynamically significant unilateral renal artery stenosis, the ipsilateral renin increment $V - A/A$ is usually approximately 0.5 or greater, whereas the contralateral kidney shows a corresponding suppression of renin secretion ($V - A/A \simeq O$). If the renin increment on the stenotic side exceeds 0.5 it indicates not that the kidney is producing renin in excess of the 50% increment required to maintain a steady rate, but rather that renal blood flow diminished. The diminished renal blood flow results in decreased dilution of the 50% renin increment secreted into the renal vein and thus produces a value spuriously greater than 0.5.

Others analyze renin values by calculating a ratio of renin secretion from the involved to the opposite kidney; a ratio of 1.5:1 or greater is assumed to be abnormal. The problem with this approach is that it assumes the contralateral kidney to be normal.

The renin confirmation of the significance of an anatomic renal artery stenosis is important; several anatomic and pathologic studies have demonstrated that patients can be normotensive in spite of having a severe renal artery stenosis. If these renin criteria are not met in unilateral renal artery stenosis, we usually perform Percutaneous Translumimal Renal Angioplasty (PTRA) only if it is necessary to preserve renal function.

Detection of Renovascular Hypertension

In our institution, all patients with suspected renovascular hypertension are evaluated according to the protocol in Fig. 5.2. Renovascular hypertension should be suspected and looked for in patients who fulfill some or all of the following clinical and laboratory criteria: (a) severe; (b) difficult to control hypertension; (c) recent onset or accelerated hypertension; (d) abdominal bruit; (e) young

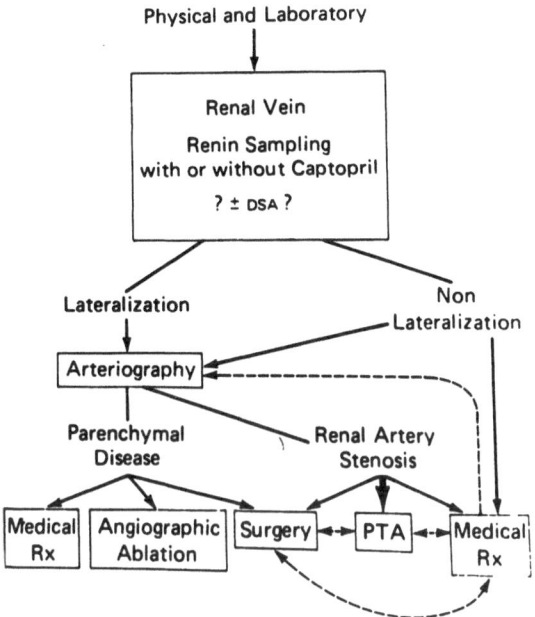

Figure 5.2. Evaluation of suspected renovascular hypertension. DSA, digital subtraction angiography; PTA, percutaneous transluminal angioplasty.

or middle age; (f) plasma renin activity; (g) positive peripheral captopril challenge test; (h) hypokalemia (Table 5.1). Confirmatory laboratory tests should start with peripheral venous blood samples for plasma renin activity (Table 5.2), captopril challenge test, and potassium, and progress in an orderly sequence toward the more complex and invasive tests based on the results of the previous screening procedures. Most biochemical screening tests for renovascular hypertension depend on measuring some component of the renin-angiotensin-aldosterone axis. Provocative tests to accentuate the differences between the involved and the normal kidney also depend on influencing this axis. Captopril, an inhibitor of the enzyme that converts angiotensin I to the active angiotensin II, can serve as a powerful clinical and laboratory testing agent. Administration of captopril to patients whose hypertension is renovascular in origin usually results in a fast and dramatic lowering of blood pressure, an increase in renin production by the abnormal kidney, and thus a rise in renal and peripheral venous plasma renin activity. If the

above tests support the suspicion or renovascular hypertension (RVHT), more invasive tests are necessary (2).

The New York Hospital–Cornell University Medical College protocol for a "peripheral" captopril challenge test is as follows:

1. Preparation
     Normal salt diet
     Off diuretics
     No antihypertensive Rx for 3 weeks
     Beta blockers OK
2. Protocol
     Baseline control
         Patient seated for 30 minutes
         BP at 20, 25, and 30 Minutes (averaged)
         Venous blood sample for Prvipheral Plasma Renin Activity (PRA) at 30 minutes
     Captopril challenge
         50 mg captopril (in 10 ml water) PO
         BP at 15, 30, 40, 45, 50, 55, and 60 minutes
         Venous blood sample for "stimulated" PRA at 60 minutes
3. Criteria for a positive test for renovascular hypertension
     "Stimulated" PRA $\geq$ 12 ng/ml/hr and
     Δ PRA $\geq$ 10 ng/ml/hr and
     Δ %PRA $\geq$ 150% or
                                     $\geq$ 400% if baseline
                                     Pra 3 ng/ml/hr

Table 5.1. Clinical findings in patients with renovascular hypertension.

1. Several hypertenision
2. Hypertension difficult to control
3. Recent onset or accelerated hypertension
4. Abdominal bruit
5. Young or middle-aged patient

Table 5.2. Laboratory findings in patients with renovascular hypertension.

1. Elevated plasma renin activity as indexed against 24-hour urinary sodium excretion (with or without captopril stimulation)
2. Hypokalemia (due to secondary hyperaldosteronism)

Radiographic Studies

Renal Vein Renin (RVR) Sampling and Assay and Intravenous Digital Subtraction Angiography (IVDSA)

Sampling of renal vein and infrarenal vena cava blood samples for assays of renin activity (RVR) and IVDSA can be performed through the same femoral or antecubital puncture site and following one another without significant additional risk, catheter manipulation, or time.

Renal vein renin samples are obtained from the left and right renal veins, each immediately followed by a control sample from the infrarenal inferior vena cava. The data obtained from RVR not only identifies the renovascular etiology and probable laterality of the lesion but also gives an indication of "surgical" curability according to the criteria listed in Table 5.3.

We routinely perform IVDSA by small volume right atrial injections of contrast material (25 ml) delivered at a high rate (32 to 35 ml/sec) through a high flow 6.5 pigtail catheter and obtain excellent opacification of the aorta and peripheral branches. We routinely obtain three views for each patient: an AP on a 9" field and the ipsilateral anterior oblique view for each kidney and renal artery also including the origin of the contralateral renal artery on a 6" field. IVDSA especially in patients being evaluated for renal artery stenosis should be followed by an abdominal radiograph which contains all of the information of the delayed film of an intravenous pyelogram (IVP), i.e., hyperconcentration, notching of ureters, and kidney size (3,4).

The two procedures are complementary rather than competitive techniques: one (IVDSA) identifies morphology, i.e., renal artery stenosis, while the other (RVR) confirms their physiological significance. In a recent review of 127 consecutive cases of combined IVDSA and RVR studies, 90% of IVDSAs were technically satisfactory. The results of IVDSA and RVR corresponded in approximately 90% of patients; however, in 10% of the cases there was disagreement. In

Table 5.3. Indicators of "surgically" curable unilateral renovascular hypertension.

1. Increased peripheral plasma renin activity indexed against 24-hour urinary sodium excretion
2. Ipsilateral hypersecretion of reinin

$$\frac{V-A}{A} \geq 50\%$$

3. Contralateral suppression of renin production

$$\frac{V-A}{A} \sim 0$$

4. Angiotensin II dependence of the hypertension (positive to captopril stimulation)

V, renin level in the renal vein; A, renin level in the renal artery.

cases where either of the two studies is inadequate or misleading, the findings of the other will alert the physician to the possibility of an error and stimulate further pursuit of the correct diagnosis. IVDSA and RVR together are, therefore, an accurate and sensitive approach to the detection of renovascular hypertension and in the follow-up of patients after renal angioplasty.

Arteriography

Patients are usually admitted to the hospital for arteriography only if the above outpatient tests confirm the presence of unilateral "surgically" curable RVHT. Two groups of patients are an exception to the above: (a) those with medically uncontrollable hypertension (who usually have bilateral renal artery and/or parenchymal disease), and (b) those with renal failure.

If arteriography is carried out to confirm the diagnosis of renal artery stenosis (Table 5.4) and PTRA is contemplated, then consent for PTRA is obtained prior to arteriography and PTRA is usually performed following the diagnostic arteriogram.

We do not routinely perform or recommend intravenous hypertensive urography for our patients as a screening test. Although this is a sensitive test, it is not highly specific. Radionuclide renal function and flow studies suffer from a similar disadvantage.

Table 5.4. Arteriographic findings in significant renal artery stenosis.

1. Stenosis $\geqq 70\%$ of luminal diameter
2. Collateral circulation
3. Poststenotic dilatation
4. Diminished velocity of flow across stenosis
5. Decreased renal size
6. Pressure gradient $\geqq 25\%$ of systolic pressure across the stenosis

Causes of Failure to Identify Renovascular hypertension by RVR

Bilateral Disease

Unfortunately, the renin criteria reliably identify only unilateral renal artery disease (Table 5.4). Patients with bilateral renal artery stenosis and/or parenchymal disease who cannot excrete the retained sodium become volume-dependent hypertensives, and may be undetectable by renin criteria. Sometimes captopril administration prior to renal vein renin sampling stimulates the more diseased kidney to significantly increase renin secretion. However, because their hypertension is difficult to control and/or they have renal failure, these patients are eventually suspected of having bilateral renovascular disease and undergo arteriography.

Incorrect Sampling of Renal Vein Renin

In branch stenosis, a sample obtained primarily from a vein draining the normal portion of the kidney gives a spurious result. This should be suspected because all samples (both renal veins and inferior vena cava) will show equal renin activity, though each of these may be abnormally but equally elevated. Equal and bilaterally suppressed renin values in both renal veins (i.e., equal to Infrarenal Inferior Vena Cava IVC) are a physiological impossibility unless there is an extrarenal renin-producing tumor or a nonsampled branch stenosis. Under such circumstances, the patient

should undergo arteriography to look for a missed branch lesion. Other causes of sampling error are erroneous sampling of a hepatic vein on the right, or sampling of the left renal vein proximal to the adrenal and gonadal veins, which produces a dilution artifact.

Other causes

Other causes of failure to identify RVHT include incorrect labeling of the sample and incorrect laboratory assay.

Conclusion

IVDSA and RVR together are accurate and sensitive approach as that complement each other in the detection of renovascular hypertension and also are useful in the follow-up of patients following renal angioplasty or surgery.

The renin confirmation of the significance of an anatomic renal artery stenosis is important; several anatomic and pathologic studies have demonstrated that patients can be normo-

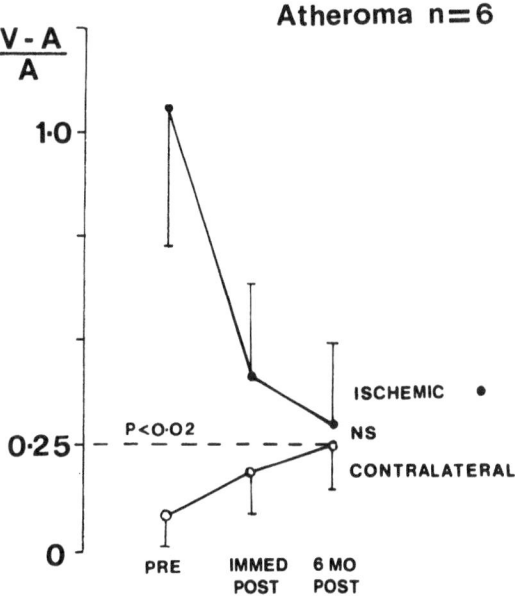

Figure 5.3. Renal vein renins after PTRA. Following successful PTRA renin secretion returns to normal from the ischemic and the contralateral kidneys in six atherosclerotic patients.

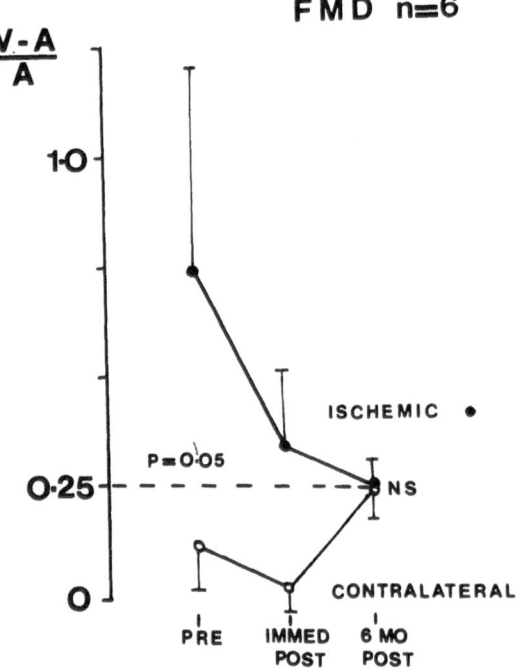

Figure 5.4. Renal vein renins after PTRA. Following successful PTRA in six patients with fibromuscular dysplasia, renal renin secretion is normalized.

tensive in spite of having a severe renal artery stenosis. If these renin criteria are not met in unilateral renal artery stenosis, we perform PTRA only if necessary to preserve renal function. We have confirmed the soundness of these criteria by analyzing renal vein renin data in six atherosclerotic (Fig. 5.3) and six fibromuscular dysplasia patients (Fig. 5.4) prior to and 6 months following successful PTRA. In each instance the ipsilateral kidney was secreting more than a 50% renin increment, while the contralateral kidney was totally suppressed prior to PTRA. After successful PTRA, renin secretion in both the ipsilateral and contralateral kidneys returned to normal.

References

1. Sos TA, et al. Diagnosis of renovascular hypertension and evaluation of "surgical curability." *Urol Radiol* 1982;3:199–203.
2. Sos TA, et al. Beneficial effects of percutaneous transluminal renal angioplasty on blood pressure in patients with renovascular hypertension due to atheroma or with fibromuscular dysplasia. *N Engl J Med* 1983;309:274–279.
3. Saddekni S, et al. Optimal injection for intravenous digital subtraction angiography: right atrial injection using small volume (25 ml) at a high rate (35 ml/sec)—animal and clinical studies. *Radiology* 1984;159:655–659.
4. Saddekni S, et al. Contrast administration and techniques of DSA performance. Radiol Clin North Am. 1985; Vol 23(2):275–292.

6

Selective Venous Sampling for Parathyroid Hormone Excess

—— *Reingard Sörensen* ——

Introduction

Up to 95% of patients with primary hyperparathyroidism can be cured by cervical parathyroidectomy with or without localization techniques (1–3). With recurrence or persistent disease, which occurs in approximately 15% after the initial procedure, reoperation is less successful and has a higher morbidity rate (4,5). In those cases, it is important to locate the remaining parathyroid tissue. (6–9). Within the last 5 years spatial resolution of noninvasive imaging systems (ultrasound, computed tomography, magnetic resonance imaging) has improved so much that venous sampling for localization of parathormone-producing tumors has been almost completely confined to postoperative cases with persistent or recurrent disease and to the localization of ectopic parathyroid tissue. This is usually found in the mediastinum. When hypercalcemia has recurred after surgery, and noninvasive imaging systems are not able to locate the excess hormone production, selective sampling is the method of choice.

Clinical Features

Hyperparathyroidism (HPT) is a generalized disorder resulting from excessive secretion of parathyroid hormone by one or more parathyroid glands or by ectopic parathyroid tissue. It is characterized by hypercalcemia, hypophosphatemia, and excessive bone resorption. Asymptomatic hypercalcemia (total serum calcium > 10.5 mg/dl) is the most frequent presentation (10). In combination with hypercalcemia, nephrolithiasis is common.

Signs and Symptoms

Clinical manifestations are constipation, anorexia, nausea, vomiting, abdominal pain, and ileus. The reversible impairment of the renal concentration mechanism leads to polyuria, nocturia, and polydipsia.

Severe elevation of serum calcium (> 12 mg/dl) is associated with emotional lability, confusion, delirium, psychosis, stupor, coma, muscular weakness, seizures, nephrolithiasis, urolithiasis, reversible acute renal failure, irreversible renal damage, nephrocalcinosis, peptic ulcers, pancreatitis, and ECG changes (shortened Q-T interval). Hypercalcemia of > 18 mg/dl may result in shock, renal failure, and death.

Osteitis Fibrosa Cystica

When hyperparathyroidism is of longer duration, increased osteoclastic activity causes rarefying osteitis with fibrous degeneration, formation of cysts, brown tumors (11), and development of fibrous nodules in the affected

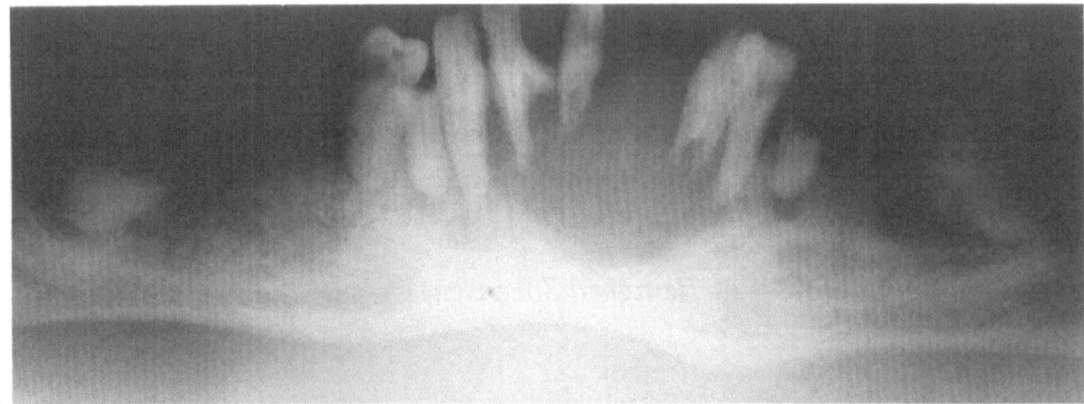

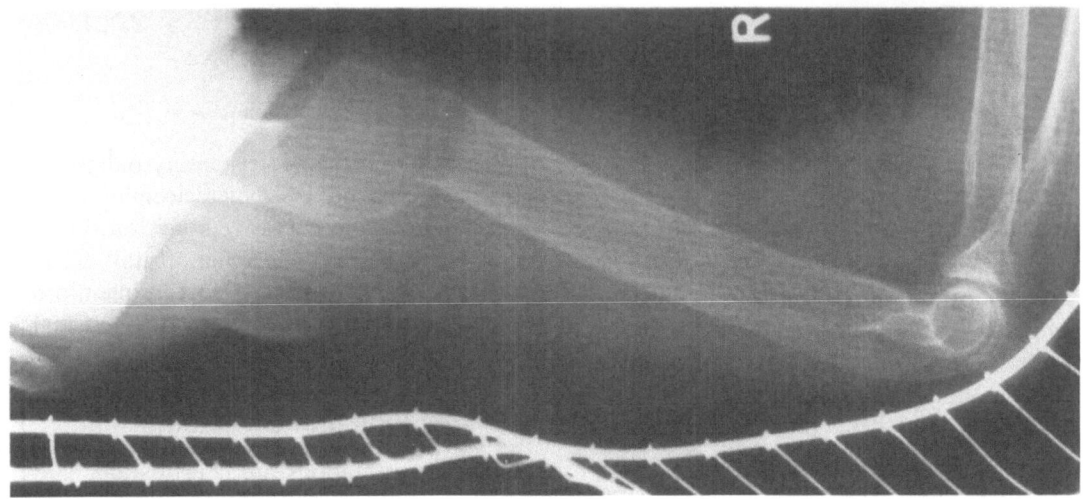

Figure 6.1. Primärer Hyperparathyroidismus: Brown Tumors. **A:** Bone destruction of the mandible in a patient with a parathyroid adenoma. **B:** Pathologic fracture of the humerus in the area of a brown tumor in a patient with a parathyroid adenoma.

bone (Fig. 6.1). This is now rarely seen, except in chronic dialysis patients with secondary HPT. Radiographic changes are bone cysts (Fig. 6.1b), "salt and pepper" appearance of the skull, subperiosteal bone resorption of the phalanges (Fig. 6.2), and the distal clavicles.

Primary Hyperparathyroidism

Primary hyperparathyroidism is the most common cause of hypercalcemia. There is a familial and a nonfamilial form. Familial forms are (a) multiple endocrine neoplasia type I (MEN-I), multiple endocrine adenomatosis type I (MEA-I), Werner's syndrome; and (b)

multiple endocrine neoplasia type II (MEN-IIA), multiple endocrine adenomatosis type II (MEA-II), Sipple's syndrome. Histology reveals a parathyroid adenoma in 90% of the patients. Sometimes it is difficult to distinguish a normal gland from an adenoma when the hypercalcemia is mild (< 12 mg/dl). A total of 10% of cases are due to hyperplasia of two or more glands (7%; 12) and parathyroid carcinoma (3%).

The syndrome of familial hypocalciuric hypercalcemia is transmitted as an autosomal dominant trait with 100% penetrance (13). It is characterized by persistent hypercalcemia, elevated levels of parathyroid hormone (PTH),

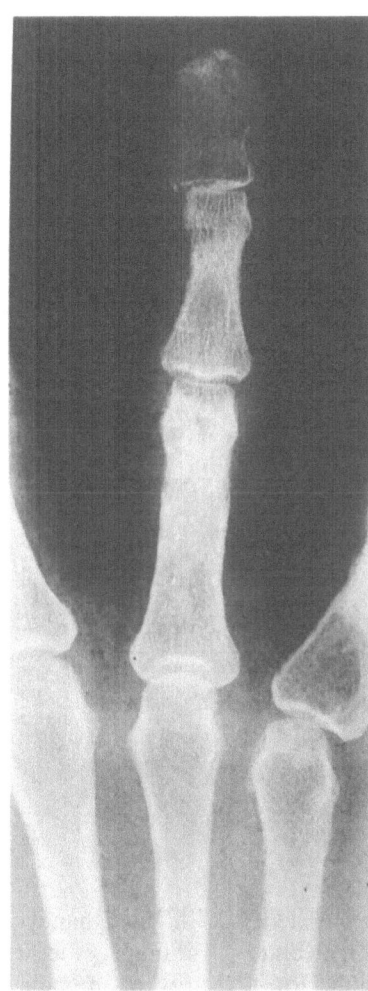

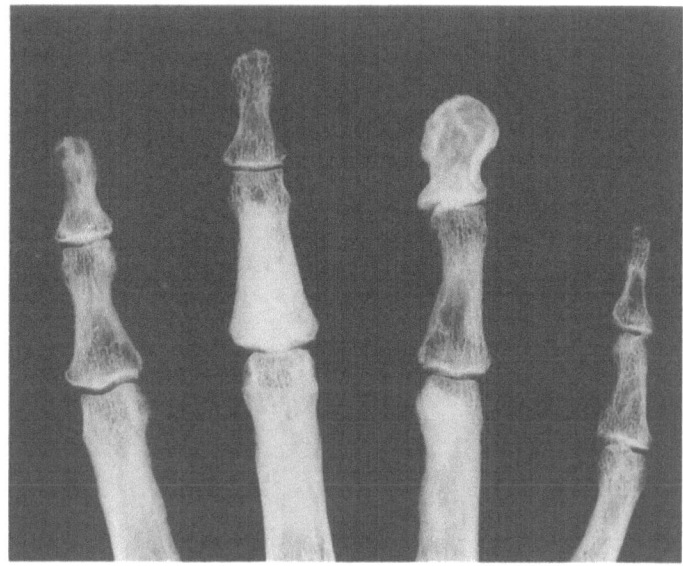

Figure 6.2. Primärer Hyperparathyroidismus. **A:** Rarefication of cortical bone with fibrous replacement. **B:** Recalcification following surgical treatment of a parathyroid adenoma.

and hypocalciuria. Hypercalcemia is usually asymptomatic, renal function is well maintained, and nephrolithiasis is unusual. Severe primary hyperparathyroidism may occur in infants of affected kindreds and in severe pancreatitis. Although parathyroid hyperplasia is consistently found in those cases, the response to subtotal parathyroidectomy generally is unsatisfactory.

Secondary Hyperparathyroidism

Secondary hyperparathyroidism refers to hypocalcemia caused by conditions that can lower the serum calcium, such as renal insufficiency and intestinal malabsorption syndromes in which increased secretion of hormone represents an adaptive response to a normal stimulus. These disorders are characterized by hypocalcemia or, less often, normocalcemia. When secondary hyperparathyroidism has been established for some time, parathyroid sensitivity to calcium may be diminished due to glandular hyperplasia and elevation of the calcium set point (the amount of calcium necessary to reduce secretion of PTH by 50%). Thus, hypersecretion of PTH may continue in the face of normocalcemia or even hypercalcemia (tertiary hyperparathyroidism).

Malignancies

Malignancies may cause hypercalcemia by several mechanisms, each of which results in

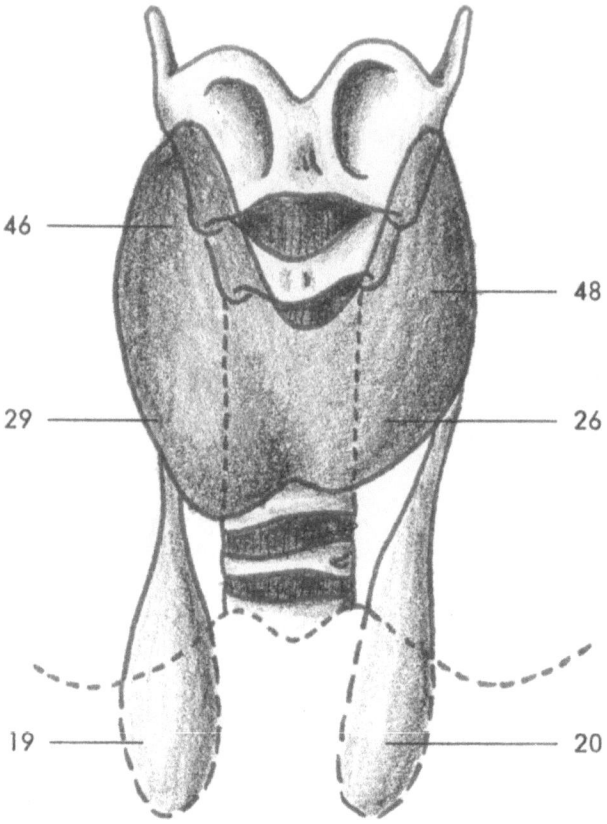

Figure 6.3. Location of Parathyroid Glands in 47 post-mortem cases according to Nathaniels. (Figure indicates the number identified)

bone resorption (14,15). Hematologic cancer such as multiple myeloma, lymphomas, and lymphosarcomas cause hypercalcemia by elaboration of an osteoclast activating factor leading to osteoclastic bone resorption with osteolytic lesions and/or diffuse osteopenia. Most frequently, hypercalcemia of malignancy occurs in breast cancer and squamous cell tumors of the lung with bone matastases. Breast cancer with bone metastases accounts for greater than 50% of patients with malignancy-associated hypercalcemia caused by local elaboration of osteoclast activating factors or prostaglandins, and/or direct bone resorption by tumor cells. Less frequently, hypercalcemia may occur in association with squamous cell carcinomas of any organ, hypernephroma, or ovarian cancer, without detectable bone metastases. Many such occurrences were formerly attributed to ectopic production of PTH. Immunoreactive PTH levels are elevated in

up to 25% of patients with malignancy-associated hypercalcemia. Although precise factors responsible for these events remain uncertain, the variable immunoreactivity of utilized antibodies to PTH are important. In any event, osteoclastic bone resorption is the main cause of hypercalcemia in these patients and may result from PTH-like substances or other tumor-elaborated factors.

Anatomy/Physiology

Human parathyroid tissue is divided into two to six portions. There are usually four glands. Figure 6.3 demonstrates where the normal glands and aberrant parathyroid tissue can be expected (16–20). PTH is secreted by parathyroid glands or by ectopic parathyroid tissue (Fig. 6.3). This is usually found in the mediastinum. The examining physician should be fami-

liar with where ectopic tissue is expected to be
found before an invasive procedure is planned.

There is no hormone to stimulate the parathyroid glands. The changing level of the
serum calcium is the primary stimulus for parathyroid hormone (PTH) secretion. The action
of PTH is the regulation and maintenance of a
normal serum calcium level. In healthy persons
this measures 9 to 11 mg %. Another important hormone maintaining the serum calcium
level is calcitonin (thyrocalcitonin). Calcitonin
is an antagonist to parathyroid hormone. It is
secreted in response to hypercalcemia, lowers
the serum calcium level, and reduces bone resorption. There is a reciprocal relationship between serum calcium and serum phosphorus so
that the product of calcium times phosphorus is
maintained at a constant level. The main actions of PTH are (a) the inhibition of phosphate resorption by the renal tubule; (b) the
resorption of calcium and phosphate from
bone, presumably by stimulating the action of
the osteoclasts; (c) the increase of calcium
absorption from the gastrointestinal tract, similar to the action of vitamin D; and (d) the
action on the renal tubule enhancing calcium
resorption.

If the parathyroid glands are not functioning, there is no readjustment; the serum calcium level will fall, below the normal threshold
of 7 mg per 100 ml, and urine calcium will be
absent. The presence of the large reservoir of
calcium in the skeleton prevents the serum calcium from falling below 5 mg per 100 ml. If
there is excessive parathyroid hormone secretion, resorption of calcium and phosphate from
the bone matrix stimulate the osteoclasts. The
response of the osteoclasts will then evoke the
osteoblasts to become active to repair bone,
with the subsequent rise of the alkaline phosphatase level in the serum.

Venous Drainage

The parathyroid glands drain into the jugular
and brachiocephalic veins by the superior, middle, and inferior thyroid veins (20,21; Fig. 6.4).
The inferior thyroid veins usually form a trunk
that drains into the left brachiocephalic vein at

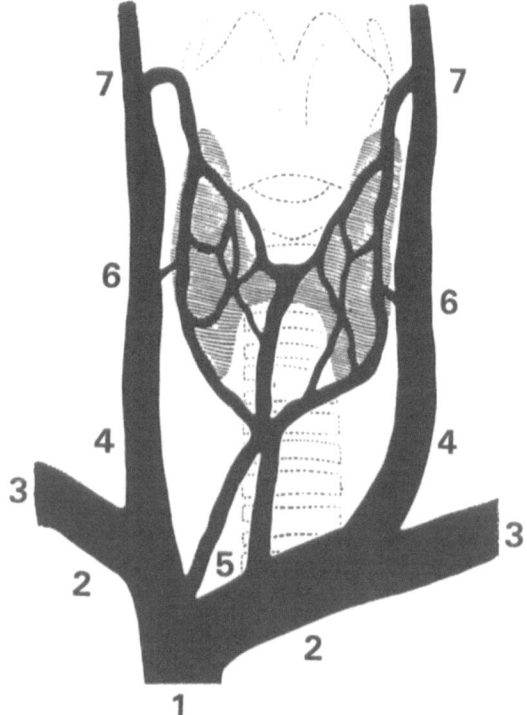

Figure 6.4. Major veins of the thyroid bed. Inter-
connections of principle veins and isthmic veins
(Doppman: Invest. Radiol 1949;4:97). (1) Superior
vena cava; (2) Brachio-cephalic veins; (3) Subclavian veins; (4) Internal jugular veins; (5) Inferior
thyroid veins, isthmic veins; (6) Middle thyroid
veins; (7) Superior thyroid veins. (From Ref. 23,
with permission.)

its superior aspect (Figs. 6.5 and 6.6). Opposite
to the thyroid trunk, the thymic veins enter
the left brachiocephalic vein (Fig. 6.7A). The
orifice of the azygos vein is found at the posterior wall of the superior vena cava (Fig.
6.7B). The right superior intercostal vein and
the mediastinal veins are drained by the azygos
system (Fig. 6.7A,B,C). The parathyroid
glands drain almost always into the ipsilateral
inferior thyroid veins, which generally join to
form a common inferior thyroid vein before
entering the left innominate vein (Fig. 6.4 and
6.5; 21–23, 24). Variations in venous anatomy
are common, especially accessory inferior thyroid veins on the left side. In addition, the inferior thyroid veins (Fig. 6.8) are frequently ligated during thyroid surgery when the gland is

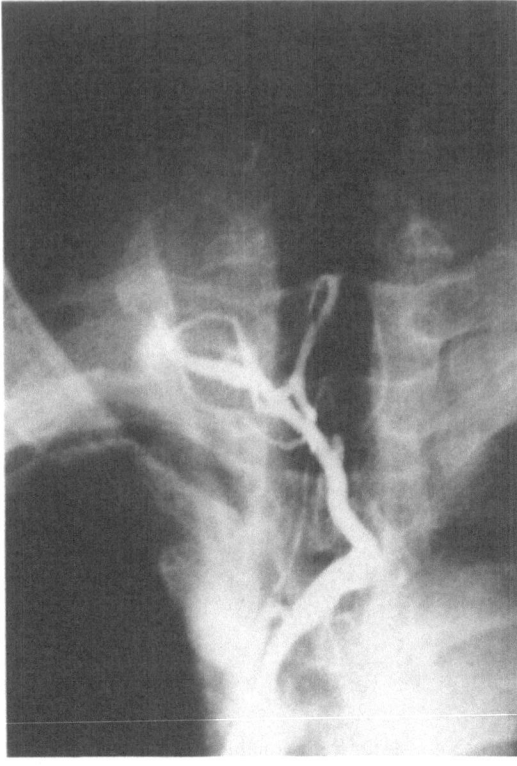 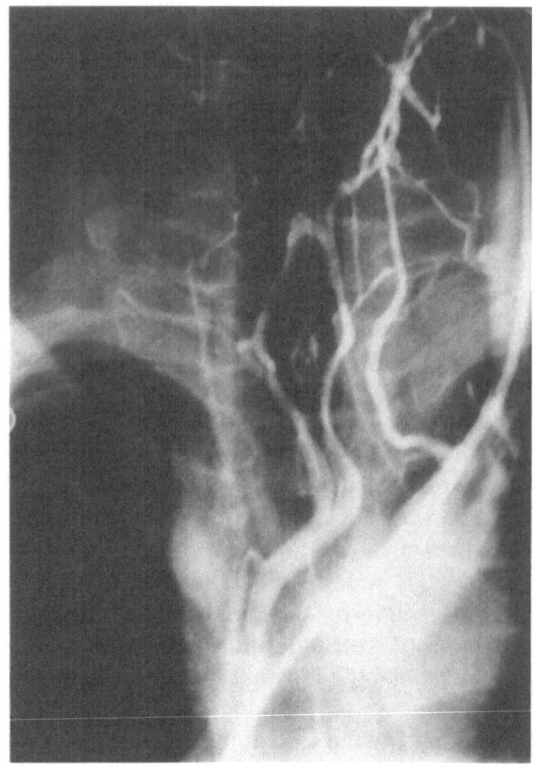

A   B

Figure 6.5. Inferior thyroid trunc. **A:** The catheter is introduced via the right femoral approach into the inferior thyroid trunc. Retrograde opacifacation of the inferior thyroid veins. **B:** There is filling of the left inferior, middle and superior thyroidal vein as well as filling of the right internal jugular vein. The left side is partially filled as well. The catheter tip is demonstrated in the left superior thyroidal vein.

mobilized (Fig. 6.9). For these reasons, a road map of the venous drainage patterns derived from delayed films following an arterial injection can be helpful.

The common inferior thyroid vein drains into the superior margin of the left innominate vein, often quite close to the junction with the right innominate vein. The catheter must be selectively advanced into both the right and left inferior thyroid veins to obtain samples for localization of the site of hormone excess. Parathyroid glands always drain into the thyroid veins descending along the lateral margin of the thyroid lobe (22; Fig. 6.4); samples from the medial lobar and the isthmic veins are of no value.

The thymic vein of Keynes drains into the inferior margin of the left innominate vein (Fig. 6.10). A PTH elevation in this vein suggests a parathyroid adenoma in the anterior mediastinum. Anastomoses between the inferior thyroid and the thymic veins are common, especially on the left side. Doppman et al. (22,23,24,25,26) have encountered PTH elevations in the thymic veins with cervical adenomas as well as PTH elevations in the cervical veins with mediastinal adenomas.

Venous drainage patterns from an arteriographic study carried out before the sampling procedure usually clarify such problems.

Laboratory Findings

Parathyroid hormone is secreted by the parathyroid glands. It is an 84-amino acid, single-chain polypeptide. Calcium (Ca) and phos-

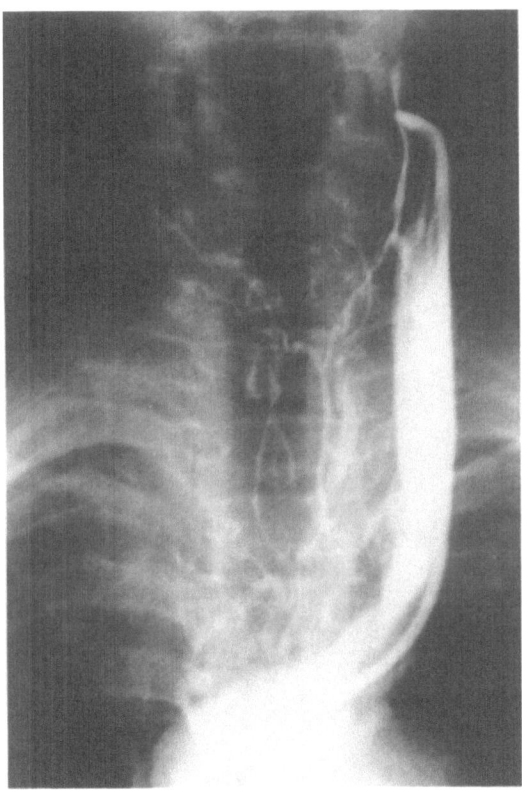

Figure 6.6. Left jugular vein with retrograde opacification of the venous network of the thyroid gland.

phorus (P) serum levels are regulated by PTH and vitamin D; their metabolic actions are interrelated. PTH promotes the active metabolite formation of vitamin D in the kidney. Conversely, with a deficiency of the vitamin or any resistance to its action, effects of these hormones are blunted. Actions of PTH are (a) the rapid mobilization of Ca and phosphate from bone and the long-term acceleration of bone resorption, (b) the increase of renal tubular resorption of Ca and Vitamin D, (c) the increase of intestinal absorption of Ca, and (d) the decrease of renal tubular resorption of phosphate (PO_4). This action accounts for most of the important clinical manifestations of PTH excess or deficiency.

In periods of calcium balance, the amount of calcium absorbed from the diet is equal to the amount of calcium excreted in the urine. The percentage of dietary calcium absorbed by the intestine increases with the decrease of the calcium intake and decreases when the dietary Ca is increased. The mechanism is vitamin D–dependent. The most active metabolite of vitamin D (1,25-dihydroxycholicalciferol; 1,25-DHCC) enhances the Ca transport within the small intestine by mediating synthesis of mucosal Ca-binding proteins. PTH also enhances intestinal Ca absorption. This action appears to be due to PTH-mediated formation of 1,25-DHCC in the kidney. Renal Ca excretion generally parallels sodium (Na) excretion. This is influenced by many of the factors that govern Na transport within the proximal tubule. Independently of Na (and vitamin D), PTH enhances renal distal tubular Ca absorption and increases renal phosphate (PO_4) excretion. PTH causes an efflux of Ca (presumably from the labile Ca pool) into the extracellular fluid within minutes after glandular release. The mechanism is not clear. Long-term increase of PTH secretion inhibits the function of osteoblasts and promotes osteolysis.

In the target organ the effects of PTH is not entirely clear. The physiologic effects of PTH upon bone are significantly influenced by the level of vitamin D being normal. In vivo, both hormones function as important regulators of bone modeling and remodeling.

Autotransplanted Parathyroid Tissue

Parathyroid autografts are performed in cases of postoperative hypoparathyroidism. Parathyroid tissue is usually transplanted into the forearm. One complication of long-term autotransplanted grafts is recurrence of the clinical signs of hyperparathyroidism due to proliferation of the transplant (27–31).

Differential Diagnosis of Hypercalcemia

The cause of hypercalcemia (Table 6.1) is often apparent from the history and associated clinical findings (excessive ingestion of calcium, milk-alkali syndrome, malignancy, Addison's

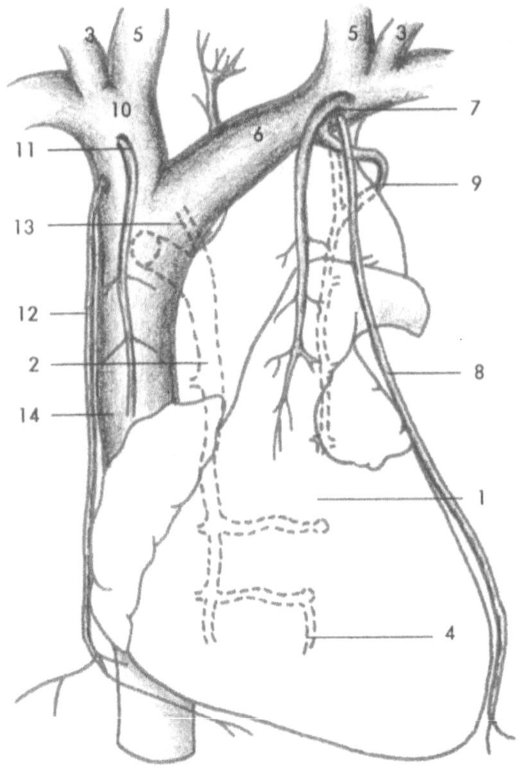

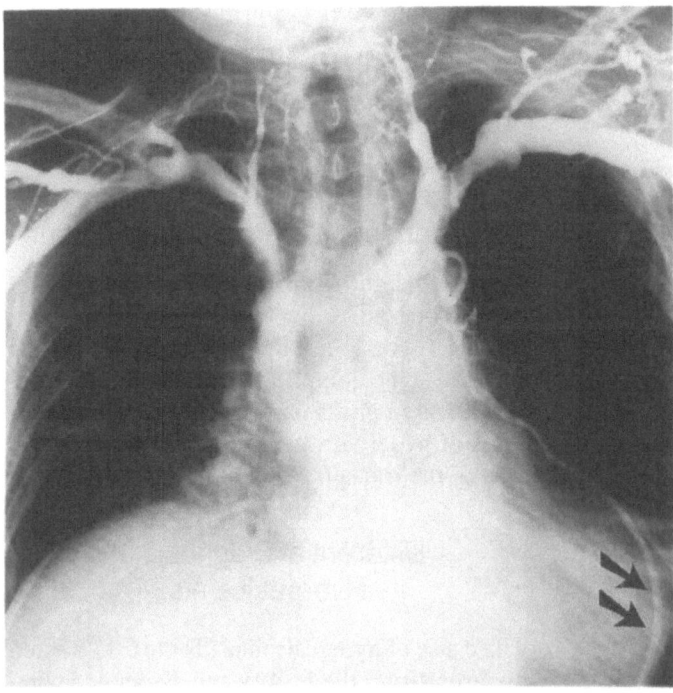

A

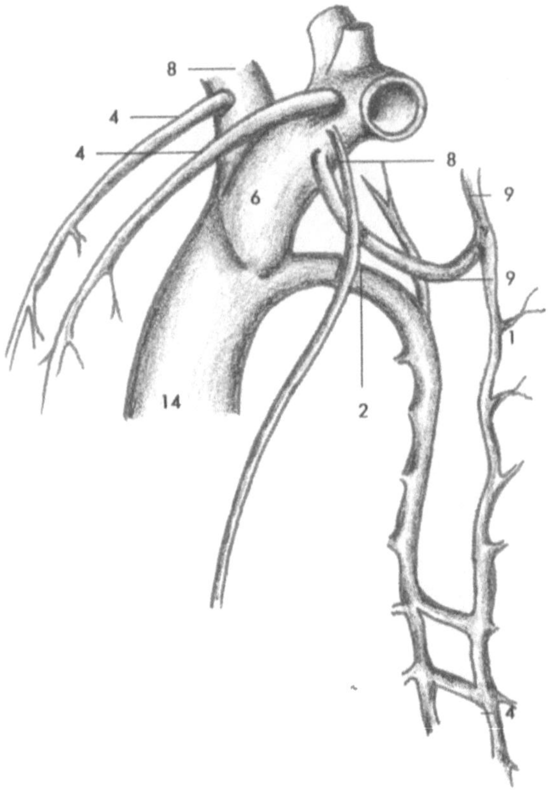

B

C

Figure 6.7. **A**: Thoracic Veins, ante-rior-posterior position. The right internal thoracic vein terminates more proximally on its brachiocephalic vein than does the left. The left pericardiophrenic vein terminates on the left brachiocephalic vein; it may also terminate on the internal thoracic or the superior intercostal vein. (1) Accessory hemiazygos vein; (2) Azygos vein; (3) External jugular vein; (4) Hemiazygos vein; (5) Internal jugular vein; **B**: Left brachiocephalic vein; (7) Internal thoracic vein; (8) Left pericardio-phrenic vein; (9) Left superior intercostal vein; (10) Right brachio-cephalic vein; (11) Right internal thoracic vein; (12) Right pericardio-phrenic vein; (13) Right superior intercostal vein; (14) Superior vena cava (from Ref. 117, with permission.) **C**: Bilateral venography of the superior vena cava. Collateral circulation in a patient with superior vena cava syndrome. Opacification of the pericardiophrenic vein (arrows).

Table 6.1. Causes of hypercalcemia.

1. Excessive osteolysis
    Parathyroid hormone excess
      Primary hyperparathyroidism
      Parathyroid carcinoma
      Hypercalciuric hypocalcemia
      Advanced secondary hyperparathyroidism
        (especially after renal transplantation)
      Malignancies with calcemia in absence of
        of bone metastases
    Malignancies with bone metastases
      Carcinoma
      Leukemias
      Lymphomas
      Myeloma
    Hyperthyroidism
    Vitamin D intoxication
    Immobilization
      In patients with rapid bone remodeling:
        Young growing individuals
        Patients with Paget's disease
        Elderly patients with osteoporosis

2. Excessive GI calcium absorption and/or intake
    Milk-alkali syndrome
    Vitamin D intoxication
    Sarcoidosis, other chronic granulomatous
      disease

3. Elevated concentration of plasma proteins

4. Uncertain mechanism
    Myxedema, Addison's disease, postoperative
    Cushing's disease
    Thiazide diuretic treatment
    Infantile hypercalcemia

5. Artifactual
    Prolonged venous stasis while obtaining
      blood sample
    Exposure of blood to contaminated
      glassware

disease). Radiographic evidence of bone disease may suggest the diagnosis (hyperparathyroidism, Paget's disease, osteolytic or osteoblastic lesions in myeloma). Patients with mild hypercalcemia are asymptomatic.

Hypercalcemia of Malignancy

The changes of PO_4 are similar to the changes of HPT (low serum PO_4, metabolic alkalosis, hypochloremia, hypoalbuminemia). Serum calcium is >12 mg/dl, circulating PTH (C-terminal or intact, midregion assay) is elevated, the simultaneous level of ionized PTH is suppressed.

Familial Hypocalciuric Hypercalcemia

Familial hypocalciuria has an early onset in life. Laboratory findings include hypermagnesemia and hypercalcemia without hypercalciuria in other family members. The fractional excretion of Ca (ratio of Ca clearance to creatinine clearance) is low ($<1\%$; 13).

Idiopathic Hypercalciuria of Infancy

There is a combination of suppressed levels of PTH, hypercalciuria, sometimes somatic abnormalities like Williams syndrome (supravalvular aortic stenosis, mental retardation, elfin facies).

Milk-Alkali Syndrome

Milk-alkali syndrome includes hypercalemia, metabolic alkalosis, azotemia, and hypocalciuria. Without alkali and Ca ingestion the blood Ca returns to normal.

Myeloma

Anemia, azotemia, and hypercalcemia are the main laboratory findings of myeloma. The diagnosis is confirmed by bone marrow examination, monoclonal gammopathy, and immunoelectrophoresis with free light chains in the serum/urine.

Other Causes of Hypercalcemia

In thyrotoxicosis and Addison's disease there exist typical laboratory findings that will establish the diagnosis.

Hypercalciuria is found in most disorders causing hypercalcemia, except familial hypocalciuric hypercalcemia, milk-alkali syndrome, Addison's disease, thiazide therapy, and renal failure. Circulating PTH (C-terminal assay) is elevated in patients with hyperparathyroidism, and is suppressed in patients with vitamin D intoxication, milk-alkali syndrome, and sarcoidosis. Immunoassays are capable of detect-

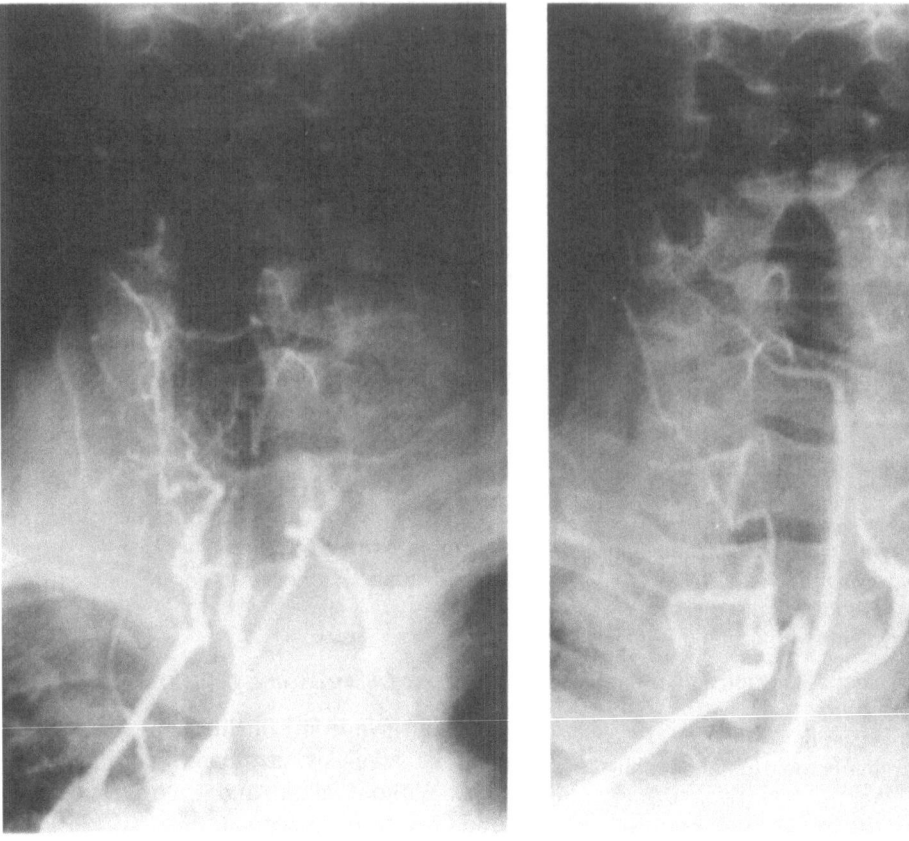

A   B

Figure 6.8. **A,B:** Retrograde filling of the vena thyreoidea veins.

ing such differences and may differentiate primary HPT from humoral hypercalcemia of malignancy (HHM).

Laboratory Tests

Physiological tests of parathyroid function largely have been supplanted by the measurement of circulating PTH levels in the plasma or serum by radioimmunoassay (RIA), and by the measurement of total urine. PTH is secreted into the circulation by the parathyroid glands as the intact hormone and as a carboxy-terminal (C-terminal) fragment. The intact hormone has a very short half-life (< 10 minutes), whereas the half-life of the C-terminal fragment is considerably longer.

It is not clear whether the amino-terminal (N-terminal) fragments circulate as such. Some evidence, however, suggests that N-terminal fragments, released by the liver after hepatic uptake of intact hormone, are taken out of the circulation by bone. Whereas intact PHT is cleared by the liver (60%) and by the kidney (40%), the kidneys are the sole route of elimination of C-terminal fragments. Clinically available RIAs for evaluation of serum PTH utilize antibodies that detect the C-terminal segment and the intact hormone, the midportion of the intact hormone, or the N-terminal segment and the intact hormone. Biological activity appears to reside in the intact hormone and the N-terminal fragment; the C-terminal segment is biologically inactive. Nonetheless, N-terminal assays have generally failed to distinguish reliably between hyperparathyroid and normal subjects, perhaps due to the short half-time of the fragment in the circulation.

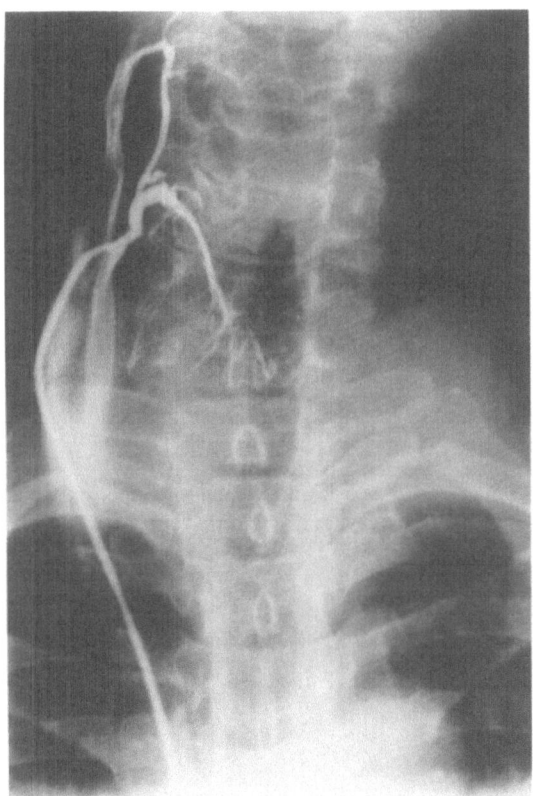

Figure 6.9. Right superior and middle thyroidal veins following partial thyroidectomy. The inferior thyroidal vein had been ligated.

Laboratory Techniques

For determination of serum parathormone, samples (1 to 5 ml) have to be transported in ice to the laboratory. Parathormone is extremely unstable. At the same time calcium and phosphate levels should be examined. The normal serum parathormone (intact) levels are 10 to 65 ng/l.

Diagnostic Procedures

Noninvasive Imaging

Despite modern imaging procedures like sonography (32–38), computed tomography (CT) (39–41), computer-assisted isotope scanning (42,43), and magnetic resonance imaging (44–46), the localization of remaining abnormal parathyroid tissue after surgery is possible in only 31% of all cases of hyperparathyroidism (47–49).

Ultrasound

Of the nonoperated patients, ultrasound is able to localize parathyroid abnormality in 70 to 80% of the patients (50,51). If it cannot be detected, it usually is ectopic and will be found either in the lower portion of the neck or in the mediastinum. Ultrasound has a very low rate of false-negative results (51–53). False-positive examinations, however, are unlikely to change the management of the patient, unless there is the suggestion of a lesion in the mediastinum that would require thoracic surgery.

The accuracy of ultrasonography in localizing hyperactive parathyroid glands has been well documented (54,55). The echogenic appearance of enlarged parathyroid glands may show a wide variation ranging from homogeneous, echo-poor, well-defined lesions to heterogeneous lesions of varying echo-density containing cystic areas, thus making discrimination from nodular and cystic thyroid lesions difficult.

Intraoperative Ultrasound. Normal parathyroid glands cannot be seen in ultrasound. Intraoperatively after the platysma muscle is

The N-terminal assays have been more suitable for detecting rapid changes in PTH secretion in response to acute changes in ionized Ca.

The C-terminal assays correlate highly with the number of osteoclasts and are useful in the diagnosis of primary hyperparathyroidism. Since the C-terminal fragments accumulate in the plasma with declining renal function, PTH levels measured by a C-terminal assay will increase progressively with decreasing renal function, limiting the usefulness of the assay. However, assays directed at both the C-terminal or intact, midregion portion of the PTH molecule have reflected the long-term activity of the parathyroid glands in patients on chronic dialysis. Whatever the RIA utilized, clinical interpretation of the PTH level is possible only in the context of the concomitantly measured serum Ca level.

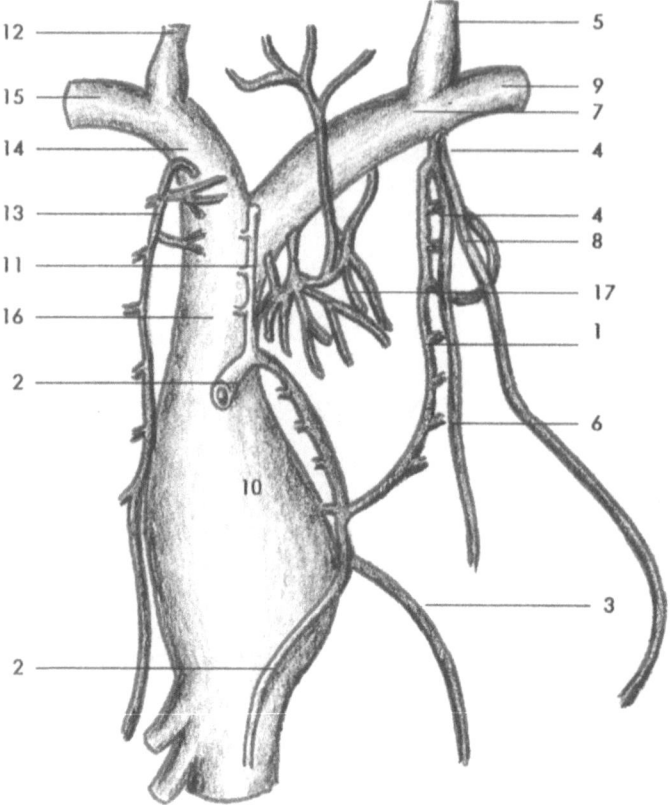

Figure 6.10. Mediastinal veins. Schematic drawing of normal venous structures of the mediastinum (according to Yune, Radiology 1972; 105:285). (1) Accessory hemiazygos vein; (2) Azygos vein; (3) Hemiazygos vein; (4) Left highest intercostal vein; (5) Left internal jugular vein; (6) Left internal mammary vein; (7) Left innominate vein; (8) Lateral mediastinal-phrenic vein; (9) Left subclavian vein; (10) Right atrium; (11) Right highest intercostal vein; (12) Right internal jugular vein; (13) Right internal mammary vein; (14) Right innominate vein; (15) Right subclavian vein; (16) Superior vena cava; (17) Thymic vein.

raised and the neck is exposed along the medial border of the sternocleidomastoid muscle, Norton et al. (56) could not find any difference in the appearance of the normal glands. Pathologic glands appear sonolucent (hypoechoic) pre- and postoperatively when examined in two planes. Comparison of both methods shows there is a high specificity rate of intraoperative ultrasound (IOUS) examinations, although it is less sensitive for superior than for inferior glands. In parathyroid reoperations, IOUS facilitates locating abnormal parathyroid tissue and leads the surgeon through dense scar tissue that is usually difficult to dissect.

Ultrasound-Guided Fine Needle Aspiration.
Ultrasound-guided fine needle aspiration in patients with biochemically confirmed hyperparathyroidism and enlarged parathyroid glands is easily performed. The parathormone content of the aspirated material can be ex-

amined and compared to an aspiration material of thyroid tissue. Fine needle aspiration for PTH is useful in patients who are suspected on sonographic examination of having parathyroid tumors in the neck. A high content of PTH is expected to be found in aspirations of parathyroid tumors.

By combining ultrasound and aspiration or CT and aspiration, a more reliable tissue diagnosis can be obtained, thus forming the basis for ultrasonically guided percutaneous inactivation of parathyroid tumors (57–62). Furthermore, a preoperative tissue diagnosis of ultrasonically suspected enlarged parathyroid glands might be helpful to the surgeons, especially in patients requiring reexplorations.

Complications.
Intraglandular hemorrhage and necrotic changes may occur following fine needle aspiration biopsy (58,62,63). These changes were found by surgeons following fine needle biopsy.

Results. The sensitivity of ultrasound (US) is reported to be between 36% and 80% (34,38,39,42,64–67). The low sensitivity (36%) in the series of Miller et al. (47) is probably due to the inclusion of mediastinal lesions in comparison with series of patients who had not had surgery before evaluation with ultrasound (35,38,68). If the adenoma is located within the neck, ultrasound is most effective; CT usually is less effective in this region. In patients who had previous total or partial thyroidectomy, however, the anatomy is disrupted and US will show a very disturbed image. US is useless for lesions within the anterior (69) mediastinum (47). The newer, improved equipment has not changed these results, except for the fact that lymph nodes can be easily identified with higher-resolution equipment (70).

Computed Tomography

The sensitivity of computed tomography in patients who had had previous surgery for parathyroid adenoma or have aberrant parathyroid tissue is reported in the literature to be between 44% and 47% (12,34,39,47,71–77). The false-positive rates are reported to be 2 to 12% (34,47,70,78–81). The tumor in relationship to the sensitivity of CT, US, magnetic resonance imaging (MRI), and scintigraphy is demonstrated by Miller (47,82).

Scintigraphy

Scintigraphy of the parathyroid glands is performed with technetium (Tc)-99m pertechnetate/thallium (Tl)-201 subtraction studies (47, 83–85). The overall sensitivity of Tc/Tl scans (patients with lesions in the neck outside the parathyroid glands, postsurgical lesions with recurrent hypercalcemia) is reported in the literature to be between 27% and 30% (47,86,87).

A focal, intense tissue accumulation of thallium-201 characterizes the classic finding of technetium-thallium scintigraphy (TTS) for parathyroid adenomas. The examination has a specificity of 97% (n = 55) in patients with an elevated level of circulating calcium and parathyroid hormone (PTH). Results were correlated with all types (chief, oxyphil, or mixture), growth patterns (solid, acinar, or cystic), cell sizes, and gland weights. Positive findings from TTS studies are found in lesions >1.5 cm in diameter. Chief cells were present in 87.5%; 76% of positive TTS studies were in patients in whom the PTH level was 1.75 of normal. The relationship of positive findings of TTS studies to histologic features appears to be multifactorial (43,88–91).

Magnetic Resonance Imaging

MRI is able to detect parathyroid adenomas as well as or even better than other imaging modalities (44–46,51,92–94). They are usually isointense or slightly hypointense when compared with the surrounding thyroid tissue on weighted pulse sequence images and isointense or slightly hyperintense on T2-weighted images (45,46,51,93,95–100). They are hyperintense to surrounding fat on T2-weighted images. Adenomas are well circumscribed, smoothly marginated, and often encapsulated or pseudo-encapsulated (50) and hyperintense on T2-weighted images. Hyperplastic glands or the rare parathyroid carcinomas also may be hyperintense on T2-weighted images. A hyperplastic gland may be isointense to the thyroid gland on T1- and T2-weighted images. Carcinomas do not always have an invasive appearance and the diagnosis requires a careful histologic evaluation. The accuracy of either CT or MRI in the evaluation or detection of mediastinal parathyroid adenomas is not known due to the lack of sufficient studies (45,46,50,51,92,93).

False-positive MRI studies occur at a higher rate, when compared with CT and ultrasound examinations, in both the initial evaluation and the postoperative state (3,29,50).

MRI is competitive with other imaging studies for the detection of parathyroid adenomas in patients with primary hyperparathyroidism and patients with end-stage renal disease who may have an adenoma. At the present time, its cost should preclude it having a primary role in patients undergoing their first surgical procedure for primary hyperparathyroidism. MRI can be used instead of CT in patients with post-operative recurrent hyperparathyroidism.

Gadolinium (Gd)-DTPA Enhanced T1-Weighted Spin-Echo (SE) Sequences.

Initial findings suggest that Gd-DPTA can enhance the signal of parathyroid adenomas on T1-weighted images combined with good anatomic depiction at a high signal-to-noise ratio and a short acquisition time. The results are still on clinical trial. Further work will define the diagnostic value of Gd-DPTA enhanced T1-weighted images versus enhanced and nonenhanced T2-weighted images. In patients who have been operated before and present with recurrent hyperparathyroidism, the evaluation of the parathyroid glands may start with MRI, CT, or a radionuclide examination. If those studies do not show the lesion, angiography [conventional with subtraction or intraarterial digital subtraction arteriography (DSA)]will be necessary to demonstrate the lesion. Venous sampling can be performed either before or after angiography. Considering that it might be possible to treat an adenoma by selective injection of contrast media alone, angiography should be performed before blood sampling.

There are several causes of unsuccessful initial neck surgery for primary hyperparathyroidism (16–19,101–103). These include failure to identify parathyroid glands in either a normal or abnormal location, and inadequate resection of a parathyroid hyperplasia.

Thermography

Thermography of the neck can detect foci of increased temperature in the neck between the suprasternal notch and the superior margin of the thyroid cartilage. These foci represent a lesion within either the thyroid or parathyroid gland and differentiation is very difficult (104,105). With the increase in quality of ultrasound, thermography is probably no longer important.

Conclusion

Noninvasive imaging studies for the evaluation of parathyroid disease are currently not always

reliable. Computed tomography, ultrasound, technetium/thallium scintigraphy, and magnetic resonance imaging are useful tools in detecting lesions after surgical intervention. The overall sensitivity of those noninvasive diagnostic methods is known to be 72% for CT, 57% for high-resolution real-time US, and 72% for computer-assisted technetium-99m/thallium-201 scintigraphy (TTS), with specificities of 92% for CT, 96% for US, and 93% for TTS. For lesions not located within the thyroid gland (thymic, tongue, mediastinum) sensitivities are 29% for CT, 20% for US, and 86% for TTS with specificities of 100% (70). TTS and CT are optimal tools to diagnose HPT with persistent or recurrent disease following exploratory surgery of the neck and for aberrant parathyroid tissue in the mediastinum. Other authors, using different equipment, describe the sensitivity of US in patients with recurrent HPT as being 82% of cervical parathyroid adenomas (38) and recommend starting the work-up of HPT with US followed by a CT or a TTS examination to evaluate the retrotracheal and mediastinal spaces, which are both difficult or impossible to reach by US.

For magnetic resonance imaging (MRI) of glandular and extraglandular parathyroid tissue the specificity is reported to be 63 to 88% (93, 103, 108). Miller et al. (107) has found that if CT, US, and scintigrapgic examinations are performed, at least one of these studies shows the lesion in 78% of cases. Two positive examinations, however, could only be achieved in 31%. These results demonstrate that there is still a good indication for invasive studies to localize remaining parathyroid tissue following surgery (106,108,109).

Invasive Diagnostic Procedures

Venous Sampling

Technique. The procedure of venous sampling is carried out under local anesthesia by the transfemoral approach (110). A vascular sheath is especially helpful in obese patients to ease exchange of catheters if necessary. A 5/7 French headhunter I or cobra-shaped catheter 100 cm in length is suitable to catheterize both

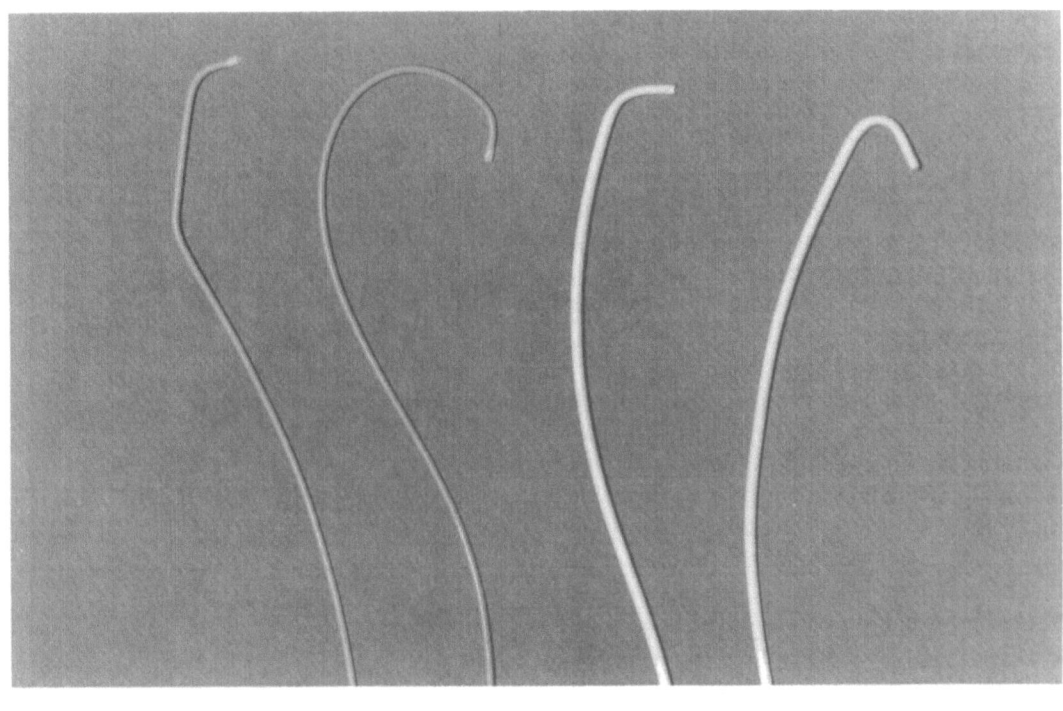

A

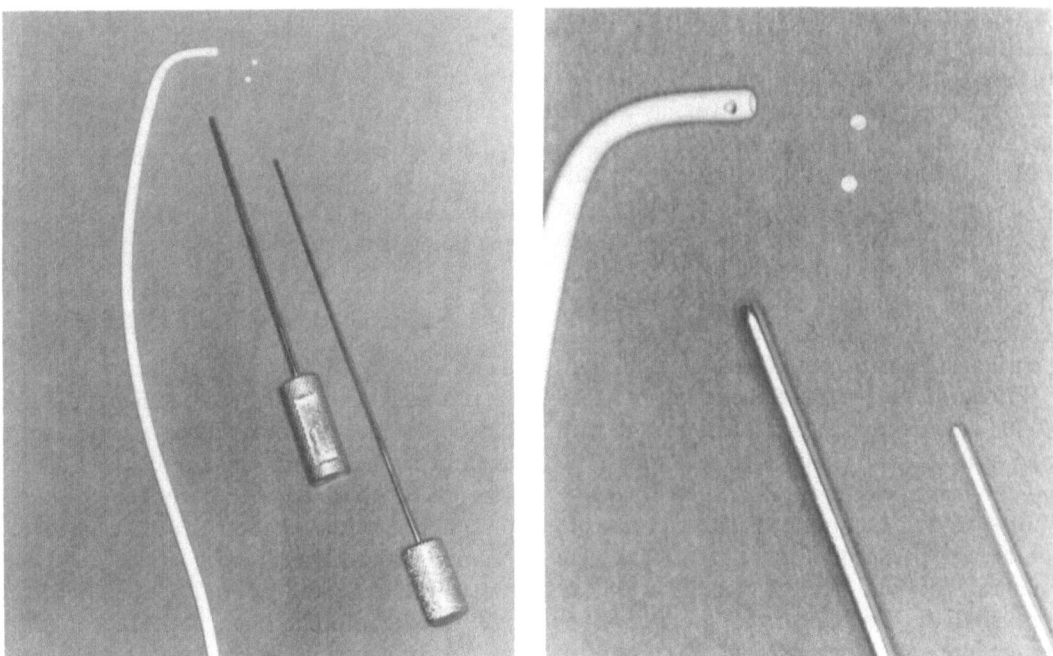

B   C

Figure 6.11. **A:** Four different shapes of catheters are suitable for parathyroid sampling procedures. (1) Haedhunter I, 100 cm, french 4–7; (2) Cobra, 80–100 cm, french 4–7; (3) Right Coronary, 100cm, french 4–7; (4) Internal mammary, 100 cm, french 4–7. **B:** All catheters should have one or two sideholes close to the tip of the catheter to ease the withdrawal of blood samples.

the left and right jugular veins and its tributaries draining the thyroid and parathyroid glands (Fig. 6.4–6.7). Blood sampling is easier, if one or two side holes are drilled close to the tip of the catheter (Fig. 6.11). The catheter is advanced through the right atrium into the brachiocephalic and jugular veins under fluoroscopic control. The patients should have ECG-monitoring during the procedure.

Thyroid and jugular veins have venous valves. These valves are often difficult to pass with a catheter. Although appearing rather delicate, the leaflets of venous valves cannot be deliberately perforated with the catheter tip without a major risk of venous wall perforation. To overcome this problem, steerable guide wires and specially coated wires (Terumo guides) almost always lead the catheter tip through the valves (Fig. 6.12). When veins are tortuous, especially in elderly patients, drinking will momentarily straighten them as the thyroid gland ascends and may permit catheter advancement. Once a catheter is well positioned, aspirating a blood sample can be equally frustrating. Gentle suction to avoid venous collapse, turning the head, or having the patient perform a Valsalva maneuver, as well as siphonage may be helpful.

The catherization procedure can be very difficult if there is an extremely wide jugular vein (Fig. 6.13). Different curved catheters have to be used to solve the problem.

The large amount of parathyroid hormone produced by an adenoma of one side will be in the ipsilateral venous sampling. In comparison, the parathormone level of the peripheral blood (or blood from the inferior vena cava) and with blood samples of the opposite side unilateral gradients can be calculated (18,21,31,111). The samples from the contralateral inferior thyroid vein are at background levels, because the remaining normal parathyroid glands are suppressed by the high PTH production of the adenoma. Primary hyperplasia results in bilateral unequally elevated PTH gradients, because hyperplasia is generally an asymmetric process. If PTH levels are more than two times the background levels (IVC, peripheral blood), they are considered to be significantly elevated (112).

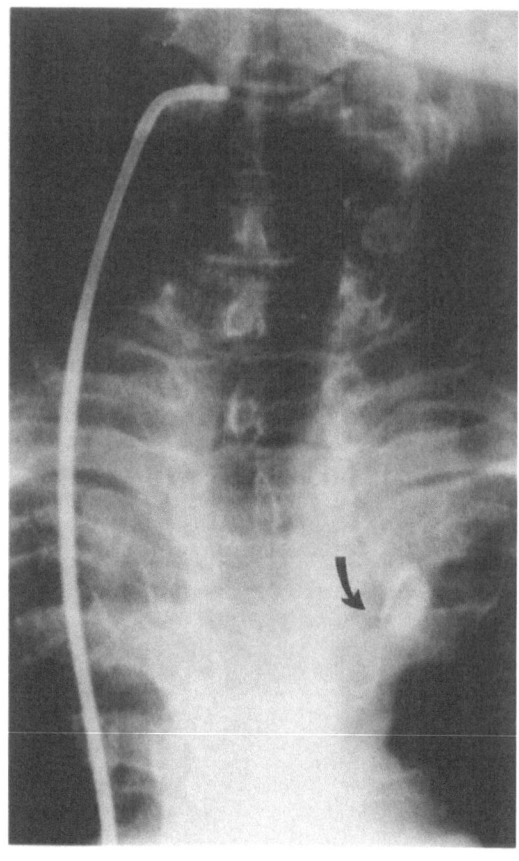

Figure 6.12. Catheter for venous sampling in the upper part of the right jugular vein. Opacification of a venous valve of the orifice of the left jugular vein from a previous injection (arrow).

Roadmapping of the Sampling

There is no need to take radiographs during the procedure, except for "roadmapping" the anatomy of the thyroid venous structures. A single radiograph with minimal contrast injection can be obtained with each sample to record the catheter position. A forceful large-volume retrograde venogram at this stage will display the complete thyroid venous bed and ease the catheterization procedure considerably. A drawing may help to ease the location of samples (Fig. 6.14).

Doppman and Hammond (20) suggest that unsuccessful surgery be followed by parathyroid arteriography, venous sampling, and computed tomography of the mediastinum (71,113). According to the authors, parathy-

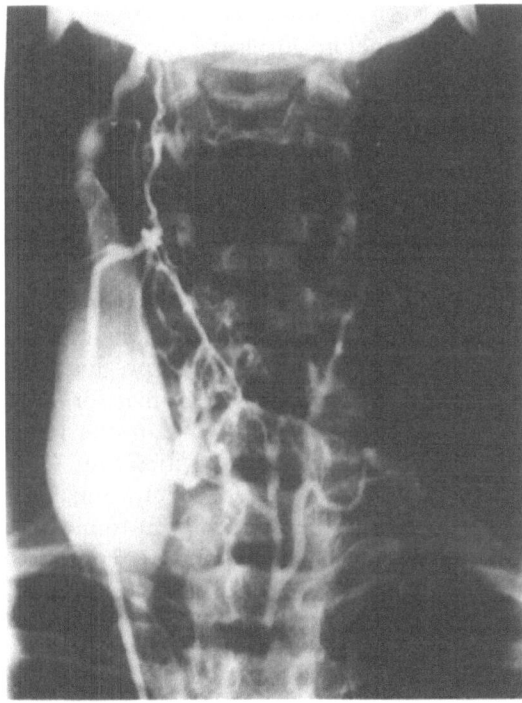

Figure 6.13. Extremely dilated right jugular vein retrograde filled via the right middle thyroeidal vein.

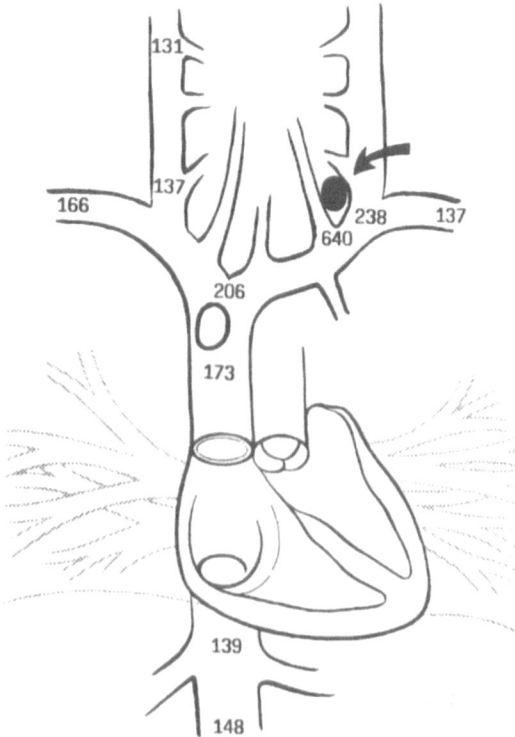

Figure 6.14. Diagram for parathyroid sampling. The drawing demonstrates the results of a sampling procedure in a patient with primary hyperparathyroidism. A parathyroid adenoma was located by intravenous selective sampling. Elevation of parathyroid hormone was found in the region of the left lower parathyroid gland (arrow). The adenoma was confirmed by surgery. The numbers demonstrate immune reactive parathormone (IPTH) in units/ml × 10 at the location of the different samples.

roid arteriography should be followed by venous sampling because normal venous anatomy is usually distorted by the surgeon and the venous phase of the arteriogram provides useful information about which veins are still intact to drain the parathyroid glands. Other authors follow different approaches and prefer sampling in the first place, followed by arteriography (114,115). Adenomas are occasionally stained by forceful retrograde venous injections. Frequently more helpful than staining has been the demonstration of a capsular or circumscribing vein surrounding the adenoma (116). When the appropriate artery cannot be catheterized, a forceful injection into the appropriate vein containing the elevated PTH level may reveal the site of the occult gland.

Technical Difficulties of Sampling— Aberrant Parathyroid Tissue and in Postoperative Anatomy

Venous sampling is the method of choice for localizing a parathyroid adenoma, aberrant parathyroid tissue, or parathyroid tissue following surgical exploration without the success of curing hyperparathyroidism. Mediastinal masses of parathyroid tissue occur in about 20% of cases examined for hyperparathyroidism (6). The accuracy of the sampling technique in predicting the site of hormone excess ranges from 50 to 90% (1,8,26,112,114, 117). Samples from the middle and superior thyroid veins are usually not helpful for localizing hormone excess unless the inferior veins have been ligated and venous drainage from the thyroid lobes comes from the upper portion of the glands. Even under such circumstances, the vertebral veins serve as collateral channels and have elevated PTH levels when the adenoma is in the neck or in the posterior superior mediastinum.

Vein samples from large vessels (jugular veins, innominate veins, superior vena cava) are generally not helpful (118). Elevation of PTH in these veins are usually very difficult to interpret in comparison to the gradients in selective veins. The interpretation of PTH gradients in the left innominate vein is particularly treacherous because the mediastinum and both sides of the neck drain into this vessel. Looking for peripheral PTH gradients following unilateral neck massage is also of no value in this group of patients (119,120,121,122).

Results of Sampling

The sensitivity of selective thyroid and thymic venous samples for parathormone assay is decreased when there are thyroid-thymic vein connections and distortion of the venous anatomy by previous surgery (5,22,32,33). The detection rate of venous sampling increases when sampling is used in combination with parathyroid arteriography (123,124,125).

A recent review of localization studies in Doppman's last 75 patients with primary hyperparathyroidism and one to four previous unsuccessful explorations showed that positive arteriographic-venographic localization was achieved in 50% and useful information (e.g., unilateral neck gradients but a negative arteriogram) was provided in 77%. False-positive localizations are extremely rare. Failure generally occured in patients who have had thyroid lobectomies, complete or subtotal, at a previous operation, because access to the thyroid/parathyroid vascular bed is denied when thyroid arteries are ligated. In addition, thyroid veins become extremely small and difficult to sample after thyroidectomy; catheter access to the parathyroid arterial and venous system is feasible only because parathyroid glands share the larger thyroid vascular system. Intrathyroid parathyroid glands, the surgeons justification for resection of thyroid tissue, are extremely rare. Doppman has encountered only six and all were correctly predicted by arteriographic localization studies (120,122). Surgeons failing to identify pathology at the initial neck ex-

ploration must be urged not to perform thyroidectomies before localizing studies can be performed.

Intraarterial DSA

Selective intraarterial DSA of the parathyroid glands is invasive and there should be strong indications before it is performed. Selective intraarterial DSA is indicated in patients with recurrent hypercalcemia after parathyroidectomy when the results of noninvasive imaging techniques are uncertain. A sensitivity of 81% can be expected (126–127, 128). In the neck and mediastinum the sensitivities are 73% (8/11) and 90% (9/10), respectively. Selective catheterization of the thyrocervical trunk, the internal mammary artery, and the superior thyroid artery is performed by the femoral approach (7,22,123,124,125,129). The procedure is/done with an nonionic contrast media, because injecting ionic contrast media into the small vessels of the thyroid gland is usually painful. If DSA is used, contrast media can be diluted 1:2 to 1:4 and still will create enough contrast to see pathology. Patients with hyperparathyroidism often have impaired renal function and therefore should be well hydrated before the procedure is started to prevent postangiographic renal failure. If vascular tortuosity prevents selective catheterization, venous sampling should be performed.

If the catheter is in a selective wedged position in the thyroid artery extensive staining may obscure pathology of the parathyroid glands. Oblique films or DSA in different positions will demonstrate the lesion.

The blood supply to a mediastinal adenoma may arise proximally from the inferior thyroid artery or from the thyrocervical trunk and may be missed by an injection distal into the vessel. With the new high-flow thin-wall catheters and the tracker catheter system that is used coaxially, very small vessels can be easily catheterized. The inferior thyroid artery may supply a contralateral parathyroid adenoma especially if the contralateral inferior thyroid artery has been ligated or after thyroidectomy.

The internal mammary artery sometimes originates from a common trunk together with the thyrocervical trunk. Multiple anterior intercostal arteries arise from the medial margin of the internal mammary artery and arc laterally to supply the anterior intercostal spaces. A prominent pericardiophrenic branch of the internal mammary artery is also common. It is important that these vessels are not taken for small thymic branches. They usually arise as second branches from the internal mammary artery and may enlarge to supply intrathymic parathyroid adenomas in the anterior mediastinum (25,76,126,129).

The vessel supplying a mediastinal adenoma can be enlarged, which makes the procedure of selective catherization much easier. The normal thymic gland does stain, especially in patients under 20 years of age, but the stain lacks the discrete margins of a parathyroid adenoma stain.

When either the inferior thyroid artery is small or the entire thyroid lobe is not stained by the inferior and superior thyroid artery injections, a search should be made for a thyroid ima artery (123,124,125). This vessel arises generally from the superior margin of the innominate artery and is ascending to supply the thyroid isthmus and the medial portions of both thyroid lobes. This vessel may enlarge following unsuccessful surgery if the normal thyroid blood supply is ligated. Doppman and Hammond (20) have detected four parathyroid adenomas supplied solely by this vessel.

Selective superior thyroid artery injections are painful and rarely disclose parathyroid pathology unless the ipsilateral inferior thyroid artery has been ligated. A proximally arising branch of the superior thyroid artery passes medially to supply the endolarynx and vocal cords, which stain densely. Coughing is often induced by this injection. This normal stain must not be confused with that of ectopic so-called parathymic parathyroid glands described by Edis et al. (67). These are undescended inferior glands lying above the upper pole of the thyroid.

Normal parathyroid glands are 1 to 2 mm in diameter and are never visualized arteriographically. Enlarged glands appear as oval or rounded areas of diffuse stain superimposed upon or lying below the thyroid lobes (84, 110,115). Doppman performs serial filming (1/sec) for 15 seconds to obtain arterial, capil-

lary, and venous phases, the latter being particularly helpful in planning the subsequent venous sampling (21). Enlarged glands as small as 4 to 5 mm can be seen on well-collimated optimally exposed films. AP and oblique projections (25° to 30°) are obtained on all inferior thyroid artery injections as the latter view will sometimes reveal posterior adenomas obscured by overlying thyroid stain. When an adenoma is demonstrated in the mediastinum, a steeply oblique or lateral projection should be obtained to distinguish anterior from posterior locations. Because areas of faint staining can be obscured by the overlying cervical spine, subtraction studies should be routine.

In patients with previous unsuccessful surgery, complete six-vessel parathyroid arteriography reveals the adenoma in about 50% of the cases. Venous gradients of parathyroid hormone are much more frequent than positive arteriographic studies in this patient group (85 to 90%), but localization by venous sampling alone has not proved to be reliable. Particularly when initial surgery has been competently performed, a parathyroid hormone (PTH) step-up in a vertebral vein or in an inferior thyroid vein stump is an insufficient basis for reexploration. For that reason arteriography with attempts actually to visualize the adenoma remains an integral part of the localization study.

Complications

The principal risk is damage to the spinal cord with quadriplegia. This results from excessive quantities of contrast material selectively injected into the costocervical trunk, which commonly provides a major radiculomedullary branch to the anterior spinal artery at the cervicothoracic level. Wedging of the catheter in this small vessel is difficult to avoid, and injection of even small amounts of contrast is likely to damage the cord. Also often incriminated in these accidents, the thyrocervical trunk rarely supplies vessels to the cord. In more than 1,000 thyrocervical trunk injections, subtracted and scrutinized for spinal cord blood supply, Doppman has encountered only three convincing examples. However, the costocervical trunk may be confused with the thyrocervical trunk on anteroposterior fluoroscopy, especially when the inferior thyroid artery has been ligated at the initial operation. In Doppman's extensive experience with parathyroid arteriography, no spinal complications have occurred (127,128).

Several instances of cortical blindness complicating parathyroid arteriography have been reported, but vision always returned within 48 hours. This complication results from excessive contrast material injected into the vertebral arteries during a prolonged search for the thoracocervical and internal mammary trunks. Patients with multiple endocrine adenomatosis may be harboring insulin or epinephrine secreting tumors that could complicate the arteriographic study.

Pheochromocytomas in multiple endocrine adenomatosis type II are frequently occult. Such risk factors should be completely evaluated prior to arteriography just as they would before any surgical procedure.

The most accurate method for localization of remaining parathyroid tissue is parathyroid arteriography (36,107). Intraarterial DSA can be performed either by nonselective injection into the aortic arch or by selective injection into the brachiocephalic arteries. Krudy et al. (125) reported 44% of 16 cases were localized by aortic injection. The sensitivity of IV DSA is 31%. Miller has reported 49% of adenomas located by arterial DSA accurately with one false-positive finding. The sensitivity for selective parathyroid DSA was 60%. Intraarterial DSA, selective arteriography, parathyroid venous sampling, and intraoperative sonography permits a localization of adenomas in 95% of the cases. In the study of Lacombe et al. (126) it was apparent that intraarterial DSA of the brachiocephalic vessels could locate most of the remaining abnormal cervical or mediastinal glands. The sensitivities of this method were 73% in the neck and 90% in the mediastinum.

Treatment

The treatment of hyperparathyroidism is surgical if the disease is symptomatic or progressive. The outcome of surgery depends on successful removal of all excess functioning tissue and on reversibility of renal damage. Renal insufficiency may progress despite cure of the underlying disease. Abnormal functioning of the parathyroid glands may be found in unusual locations and experience is required to find them. Preoperative localization of parathyroid tissue is possible by ultrasound or computed tomography. Abnormal function may be confirmed by immunoassay of the thyroid venous drainage. Such procedures are mandatory in all patients having had previous unsuccessful parathyroid surgery. Indications for surgery in patients with mild, asymptomatic primary HPT are yet to be clarified. Current data suggest that such patients be managed conservatively in the absence of progressive hypercalcemia or other complications. When HPT is mild no special preoperative precautions are required. The elevated serum Ca level drops to just below normal within 24 to 48 hours following surgery. In patients with severe osteitis fibrosa, prolonged symptomatic hypocalcemia may occur and require large doses of Ca together with vitamin D, usually for 1 to 3 months.

Transcatheter Therapy

Transcatheter ablation (22,62,107,127,128) of parathyroid adenomas can be performed, if selectivity of the feeding vessel is possible.

Ultrasound-Guided Percutaneous Treatment of Parathyroid Tumors

Nonoperative ablation of parathyroid adenomas by ultrasound-guided percutaneous direct injection of ethanol (96%) into the tumor in patients with uremia and secondary hyperparathyroidism has been performed by Solbiati et al. (63). This treatment is performed under ultrasound guidance with a fine needle (23 gauge, 0.6 mm). The procedure can be done on an outpatient basis under local anesthesia with 0.4 to 1.0 ml (58). Following the treatment, biochemical parameters decrease in PTH, and ionized calcium serum levels are expected to be observed immediately and up to 5 months (58). Complications have not been described so far;

however, small areas of hemorrhage and necrosis have been found following needle aspiration biopsy (40,63), and theoretically damage to the recurrent laryngeal nerve is possible (58).

Patients who were treated for hyperparathyroidism can be followed by examining the serum levels of parathormone or determining the bone mineral content (181).

References

1. Satava RM, Beahres OH, Scholz DA. Success rate of cervical exploration for hyperparathyroidism. *Arch Surg* 1975;110:625–628.
2. Dubost CI, Boucaut PH. Hyperparathyroide primaire: ètude rétrospective de 500 cas. *Presse Med* 1982;11:443–446.
3. Brennan MF, Norton JA. Reoperation for persistent and recurrent hyperparathyroidism. *Ann Surg* 1985;201:40–44.
4. Brennan MF. Reoperation of suspected hyperparathyroidism. In: Dudley HAF, De Cosse JJ, Morris PJ *Clinical Surgery International, vol. 4. Surgery of the Thyroid and the Parathyroid Glands*. Edinburgh, New York: Churchill-Livingstone, 1983:168–176.
5. Wang CA. Parathyroid re-exploration. A clinical and pathological study of 112 cases. *Ann Surg* 1977;186:140–145.
6. Nathaniels EK, Nathaniels AM, Wang C. Mediastinal parathyroid tumors: a clinical and pathological study of 84 cases. *Ann Surg* 1970;171:165–170.
7. Doppman JL. Parathyroid localisation: arteriography and venous sampling. *Radiol Clin North Am* 1976;46:403–418.
8. O'Riordan JLH, Kendall BE, Woodhead JS. Preoperative localisation of parathyroid tumors. *Lancet* 1971;2:1172–1175.
9. Levin KE, Gooding GAW, Okerlund M, Higgins CB, Norman D, Newton TH, Duh QY, Arnaud CD, Siperstein AE, Zeng QH, Clark OH. Localization studies in patients with persistent or recurrent hyperparathyroidism. *Surgery* 1987;102:917–925
10. Christensson T, Hellström K, Wengle B, Alveryd A, Wikland B. Prevalence of hypercalcemia in health screening in Stockholm. *Acta Med Scand* 1976;200:131–137.
11. Doppman JL, Marx S, Spiegel A, Brown E, Downs R, Brennan MF, Aurbach GD. Differential diagnosis of brown tumor versus

cystic osteitis by arteriography and computed tomography. *Radiology* 1979;131:339–340.
12. Roth SI. Recent advances in parathyroid pathology. *Am J Med* 1971;50:612–621.
13. Marx SJ, Stock JL, Attie MF, Downs RW Jr, Gardner DG, Brown EM, Spiegel AM, Doppman JL, Brennan MF. Familial hypercalciuric hypercalcemia: recognition among patients referred after unsuccessful parathyroid exploration. *Ann Intern Med* 1980;92:351–356.
14. Mallette LE, Bilezikian JP, Heath DA, Aurbach GD. Primary hyperparathyroidism: clinical and biochemical features. *Medicine (Baltimore)* 1974;53:127–146.
15. Van Heerden, JA, Weiland LH, ReMine WH, Walls JT, Purnell DC. Cancer of the parathyroid glands. *Arch Surg* 1979;114:475–480.
16. Akerström G, Malmaeus J, Bergström R. Surgical anatomy of the human parathyroid glands. *Surgery* 1984;95:14–21.
17. Wang CA, Mahaffey J, Axelrod L, Perlman JA. Hyperfunctioning supernumerary parathyroid glands. *Surg Gynecol Obstet* 1979; 148:711–714.
18. Thompson NW, Eckhauser FE, Harness JH. The anatomy of primary hyperparathyroidism. *Surgery* 1982;92:814–821.
19. Doppman JL. Parathyroid angiography In: Abrams HL, ed. *Abrams' Angiography*. Boston: Little, Brown; 1983:977–999.
20. Doppman JL, Hammond WG. The anatomic basis of parathyroid venous sampling. *Radiology* 1970;95:603–610.
21. Doppman JL, Hammond WG, Melson GI, Evens RG, Ketcham AS. Staining of parathyroid andenomas by selective arteriography. *Radiology* 1969;92:527–530.
22. Shimkin PM, Doppman JL, Pearson KD, Powell D. Anatomic considerations in parathyroid venous sampling. *AJR* 1973;118:654–662.
23. Doppman JL, Melson GL, Evens RG, Hammond WG. Selective superior and inferior thyroid vein catheterization. *Invest Radiol* 1969;4:97–99.
24. Öffermann G, Opitz A, Sörensen R. Localization of parathyroid adenomas in primary hyperparathyroidism. *Dtsch Med Wochenschr* 1974;99:1308–1312.
25. Doppman JL, Mallette LE, Marx S, Monchik J, Broadus A, Spiegel A, Beazley R, Aubach G. The localization of abnormal mediastinal parathyroid glands. *Radiology* 1975;115:31–34.

26. Doppman JL, Brennan MF, Brown EM. Tracheal overlap: Arteriograhic sign of parathyroid adenomas in the posterior superior mediastinum. *AJR* 1978;130:1197–1199.

27. Brennan MF, Doppman JL, Marx SJ, Spiegel AM, Brown EM, Aurbach GD. Reoperative parathyroid surgery for persistent hyperparathyroidism. *Surgery* 1978;83:669–676.

28. Brennan MF, Brown EM, Spiegel AM, Marx SJ, Doppman JL, Jones DC, Aurbach GD. Autotransplantation of cryopreserved parathyroid tissue in man. *Ann Surg* 1979;189:139–142.

29. Brennan MF, Brown EM, Marx SJ, Spiegel AM, Broadus AE, Doppman JL, Weber B, Aurbach GD. Recurrent hyperparathyroidism from an autotransplanted parathyroid adenoma. *N Engl J Med* 1978;299:1057–1059.

30. Haase GM, Luce JM, Lock JP, Hammond WS, Penn I. Hyperparathyroidism following parathyroid autotransplantation. *Surgery* 1979;86:694–697.

31. Wells SA Jr., Ellis JG, Gunnels JC, Schneider AB, Sherwood LM. Parathyroid autotransplantation in primary parathyroid hyperplasia. *N Engl J Med* 1976;295:57–62.

32. Brennan MF, Doppman JL, Kurdy AG, Marx SJ, Spiegel AM, Aurbach GD. Assessment of techniques for preoperative parathyroid gland localization in patients undergoing reoperation for hyperparathyroidism. *Surgery* 1982;91:6–12.

33. Clark OH. Parathyroid cysts *Am J Surg* 1978;135:395–402.

34. Clark OH, Okerlund MD, Moss AA, Stark D, Norman D, Newton TH, Duh QY, Arnaud CD, Harris S, Gooding GAW. Localization studies in patients with persistent or recurrent hyperparathyroidism. *Surgery* 1985;98:1083–1094.

35. Clark OH, Stark DD, Gooding GAW. Localization procedures in patients requiring reoperation for hyperparathyroidismus. *World J Surg* 1984;8:509–525.

36. Krudy AG, Doppman JL, Brennan MF, Marx SJ, Spiegel AM, Stock JL, Aurbach GD. The detection of mediastinal parathyroid glands by computed tomography, selective arteriography, and venous sampling. *Radiology* 1981;140:739–744.

37. Reading CC, Charboneau JW, James EM. High-resolution parathyroid sonography. *AJR* 1982;139:539–546.

38. Reading CC, Charboneau JW, James EM. Postoperative parathyroid high-frequency sonography: evaluation of persistent or recurrent hyperparathyroidism. *AJR* 1985;144:399–402.

39. Stark DD, Gooding GAW, Moss AA, Clark OH, Ovenfors CO. Parathyroid imaging: comparison of high-resolution CT and high-resolution sonography. *AJR* 1983;141:633–638.

40. Doppman JL, Shawker TH, Krudy AG. The parathymic parathyroid: CT, US, and angiographic findings. *Radiology* 1985;157:268–281.

41. Doppman JL, Krudy AG, Marx SJ, Saxe A, Schneider P, Norton JA, Spiegel AM, Downs RW, Schaaf M, Brennan ME, Schneider AB, Aurbach GD. Aspiration of enlarged parathyroid glands for hormone assay. *Radiology* 1983;148:31–35.

42. Winzelberg GG, Hydovitz JD, O'Hara KR, Anderson KM, Turbiner E, Danowski TS, Lippe RD, Melada GA, Harrison AM. Parathyroid adenomas evaluated by Tl-201/Tc-99m pertechnetate subtraction scintigraphy and high-resolution ultrasonography. *Radiology* 1985;155:231–235.

43. Percifal RC, Blake GM, Urwin GH, Talbot CH, Williams JL, Kanis JA, Path MR. Assessment of thallium-pertechnetate subtraction scintigraphy in hyperparathyroidism. *Br J Radiol* 1985;58:131–135.

44. Kier R, Herfkens RJ, Blinder RA, Leigth GS, Utz JA, Silverman PM. MRI with surface coils for parathyroid tumors: preliminary investigation. *AJR* 1986;147:497–500.

45. Kier R, Blinder RA, Herfkens RJ, Leight GS, Spritzer CE, Carroll BA. MR imaging with surface coils in primary hyperparathyroidism. *J Comput Assist Tomofr* 1987;11:863–868.

46. Spritzer CE, Gefter WB, Hamilton R, Greenberg BM, Axel L, Kressel HY. Abnormal parathyroid glands: high resolution MRI. *Radiology* 1987;162:487–491.

47. Miller DL, Doppman JL, Shawker TH, Krudy AG, Norton JA, Vucich JJ, Morrish KA, Marx SJ, Spiegel AM, Aurbach GD. Localisation of parathyroid ademomas in patients who have undergone surgery. Part I. Noninvasive imaging methods. *Radiology* 1987; 162:133–137.

48. Miller DL, Doppman JL, Krudy AG, Norton JA, Vucich JJ, Morrish KA, Marx SJ, Spiegel AM, Aurbach G. Localisation of parathyroid adenomas in patients who have undergone

surgery. Part II. Invasive procedures. *Radiology* 1987;162:138–141.
49. Okerlund MD, Sheldon K, Corpuz S, O'Connell W, Faulkner D, Clark 0, Galante M. A new method with high sensitivity and high specificity for localization of abnormal parathyroid glands. *Ann Surg* 1984;200:381–388.
50. Mancuso AA, Dillon WP. MRI of the head and neck. The neck. *Radiol Clin North Am* 1989;27:407–434.
51. Sample WF, Michell SP, Bledsoe RC. Parathyroid ultrasonography. *Radiology* 1978; 127:485–490.
52. Takebayashi S, Matsui K, Onohara Y. Sonography for early diagnosis of enlarged parathyroid glands in patients with secondary hyperparathyroidism. *AJR* 1987;148:911–914.
53. Buchwach KA, Mangum WB, Hahn FW. Preoperative localization of parathyroid adenomas *Laryngoscope* 1987;97:13–15.
54. Butch RJ, Simeone JF, Mueller PR. Thyroid and parathyroid ultrasonography. Radiol Clin North Am 1985;23:57–71.
55. Zocholl G, Kuhn FP, Kraus WG, Wagner P. High resolution 7.5/10 MHz-B-scan sonography for the localization of parathyroid tumors. *Fortschr Röntgenstr* 1986;144:422–427.
56. Norton JA, Shawker TH, Bonnie LJ, Spiegel AM, Marx SJ, Fitzpatrick L, Aurbach GD, Doppman JL. Intraoperative ultrasound and reoperative parathyroid surgery: an initial evaluation. *World J Surg* 1986;10:631–639.
57. Karstrup S, Hegedüs L. Concomitant thyroid disease in hyperparathyroidism: reasons for unsatisfactory ultrasonographical localization of parathyroid glands. *Eur J Radiol* 1986;6: 149–152.
58. Karstrup S, Holm HH, Torp-Pedersen S. Ultrasonically guided inactivation of parathyroid tumors. *Br J Radiol* 1987;60:667–670.
59. Karstrup S, Glenthoj A, Torp-Pedersen S. Ultrasonically guided fine needle aspiration of suggested enlarged parathyroid glands. *Acta Radiol* 1988;29:213–216.
60. Karstrup S, Glenthoj A, Torp-Pedersen S, Hegedüs L, Holm HH. Ultrasonically guided fine needle aspiration of suggested enlarged parathyroid glands. *Acta Radiol* 1988;29:213–216.
61. Solbiati G, Montali G, Croce F, Belloti E, Giangrande A, Ravetto C. Parathyroid tumors detected by fine-needle aspiration biopsy under ultrasonic guidance. *Radiology* 1983; 148:793–797.
62. Doppman JL, Adrian GK, Stephan JM, Saxe A, Schneider P, Norton JA, Spiegel AM, Downs RW, Schoof N, Brennan ME, Schneider AB, Auerbach GD. Aspiration of enlarged parathyroid glands for hormone assay. *Radiology* 1983;148:31–35.
63. Solbiati L, Giangrande A, De Pra L, Bellotti E, Cantu P, Ravetto C. Percutaneous ethanol injection of parathyroid tumors under ultrasound guidance. Treatment for secondary hyperparathyroidism. *Radiology* 1985;155: 607–611.
64. Rastad J, Lindgren PG, Ljunghall S, Johansson H, Malmaeus J, Rudberg C, Akerström G. Ultrasound scanning for preoperative location of parathyroid tumors. *Acta Chir Scand* 1984:150:199–204.
65. Krudy AG, Doppman JL, Miller DL, Norton JA, Marx SJ, Spiegel AM, Santora AC, Aurbach GD, Schaaf M. Detection of mediastinal parathyroid glands by nonselective digital arteriography. *AJR* 1984;142:693–695.
66. Edis AJ, Evans TC. High-resolution, real-time ultrasonography in the preoperative localization of parathyroid tumors. *N Engl J Med* 1979;301:532–534.
67. Edis AJ, Purnell DC, Van Heerden JA. The undescended "parathymus": an occasional cause of failed neck exploration in hyperparathyroidism. *Ann Surg* 1979;190:64–68.
68. Graif M, Itzchak Y, Strauss S. Parathyroid sonography: diagnostic accuracy related to shape, location and texture of the gland. *Br J Radiol* 1987;60:439–443.
69. Randel SB, Gooding GAW, Clark OH, Stein RM, Winkler B. Parathyroid variants: US evaluation. *Radiology* 1987;165:191–194.
70. Krubsack AJ, Wilson SD, Lawson TL, Collier BD, Hellman RS, Isitman AT. Prospective comparison of radionuclide, computed tomography, and sonographic localisation of parathyroid tumors. *World J Surg* 1986;10:579–585.
71. Bilezikian JP, Doppman JL, Shimkin PM, Powell D, Wells SA, Heath DA, Ketcham AS, Onchik J, Mallette LE, Potts J Jr, Aurbach GD. Preoperative localisation of abnormal parathyroid tissue: cumulative experience with venous sampling and arteriography. *Am J Med* 1973;55:505–514.
72. Ovenfors CO, Stark D, Moss A, Goldberg H, Clark 0, Galante M. Localization of parathyroid adenoma by computed tomography. *J Comput Assist Tomogr* 1982;6:1094–1098.

73. MacFarlane SD, Hanelin LG, Taft DA, Ryan JA Jr., Fredlund PN. Localization of abnormal parathyroid glands using thallium-201. *Am Surg* 1984;148:7–13.

74. Doppman JL, Brennan MF, Koehler JO, Marx SJ. Computed tomography for parathyroid localisation. *J Comput Assist Tomogr* 1977; 1:30–37

75. Cates JD, Thorsen MK, Lawson TL. CT evaluation of parathyroid adenomas: diagnostic criteria and pitfalls. *J Comput Assist Tomogr* 1988;12:626–631.

76. Doppman, JL, Marx SJ, Brennan MF, Beazly RM, Geelhoed G, Aurbach GD. The blood supply of mediastinal parathyroid adenomas. *Ann Surg* 1977;185:488–490

77. Sommer B, Welter HF, Spelsberg F, Scherer U, Lissner J. Computed tomography for localizing enlarged parathyroid glands in primary hyperparathyroidism. *J Comput Assist Tomogr* 1982;6:521–526.

78. Awwad EE, Archer CR, Krebs FJ. Parathyroid adenomas; computed tomographic imaging and the importance of preoperative localization. *Comput Med Imaging Graph* 1988;12:305–309.

79. Takagi H, Tominaga Y, Uchida K, Yamada N, Ishii T, Morimoto T, Yasue M. Preoperative diagnosis of secondary hyperparathyroidism using computed tomography. *J Comput Assist Tomogr* 1982;6:527–528.

80. Lineaweaver W, Clore F, Mancuso A, Hill S, Rumley T. Calcified parathyroid glands detected by computed tomography. *J Comput Assist Tomogr* 1984;8:975–977.

81. Silverman PM, Newman GE, Korobkin M, Workman JB, Moore AV, Coleman RE. Computed tomography in the evaluation of thyroid disease. *AJR* 1984;141:897–902.

82. Whitley NO, Bohlman M, Connor TB, McCrea ES, Mason GR, Whitley JE. Computed tomography for localization of parathyroid adenomas. *J Comput Assist Tomogr* 1981;5:812–817.

83. Blake GM, Percival RC, Kanis JA. Thallium-pertechnetate subtraction scintigraphy: a quantitative comparison between adenomatous and hyperplastic parathyroid glands. *Eur J Nucl Med* 1986;12:31–36.

84. Al-Suhaili AR, Lynn J, Lavender JP. Intrathyroidal parathyroid adenoma: preoperative identification and localization by parathyroid imaging. *Clin Nucl Med* 1988;13:512–515.

85. Wells SA Jr., Ketcham AS, Marx SJ, Powell D, Bilezikian JP, Shimkin PM, Potts JT Jr., Pearson KD, Doppman JL. Preoperative localization of hyperfunctioning parathyroid tissue: radioimmuniassay of parathyroid hormone in plasma from selectively catheterized veins. *Ann Surg* 1973;177:93–98.

86. Maslack MM, Brosbe RJ. Dual isotope parathyroid imaging. *Clin Nucl Med* 1986;11:622–625.

87. Fine EJ. Parathyroid imaging: its current status and future role. *Semin Nucl Med* 1987; 17:350–359.

88. Manni A, Basarab RM, Plourde PV, Koivunen D, Harrison TS, Santen RJ. Thallium-Technetium parathyroid scan. *Arch Intern Med* 1986;146:1077–1080.

89. Picard D, D'Amour P, Carrier L. Localization of abnormal parathyroid gland(s) using thallium-201/iodine-123 subtraction scintigraphy in patients with primary hyperparathyroidism. *Clin Nucl Med* 1987;12:60–64.

90. Gooding GAW, Okerlund MD, Stark DD, Clark OH. Parathyroid imaging: comparison of double-tracer (T1-201, Tc-99m) scintigraphy and high-resolution US. *Radiology* 1986;161: 57–64.

91. Skibber JM, Reynolds JC, Spiegel AM, Marx SJ, Fitzpatrick LA, Aurbach GD, Wesley RA, Norton JA. Computerized technetium/thallium scans and parathyroid reoperation. *Surgery* 1985;98:1077–1082.

92. Auffermann W, Gooding GAW, Okerlund MD. Diagnosis of recurrent hyperparathyroidism: comparison of MR imaging and other imaging techniques. *AJR* 1988;150:1027–1033.

93. Auffermann W, Guis M, Taveras NJ, Clark OH, Higgins CB. MR signal intensity of parathyroid adenomas: correlation with histopathology. *AJR* 1989;153:873–876.

94. Peck WW, Higgins CB, Fisher MR, Ling M, Okerlund MD, Clark OH. Hyperparathyroidism: comparison of MR imaging with radionuclide scanning. *Radiology* 1987;163:415–420.

95. Kang EH, Schiebler ML, Gefter WB. MR demonstration of bilateral intrathyroidal parathyroid glands. *J Comput Assist Tomogr* 1988;12:349–352.

96. Sandler MP. High-resolution MR imaging of abnormal parathyroid glands. *Radiology* 1988; 166:582.

97. Higgins CB, Auffermann W. MR imaging of thyroid and parathyroid glands: a review of the current status. *AJR* 1988;151:1085–1106.

98. Seelos CS, DeMarco R, Clark OH, Higgins

CB. Persistent and recurrent hyperparathyroidism: assessment with gadopentetate dimeglumine-enhanced MR imaging. *Radiology* 1990;177:373–378.

99. Robinson JD, Crawford SC, Teresi LM. Extracranial lesions of the head and neck: preliminary experience with Gd-DTPA-enhanced MR imaging. *Radiology* 1989;172:165–170.

100. Hamilton R, Greenberg BM, Gefter W, Kressel H, Spritzer C. Successful localization of parathyroid adenomas by magnetic resonance imaging. *Am J Surg* 1988;155:370–373.

101. Mitchell DG, Vinitski S, Rifkin MD, Burk DL. Sampling bandwidth and fat suppression. *AJR* 1989;153:419–425.

102. Wang CA. The anatomic basis of parathyroid surgery. *Ann Surg* 1976;271:271–275.

103. Kneeland JB, Krubsack AJ, Lawson TL, Wilson SD, Collier BD, Froncisz W, Jesmanowicz A, Hyde JS. Enlarged parathyroid glands: high resolution local coil MR imaging. *Radiology* 1987;162:143–146.

104. Samuels BI, Dowdy AH, Lecky JW. Parathyroid thermography. *Radiology* 1972;104:575–578.

105. Samuels BI. The present status of parathyroid thermography. *JAMA* 1975;233:907–908.

106. Vogel T, Hefele B, Hahn D, Nieden Z, Mühlig HP. A comparitive study of MR, CT, and sonography in patients with primary hyperparathyroidism. *Fortschr Röntgenstr* 1986;145:167–172.

107. Miller DL, Doppman JL, Chang R, Simmons JT, O'Leary TJ, Norton JA, Spiegel AM, Marx SJ, Aurbach GD. Angiographic ablation of parathyroid adenomas: lessons from a 10 year experience. *Radiology* 1987;165:601–606.

108. Von Schulthess GK, Weder W, Goebel N, Buchmann P, Gadze A, Augustiny N, Largiadèr F. 1.5 T MRI, CT, ultrasonography, and scintigraphy in hyperparathyroidism. *Eur J Radiol* 1988;8:157–164.

109. Erdmann WA, Breslau NA, Weinreb JC. Noninvasive localization of parathyroid adenomas: a comparison of x-ray computerized tomography, ultrasound, scintigraphy and MRI. *Magn Reson Imaging* 1989;7:187–194.

110. Seldinger SI. Localization of parathyroid adenomata by arteriography. *Acta Radiol (Stockh)* 1954;42:353–366.

111. Hjern B, Almquiost S, Granberg PO, Lindvall N, Wästhed B. Pre-operative localization of parathyroid tissue by selective neck vein catheterization and radioimmunoassay of para-

thyroid hormone. *Acta Chir Scand* 1975; 141:31–39.

112. Powell D, Shimkin PM, Wells S, Aurbach GD, Marx SJ, Kecham AS, Potts JT Jr. Primary hyperparathyroidism: Preoperative tumor localization and differentiation between adenoma and hyperplasia. *N Engl J Med* 1972; 286:1169–1175.

113. Doppman JL, Wells SA, Shimkin PM, Pearson KD, Bilezikian JP, Heath DA, Powell D, Ketcham AS, Aurbach GD. Parathyroid localization by angiographic techniques in patients with previous neck surgery. *Br J Radiol* 1973;46:403–418.

114. Eisenberg H, Pallotta J, Sherwood LM. Selective arteriography, venography and venous hormone assay in diagnosis and localization of parathyroid lesions. *Am J Med* 1974;56:810–820.

115. Newton TH, Eisenberg E. Angiography of parathyroid adenomas. *Radiology* 1966;86:843–850.

116. Doppman JL, Brennan MF, Kahn CR, Marx SJ. The circumscribing or per-adenomal vessel: a helpful angiographic finding in certain islet cell and parathyroid adenomas. *AJR* 1981;136:163–165.

117. Godwin JD, Chen JTT. Thoracic venous anatomy. *AJR* 1986;147:674–684.

118. Reitz RE, Pollard JJ, Wang CA, Fleischli DJ, Cope O, Murray TM, Deftos LJ, Potts JT Jr. Localization of parathyroid adenomas by selective venous catheterization and radioimmunoassay. *N Engl J Med* 1969;281:348–351.

119. Reiss E, Canterbury JM. Primary hyperparathyroidism: application of radioimmunoassay in differentiation of adenoma and hyperplasia and preoperative localization of hyperfunctioning parathyroid glands. *N Engl J Med* 1969;280:1381–1385.

120. Spiegel AM, Marx SJ, Doppman JL, Beazley RM, Ketcham AS, Kasten B Aurbach GD. Intrathyroidal parathyroid adenoma or hyperplasia: an occasional overlooked cause of surgical failure in primary hyperparathyroidism. *JAMA* 1975;234:1029–1033.

121. Spiegel AM, Doppman JL, Marx SJ, Brennan MF, Brown EM, Downs RW, Garner DG, Attie M, Aurbach GD. Preoperative localization of abnormal parathyroids: neck massage vs. arteriography and selective venous sampling. *Ann Intern Med* 1978;89:935–936.

122. Spiegel AM, Adamson RH, Mallette LE, Doppman JL, Beazley RM, Ketcham AS, Kas-

ten B, Aurbach GD. Intrathyroid parathyroid tumors: a seldom recognized cause of surgical failure in primary hyperparathyroidism. *JAMA* 1975;234:1029–1033.

123. Krudy A, Doppman JL, Brennan MF. The significance of the thyroidea ima artery in arteriographic localization of parathyroid adenomas. *Radiology* 1980;136:51–55.

124. Krudy AG, Doppman JL, Brennan MF, Saxe AW, Marx SJ. Arteriographic localization of parathyroid adenoma in the presence of lingual thyroid. *AJR* 1981;136:1227–1230.

125. Krudy AG, Doppman JL, Miller DL, et al. Work in progress—abnormal parathyroid glands: comparison of nonselective arterial digital subtraction arteriography, selective parathyroid arteriography, and venous digital arteriography as methods of detection. *Radiology* 1983;148:23–29.

126. Lacombe P, Foster D, Dubost C, Schouman-Clays E, Frija G, Assens P, Bismuth V. Selective intraarterial DSA of the parathyroid glands in patients with hyperparathyroidism after parathyroidectomy. *AJR* 1987;149:479–483.

127. Doppman JL, Marx SJ, Spiegel A, Mallette LE, Wolfe BA, Aurbach GD, Geelhoed G. Treatment of hyperparathyroidism by percutaneous embolization of a mediastinal adenoma. *Radiology* 1975;115:37–42.

128. Doppman JL, Brown EM, Brennan MF, Spiegel A, Marx SJ, Aurbach GD. Angiographic ablation of parathyroid adenomas. *Radiology* 1979;130:577–582.

129. Rossi P, Carillo FJ, Johnston B. Angiography in the diagnosis of parathyroid carcinoma. *N Engl J Med* 1971;284:198–201.

130. Yune, HY, Klatte EC. Mediastinal Venography Subselective Transfemoral Catheterization Technique. *Radiology* 1972;105:285–291.

131. Richardson ML, Pozzi-Mucelli RS, Kanter AS, Kolb FO, Ettinger B, Genant HK. Bone mineral changes in primary hyperparathyroidism. *Skeletal Radiol* 1986;15:85–95.

7

Clinical and Laboratory Evaluation of Endocrine Diseases

—— Claudio E. Kater and Jose Gilberto H. Vieira ——

Introduction

Despite what the title may imply, it is beyond the scope of this chapter to present extensive clinical and laboratory data on endocrine diseases. Not even an entire separate textbook would suffice. Thus, our purpose in this review is to concentrate on those relevant endocrine syndromes for which, as part of the investigative strategy, a percutaneous venous blood sampling might help in determining a final diagnosis.

Adrenal and Ovarian Hormones

The adrenal cortex produces a variety of steroid hormones. The most important are the glucocorticoids (cortisol and corticosterone), the mineralocorticoids [aldosterone and deoxycorticosterone (DOC)], and the sex hormones, especially adrenal androgens [dehydroepiandrosterone (DHEA) and its sulfate (DHEA-S)] (1). Depending on the steroid hormone produced in excess, a distinct clinical syndrome will develop: cortisol excess results in Cushing's syndrome; aldosterone excess in primary aldosteronism (Conn's syndrome), and excess androgens lead to syndromes of hirsutism and virilization in the adult woman and precocious puberty (iso- or heterosexual) in prepubertal children. Occasionally, excess production of adrenal estrogens will result in a syndrome of feminization in men. Not infrequently, excess production of different steroid hormones manifests as combined syndromes.

Since the ovaries produce not only estrogens (estradiol and estrone) but also androgens (testosterone and androstenedione), immediate precursors for estrogen formation, syndromes of virilization in women and children have to be evaluated with regard to the origin of the excessive androgen production. Similarly, syndromes of feminization in men result from estrogen excess either from adrenal or testicular source (due to the potential of the Leydig cell to transform androgens in estrogens).

Therefore, data will be presented according to each steroid hormone produced in excess and its respective clinical syndrome.

Cortisol and Cushing's Syndrome

Excessive and continuous production of cortisol by the adrenal cortex zona fasciculata, and prolonged administration of pharmacologic doses of synthetic glucocorticoid analogues (prednisone and dexamethasone) lead to the classic stigmata of Cushing's syndrome, whose main clinical manifestations are centripetal obesity; round facies with plethora ("moon facies"); dorsocervical ("buffalo hump") and supraclavicular fat deposition; muscle atrophy;

purple striae in the lower abdomen, thighs, axillae, buttocks, and breasts; thinning of the skin; arterial hypertension; glucose intolerance and diabetes mellitus; easy bruisability; osteoporosis; and menstrual abnormalities (oligomenorrhea and amenorrhea) (2,3).

Cortisol can be secreted autonomously by a unilateral adrenocortical neoplasm (adenoma or carcinoma), in which case Cushing's syndrome is said to be primary or of adrenal origin; on the other hand, it can be secreted by both adrenals in response to continuous stimulation by adrenocorticotropic hormone (ACTH) of pituitary origin (pituitary micro- or macroadenoma) or from an ectopic source (the "ectopic ACTH syndrome"), most commonly due to a malignancy of the lung, pancreas, or thymus (4–6). In this condition, known as secondary Cushing's syndrome, both adrenal cortices are hyperplastic. Pituitary Cushing's syndrome is also referred to as Cushing's disease in honor of Harvey Cushing's distinct description of this pathology in 1932 (7).

Cushing's disease may seldom originate from abnormal pituitary secretion of ACTH due to hypothalamic dysregulation in corticotropin releasing hormone (CRH) secretion (hypothalamic neurosecretory dysfunction of CRH) (8); rare cases of ectopic CRH secretion by nonendocrine malignancies have also been reported (9). Primary Cushing's syndrome can occasionally be associated with tumors of embryonic rests or with primary nodular ("pigmentosa") adrenocortical dysplasia or hyperplasia (10).

Two-thirds of Cushing's syndrome cases are due to ACTH-producing pituitary micro/macroadenomas (Cushing's disease), whereas ectopic ACTH-producing tumors cause 12% of cases; Cushing's syndrome due to autonomous cortisol production by adrenocortical tumors has an incidence of about 18% (equally distributed between adenoma and carcinoma). Less than 5% of the cases are due to other abovementioned causes.

Laboratory diagnosis of Cushing's syndrome is aimed at both establishing unequivocal cortisol excess and identifying the etiology of the syndrome. Although the first step is usually accomplished by simple plasma and/or urinary determinations, the second step involves several maneuvers that, not infrequently, are deceptive in establishing the differential diagnosis of Cushing's syndrome. In addition, radiologic or imaging procedures are always necessary to confirm the anatomic lesion.

The following biochemical routine procedures and dynamic tests are used for the diagnosis of Cushing's syndrome:

Determination of Urinary Free Cortisol Excretion Rate

The 24-hour urinary excretion rate of free cortisol correlates very accurately with its daily secretion rate, which is normally between 20 and 30 mg/24 hr (11); 24-hour urinary free cortisol excretion greater than 100 μg/24 hr is indicative of endogenous hypercortisolism (12). False-positive results may occur in association with acute or chronic illnesses, other stressful situations, alcohol abuse, and endogenous depression.

To avoid the inaccurate 24-hour urinary volume collection, especially in children, which causes misleading false-negative results, free cortisol concentration (as well as any hormones to be measured in a 24-hour urine specimen) should be expressed per gram of creatinine simultaneously excreted (24-hour urinary creatinine excretion correlates very well with body weight and body surface area), provided the patient's renal function is normal (12).

Determination of Plasma/Serum Cortisol Levels

Cortisol can be measured in plasma or serum by several laboratory methods [fluorometry, competitive protein (CBG)-binding assay, radioimmuno- or enzyme-assay, radioreceptorassay and UV detection during high-performance liquid chromatography (HPLC) separation]. Radioimmunoassay (RIA) is the most commonly available method; it is known for its simplicity and high specificity and accuracy. The above procedures determine total circulating cortisol (both free and protein-bound fractions). RIA can performed with 100 to 200 μl of plasma or serum; no special care is needed for blood collection or storage (13).

Figure 7.1. Individual serum cortisol levels determined three times
daily (between 8 and 10 A.M., 4 and 6
P.M., and 10 P.M. and 12 midnight) in
34 patients with Cushing's syndrome
(Cushing's disease, $n = 23$ [●];
adrenal adenoma, $n = 5$ [○]; adrenal
carcinoma, $n = 6$ [△]). Stippled areas
represent the normal range (mean ±
2 SD).

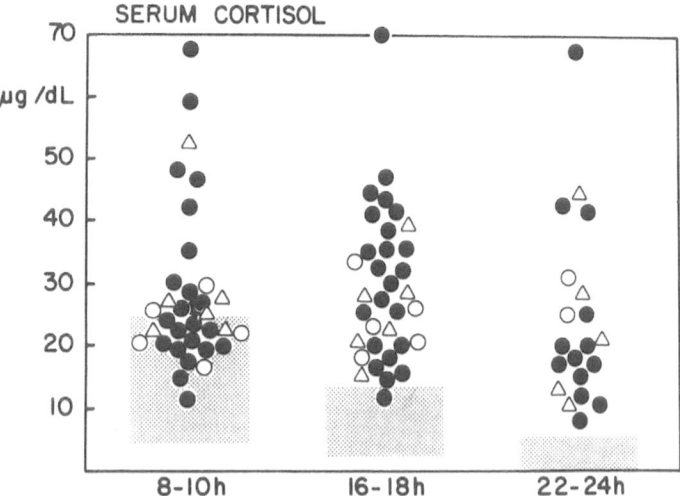

Plasma free cortisol can be determined after
equilibrium dialysis but does not necessarily
add significant information for the diagnosis.

In physiologic conditions, adrenocortical
secretion of cortisol follows a characteristic 24-
hour rhythmic pattern, the so-called circaadian
or nyctohemeral rhythm. This phenomenon is
inherent to the autonomic nervous system and
associated with the individual sleep-awake
habitus; it influences adrenocortical production
of cortisol via ACTH and typically presents
higher plasma levels during the early morning
hours, gradually decreasing during the day,
and reaching its nadir by bedtime. Absence of
the circadian rhythm is one of the initial and
most consistent biochemical abnormalities in
Cushing's syndrome (8,11); plasma/serum cortisol levels are fixed and frequently (but not
necessarily) elevated throughout the day.

Thus, simple baseline determinations of
plasma/serum cortisol should take into consideration the time of the day. We sample the
suspected patient usually three times daily: between 8 and 10 A.M., 4 and 6 P.M., and 10 P.M.
and midnight. Evaluation of the plasma/serum
cortisol rhythm is a high-sensitivity lowspecific-
ity test since a variety of different stimuli
(stress, alcoholism, depressive syndromes)
may produce false-positive responses. Figure
7.1 shows the results of serum cortisol obtained
three times a day in 34 patients with Cushing's
syndrome of different etiologies.

Overnight 1-mg Dexamethasone Suppression Test (DST)

This simple procedure is performed either as a
complement of the previous test (evaluation of
the absence of circadian cortisol rhythm) or as
the initial screening test for the diagnosis of
Cushing's syndrome. Dexamethasone (1 mg
PO) is administered between 11 P.M. and 12
midnight and a blood sample for cortisol determination is drawn the next morning (14– 16).

In normal subjects, pituitary secretion of
ACTH is regulated by peripheral cortisol levels
through the negative feedback mechanism.
Supraphysiologic doses of a potent synthetic
glucocorticoid analogue such as dexamethasone, administered to normal subjects, will
suppress ACTH secretion that would occur
during the early morning hours, thus impairing
parallel elevation in plasma/serum cortisol
levels. Dexamethasone does not interfere with
the RIA determination of plasma/serum cortisol or its urinary metabolites.

In patients with Cushing's syndrome,
plasma/serum cortisol levels do not suppress
due to (a) autonomy of cortisol production in
the primary (adrenal) disease, or (b) an abnormality in the negative feedback in Cushing's
disease characterized by corticotroph resistance to reduce ACTH secretion with only
slightly elevated glucocorticoid (dexamethasone) levels. A fall the next morning in plasma/

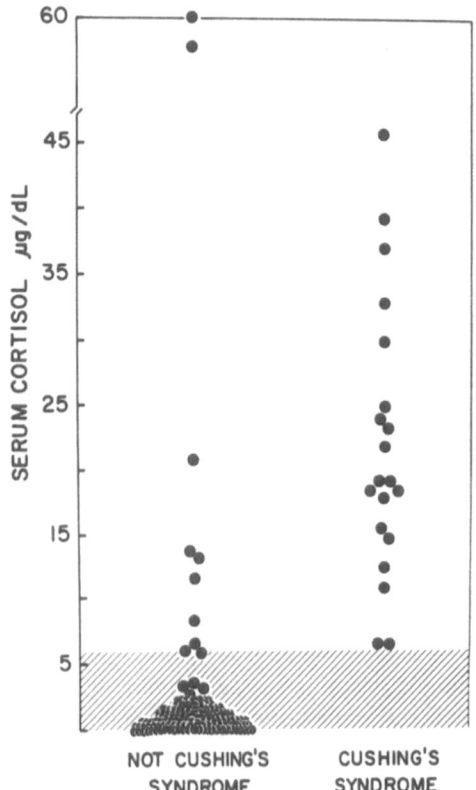

Figure 7.2. Individual serum cortisol levels determined at 8:00 A.M. after overnight 1-mg dexamethasone suppression in 20 patients with surgically confirmed Cushing's syndrome of different etiologies and 149 suspected patients in whom the diagnosis was subsequently ruled out. Hatched area represents the upper limit of normal (6 µg/dl).

bolism of dexamethasone (such as phenytoin, phenobarbital, or primidone), obesity, pregnancy or use of oral contraceptives (which increase CBG), acute and chronic illnesses, stress, depressive syndromes, and alcoholism (17).

"Classic" Dexamethasone Suppression Test (Liddle's Test)

Although designed in 1960 (18), Liddle's classic DST still is the reference test for the functional and differential diagnosis of Cushing's syndrome. It is performed in two stages:

The 2-Day Low-Dose Test. After a basal 24-hour urinary specimen and/or a blood sample is collected, respectively, for 17-hydroxycorticosteroids (17-OHCS) or urinary free cortisol and for plasma/serum cortisol, dexamethasone (0.5 mg PO every 6 hours) is given for 48 hours beginning at 12 noon. A second 24-hour urine specimen is collected during the second day of dexamethasone administration and/or a blood sample is drawn in the morning, at the end of the test, 2 hours after the last dose of dexamethasone. Normal responses are suppression of the urinary excretion of 17-OHCS to less than 4 mg/24 hr (or urinary free cortisol to less than 25 µg/24 hr) and plasma/serum cortisol to less than 5 µg/dl. Postdexamethasone values above these levels establish the diagnosis of endogenous hypercortisolism. False-positive and false-negative results are uncommon.

The 2-Day High-Dose Test. The procedure above is repeated now with a higher dexamethasone dose (2 mg PO every 6 hours for an additional 2 days), in an attempt to suppress ACTH in the ACTH-dependent Cushing's disease. Patients with Cushing's disease (pituitary hypersecretion of ACTH) usually suppress urinary 17-OHCS excretion (or urinary free cortisol) and plasma/serum cortisol levels to values less than 50% of baseline, whereas those with primary adrenal disease maintain elevated levels identifying the autonomy of cortisol production by the adrenal tumors. Also, the ectopic ACTH syndrome is resistant to suppression. Occasionally, even higher

serum cortisol to values below 6 µg/dl is considered a normal response (16).

Figure 7.2 shows individual serum cortisol responses obtained after overnight 1-mg DST in 20 surgically confirmed cases of Cushing's syndrome and 149 patients in whom the pathology was ruled out with subsequent testing. A sensitivity of 100% with specificity of 94.6% qualify the overnight DST as the best screening procedure for the diagnosis of Cushing's syndrome owing to its simplicity and high accuracy (16). False-positive results (absence of suppression in patients who do not have Cushing's syndrome) may occur due to failure in the ingestion or absortion of dexamethasone, previous use of drugs that accelerate hepatic meta-

doses of dexamethasone (16 or 32 mg/day) may be necessary to suppress ACTH and cortisol in the hypothalamic-pituitary disease due to singular corticotroph resistance (higher set-point for the negative feedback) (17).

The Overnight High-Dose Test.

It has been recently shown that overnight administration of a single 8-mg dose of dexamethasone at 11 P.M., followed by a blood collection for plasma/serum cortisol the next morning, aside from its simplicity, has an even higher sensitivity (92% versus 79%) and accuracy (93% versus 83%) as compared to the classic 2-day high-dose test (19). In the last 4 years it has been our policy to utilize the overnight instead of the 2-day high-dose DST.

Diagnostic procedures involving the determination of plasma ACTH in Cushing's syndrome are presented below (see Pituitary Hormones).

Aldosterone and Primary Aldosteronism (Conn's Syndrome)

Primary hyperaldosteronism is clinically characterized by hypertension and hypokalemia (20); additionally, expansion of the extracellular (plasma) fluid volume and increase in total body sodium result in renin-angiotensin suppression. Additional clinical features include metabolic alkalosis, glucose intolerance, and resistance to antidiuretic hormone action (vasopressin-resistant diabetes insipidus), all consequences of chronic hypokalemia (21,22).

Primary aldosteronism is due to an aldosterone-producing adrenocortical adenoma (APA) in 60 to 70% of cases; 30% are due to micro/macronodular adrenocortical hyperplasia, also called idiopathic hyperaldosteronism (IHA) (23). The remaining 5 to 10% encompasses cases of adrenocortical carcinoma (24,25), "primary adrenal hyperplasia" (an entity similar to the adrenocortical nodular dysplasia of Cushing's syndrome) (26,27), angiotensin-responsive adenomas (28–30), and ectopic aldosterone production by nonadrenal tumors (mainly from ovarian origin) (31,32).

The diagnosis of primary aldosteronism is based on the presence of spontaneous hypo-

kalemia in the hypertensive patient, usually a woman between 25 and 45 years. Hormonal measurements and diagnostic maneuvers should only be performed after discontinuing any previous medications for at least 3 weeks, especially diuretics, glucocorticoids, and oral contraceptives. Other treatable causes of hypertension, such as Cushing's syndrome, pheochromocytoma, coarctation of the aorta, renal artery stenosis, and parenchymal kidney disease, should be excluded. It is advisable to conduct any detailed biochemical investigation after the patient has been equilibrated on a fixed metabolic diet containing 120 to 150 mEq of sodium (Na) and 60 to 80 mEq of potassium (K) per day (33).

Determination of Plasma/Serum Electrolytes

A common biochemical feature of mineralocorticoid excess is metabolic alkalosis and particularly hypokalemia due to prolonged renal K wasting. Since K and hydrogen ions are excreted in the urine in exchange for the actively reabsorbed Na, both hypokalemia and alkalosis may not be manifested in primary aldosteronism if the patient is ingesting a diet with reduced Na content (which is not an uncommon practice among hypertensive people). Thus, before investigation proceeds, the outpatient should be oriented to increase Na content of his/her diet; addition of $\frac{1}{3}$ teaspoon (1 to 2 g) of table salt (sodium chloride) to each meal represents an adequate Na intake (33,34). Plasma Na concentration is high normal, usually greater than 142 mEq/1, in patients with an APA, whereas the average K level is 2.9 mEq/1, ranging from 1.7 to 3.8 mEq/1, in our experience. Patients with IHA have similar but less obvious abnormalities.

Determination of Plasma Renin Activity or Concentration

Primary mineralocorticoid excess produces Na and fluid retention by the renal tubules (and other aldosterone-responsive cells), resulting in expansion of the extracellular (plasma) fluid volume and suppression of renin production (35).

Plasma renin activity (PRA) is an indirect measurement of circulating renin; it is determined by the RIA of angiotensin I generated in standard laboratory conditions (36). If the RIA is performed in presence of excess renin substrate (angiotensinogen, obtained from previously nephrectomized sheep) the resulting angiotensin I generated in the assay is used as an expression of plasma renin "concentration" (PRC). A direct RIA for renin has only recently been developed but is not available routinely. Blood samples for PRA determinations should be carefully handled: plastic syringes and tubes containing EDTA and aprotinin should be kept on ice; samples should be centrifuged (under refrigeration) within 30 to 60 minutes from collection and stored at −20°C (for details see Renal Hormones, below).

PRA is often undetectable in primary aldosteronism, whereas PRC values are very low (PRC values are approximately four times greater than corresponding PRA levels) (21, 37). Therefore, stimulation maneuvers are routinely employed to evaluate the degree of renin suppression.

Low-Sodium Diet/Diuretic Administration. A 10 to 20 mEq Na per day diet for 3 to 5 days or, alternatively, acute administration of furosemide (40 to 80 mg PO or IV) will enhance discrimination of patients with primary aldosteronism from those with essential hypertension or normal subjects. Blood for PRA/PRC is drawn in recumbency and after 2 hours in the upright position, on the 4th to 5th day of the low Na diet or 2 to 4 hours after diuretic administration. Although PRA/PRC maintains subnormal levels in the former, it increases three to five fold in the latter groups (38,39). Figure 7.3 shows PRC responses to postural stimulation in normal subjects, in essential hypertension, and in primary aldosteronism.

Determination of Plasma and Urinary Aldosterone Levels

In normal subjects, plasma aldosterone concentration and 24-hour urinary aldosterone excretion rates, both measured by RIA, vary significantly, depending upon Na balance. Thus, similarly to PRA/PRC, determination of plasma aldosterone or urinary excretion of

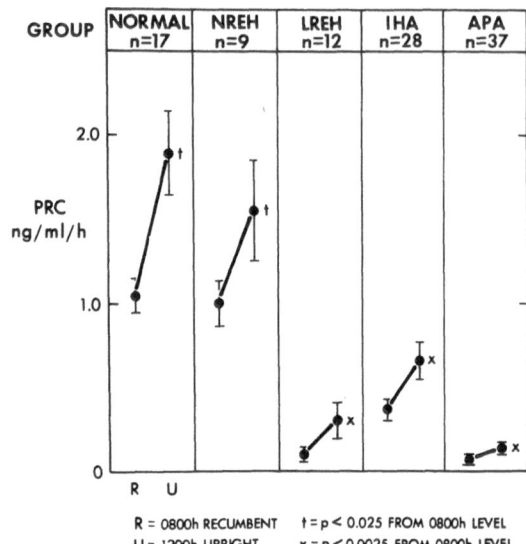

PRC IN HYPERTENSIVE GROUPS

Figure 7.3. Plasma renin concentration (PRC) in response to 4-hour postural stimulation in normal subjects, essential hypertension [with normal (NREH) and low-renin (LREH)], and primary aldosteronism. IHA, idiopathic hyperaldosteronism; APA, aldosterone-producing adenoma.

one of its metabolites (tetrahydroaldosterone or aldosterone 18-glucuronate), should be performed under strict dietary conditions, fixing electrolyte intake for a few days before sampling. If not possible, PRA/PRC and plasma or urinary aldosterone should be compared with concurrent 24-hour urinary Na excretion, using standard nomograms for this correlation (39,40).

Autonomous aldosterone production by an adenoma or adrenal hyperplasia is typically associated with elevated basal plasma and urinary aldosterone levels. Not infrequently, however, aldosterone production in primary aldosteronism is somewhat restrained by the prevailing hypokalemia resulting in "normal" plasma and urinary levels; nevertheless, values in the normal range are inappropriately elevated for the suppressed renin levels.

Postural Stimulation Test

Two to four hours in the standing or upright position increases substantially both PRA/PRC (by 200 to 300%) and plasma aldosterone in

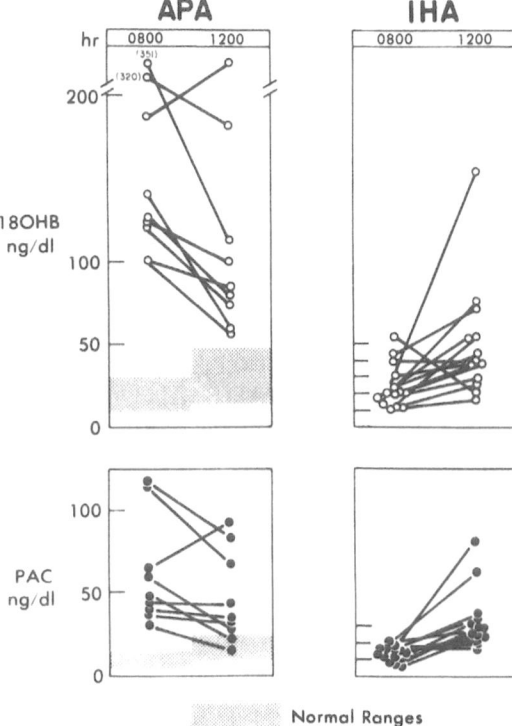

Figure 7.4. Individual plasma aldosterone (PAC) and 18-hydroxycorticosterone (18-OHB) concentrations in response to 4-hour postural stimulation in patients with primary aldosteronism. APA, aldosterone-producing adenoma, $n = 9$; IHA, idiopathic hyperaldosteronism, $n = 14$.

normal subjects (41). Also, patients with IHA (adrenal hyperplasia) increase plasma aldosterone markedly without significantly increasing PRA/PRC levels; however, plasma aldosterone does not change and even falls in response to posture in patients with an APA (42–44). This discrepancy is due to a significant reduction in the number and affinity of angiotensin II receptors in the adenoma cell (45), whereas sensitivity to angiotensin II is even increased in IHA (46–48). Aldosterone production in APA is influenced by the prevailing ACTH levels that are gradually decreasing during the day. The postural stimulation test is one of the most valuable discriminatory maneuvers to differentiate APA from IHA. Figure 7.4 depicts individual values of plasma aldosterone and 18-hydroxycorticosterone (18-OHB, see below) in APA and IHA, in response to posture.

Aldosterone Suppression Tests

The degree of renin autonomy in aldosterone production can be evaluated with maneuvers designed to expand chronically or acutely the plasma volume (the extracellular fluid compartment) and increase total body Na content, thereby suppressing the renin-angiotensin system.

The Deoxycorticosterone Acetate (DOCA) Suppression Test. DOCA is a potent synthetic mineralocorticoid that is able to retain Na and fluid, expand the extracellular fluid volume and suppress the renin-angiotensin system (49,50). The procedure (10 mg IM every 12 hours for 3 consecutive days) is similar to the dexamethasone suppression test for cortisol in Cushing's syndrome. Twenty-four-hour urine specimens are collected before and during the 3rd day of DOCA administration for aldosterone determinations. Normal subjects and patients with essential (low renin) hypertension will suppress PRA/PRC and, accordingly, reduce urinary aldosterone levels by more than 50% from baseline (50). A unique subtype of primary aldosteronism and adrenal hyperplasia, called "indeterminate (or DOCA-suppressible) hyperaldosteronism," will also present similar responses (33,40). In APA and IHA, the absence of suppression with DOCA characterizes aldosterone autonomy from renin in these patients. Figure 7.5 depicts urinary aldosterone responses to the DOCA suppression test in primary aldosteronism, essential hypertension, and normal subjects. Instead of intramuscular DOCA, one may give oral fludrocortisone acetate (Florinef, 0.2 mg every 12 hours for 3 consecutive days) and obtain similar results.

The Saline Infusion Test. Intravenous infusion of isotonic saline (0.9% sodium chloride solution), 2 l during 4 hours (or 1.5 l in 2 hours), will acutely expand the ECFV ad suppress renin-angiotensin levels (51). Blood is drawn immediately before and at the end of infusion for plasma aldosterone and cortisol determinations. Similarly to the DOCA test, patients with primary aldosteronism do not significantly reduce plasma aldosterone levels. Additionally, if the ratio of plasma aldosterone

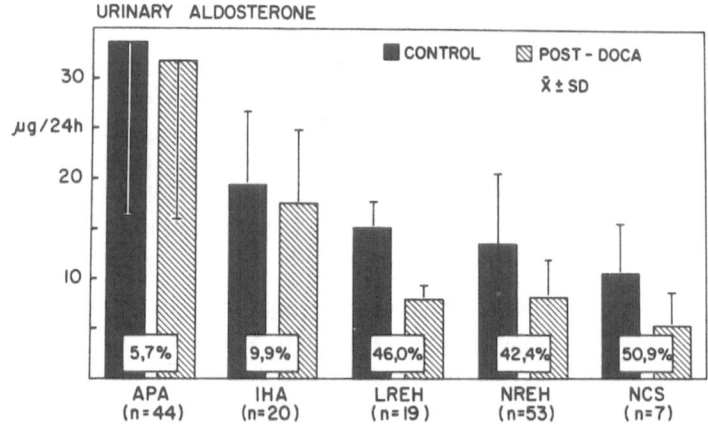

Figure 7.5. Twenty-four-hour urinary aldosterone excretion rates in response to deoxycorticosterone acetate (DOCA) administration (10 mg IM every 12 hour for 3 days) in primary aldosteronism. APA, aldosterone-producing adenoma; IHA, idiopathic hyperaldosteronism; essential hypertension [with normal (NREH) and low-renin (LREH)], and normal control subjects (NCS). Values in the insets at the bottom of the columns represent the percentage suppression from control levels in each group.

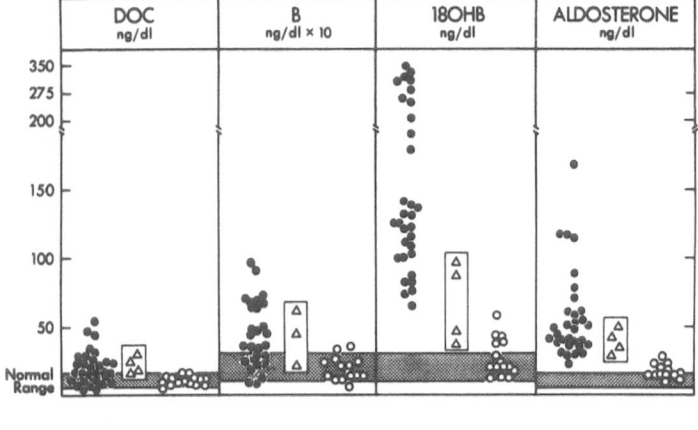

Figure 7.6. Individual basal levels of plasma corticosterone (B), deoxycorticosterone (DOC), 18-hydroxycorticosterone (18-OHB), and aldosterone in patients with primary aldosteronism. APA, aldosterone-producing adenoma, $n = 32$; IHA, idiopathic hyperaldosteronism, $n = 15$; PAH, primary adrenal hyperplasia, $n = 4$.

(in ng/dl) to plasma cortisol (in μg/dl) is used to interpret the test, it is possible to discriminate between APA and IHA: values greater than 2.0 after infusion are suggestive of the former, whereas in IHA the ratio remains below this level. Determining the ratio between 18-OHB in ng/dl (see below) and cortisol (in μg/dl), would be even more accurate if 3.0 is used as the cutoff point (51).

Determination of Plasma Aldosterone Precursors

Profiling of plasma aldosterone precursors, corticosterone (compound B), DOC, and 18-OHB can be a valuable tool to differentiate APA from IHA. Basal levels of these steroids are consistently elevated in APA, but not in

IHA (52,53). 18-OHB is the immediate precursor of aldosterone in the zona glomerulosa biosynthetic pathway and is a more important "marker" of zona glomerulosa hyperfunction than aldosterone itself (53,54); basal plasma 18-OHB is invariably increased in patients with an APA, to levels greater than 80 ng/dl and shows (differently from plasma aldosterone) no overlap with the normal or slightly elevated values of this steroid in patients with IHA (53,55). RIAs for B and DOC are commonly available; however, the technique to measure 18-OHB, is not routinely available. Figure 7.6 shows the individual basal values of plasma aldosterone, 18-OHB, DOC, and B in patients with APA, IHA, and those with the biochemical APA-like characteristics, PAH (primary adrenal hyperplasia) (28,30).

Response to Spironolactone Trial

Spironolactone (SPL; Aldactone, MS&D) is a synthetic progestogen that has antimineralocorticoid activity by competing with aldosterone receptor binding sites at the renal tubule cells (56). Administration of SPL (100 to 300 mg per day) for several weeks completely corrects hypertension and normalizes plasma K levels in patients with primary aldosteronism, especially those with an APA (57). After 2 to 3 months PRA/PRC also returns to normal levels. At this point, when renin and K have returned to normal, ECFV has contracted back, and total body Na\surfeit has been eliminated, and divergent responses of plasma and urinary aldosterone are seen in patients with APA and IHA, which permits additional discrimination between both groups: plasma and urinary aldosterone increase significantly in patients with IHA, whereas they remain at the same (or even lower) pretreatment levels in APA (58). Although not completely understood, this event may possibly represent a direct inhibiting effect of SPL at the adrenal level, blocking the renin- and K-mediated stimulation of aldosterone in the adenomatous cells (58).

Figure 7.7 shows data on plasma and urinary aldosterone, PRC and plasma K in response to SPL therapy in patients with primary aldosteronism. As mentioned previously, aldosterone production in APA is unresponsive to endogenous renin stimulation and also to exogenous infusion of graded doses of angiotensin II. A particular subtype of APA, known as APA-RA (aldosterone-producing angiotensin- responsive adenoma) (30), retains sensitivity to angiotensin and behaves biochemically like IHA, whereas PAH (28,30), different from other hyperplasias (IHA and IndHA), behaves biochemically like an adenoma.

Androgens and Syndromes of Hirsutism and Virilization

Mild androgen excess in adult women results in hirsutism, acne, and oily skin. Severe hyperandrogenism is associated with signs of defeminization and virilization, including breast atro-

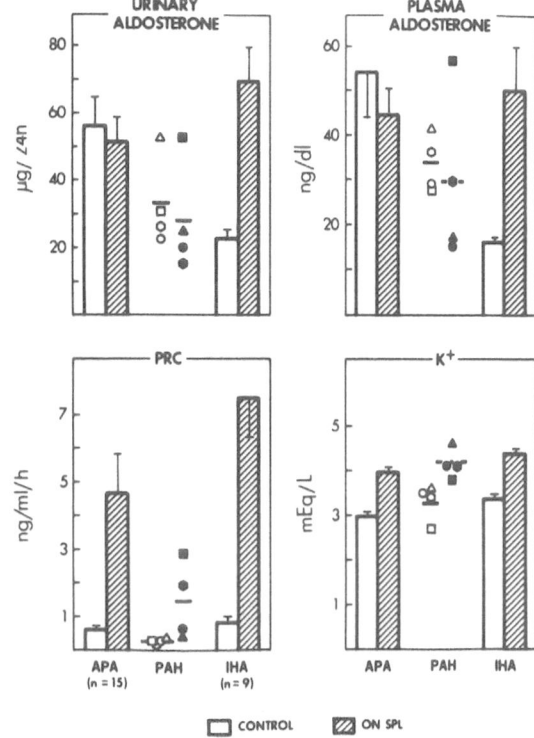

Figure 7.7. Urinary and plasma aldosterone, plasma renin concentration (PRC), and plasma potassium (K+) levels in response to spironolactone (SPL) therapy (100 to 300 mg PO for an average period of 3 months) in patients with primary aldosteronism. APA, aldosterone-producing adenoma, $n = 15$; IHA, idiopathic hyperaldosteronism, $n = 9$; PAH, primary adrenal hyperplasia, $n = 4$.

phy, increased muscular mass, temporal recess and male pattern baldness, clitoral enlargement, deepening of the voice, masculine habitus, and amenorrhea (59).

Hirsutism and virilization in the adult women and children of both sexes, are a consequence of:

1. excessive androgen production by the adrenal glands and/or the ovaries (occasionally by the testes in boys),
2. marked peripheral conversion of androgen precursors,
3. increased target cell sensitivity, and
4. prolonged administration of synthetic androgens or analogues.

The zona reticularis of the adrenal cortex secretes predominantly DHEA, DHEA-S, and androstenedione, sex steroids with reduced intrinsic androgenic activity; however, peripheral conversion to the more potent androgens, testosterone and dihydrotestosterone (DHT), results in a clinically significant hyperandrogenic state.

Plasma concentration of androgens are elevated in most cases with hirsutism and/or menstrual abnormalities and in virtually all patients with virilization (59,60). A few cases may have normal plasma androgen concentration but increased peripheral conversion and/or hypersensitivity of the target tissue.

Diagnostic laboratory procedures for the syndromes of hyperandrogenism are based on the biochemical confirmation of androgen excess followed by an attempt to determine its source.

Idiopathic Hirsutism

This is, essentially, a diagnosis of exclusion; idiopathic hirsutism is a common disorder in which plasma androgen levels are slightly to moderately elevated but the origin of the abnormal production is difficult to ascertain. Thus, either the adrenal or the ovary (or both) may be contributing to the excess androgen state.

The diagnostic maneuvers designed to solve this question, thereby permitting a more specific therapy, are based on the degree of androgen suppression by glucocorticoids or estrogens. The rationale for the "dexamethasone suppression test" in hyperandrogenism is that supraphysiologic doses of synthetic glucocorticoids for an appropriate period of time will suppress ACTH secretion [or a putative cortical androgen stimulating hormone (CASH)] and, consequently, reduce adrenal androgen production; alternatively, pharmacologic doses of estrogens will suppress pituitary luteinizing hormone (LH) secretion, reducing ovarian androgen formation. The magnitude of the androgen suppression will facilitate, within certain limits, establishing the adrenal, ovarian, or combined origin of the hyperandrogenism. Acceptance of these tests is not universal, since it has been demonstrated that dexamethasone may also reduce ovarian androgen

production, whereas pituitary LH may also stimulate adrenocortical androgen synthesis.

Determination of Plasma/Serum Androgen Profile.

In adult women, plasma or serum concentrations of the sexual steroids oscillate both during the menstrual cycle and within the 24-hour day; thus, determination of normal plasma androgen concentrations should consider the time of day and, especially, the phase of the menstrual cycle from which the sample is drawn. Our experience, and that of others, show that a pool of three morning blood samples drawn 10 to 15 minutes apart is more representative than a single sample. Likewise, although special conditions may suggest a different approach, plasma androgen profiling in hirsutism is best evaluated in the early follicular phase (between days 1 and 5) in women that have normal menstrual periods. Patients with menstrual abnormalities, such as oligomenorrhea and amenorrhea, should preferably be evaluated also in the early follicular phase of an artificially induced (with oral progestins) menstrual bleeding. Amenorrheic patients who fail to menstruate after oral progestins may be studied at any period.

The plasma/serum androgen profiling includes hormonal determinations of total or free testosterone, dihydrotestosterone (DHT; if available), androstenedione, and DHEA or DHEA-S. If available, plasma or urinary levels of 3-alpha-androstenediol glucuronate (a metabolite of DHT) should also be added, since it appears to be one of the most consistent "markers" of the peripheral androgenic activity. Approximately 85 to 90% of hirsute or virilized women will have elevation of at least one of these plasma androgens; testosterone is the most consistently elevated androgen, present in more than 90% of cases (60). Plasma testosterone levels greater than 200 ng/dl are suggestive of the presence of an ovarian (or adrenal) tumor (61); elevated DHEA-S levels are characteristic of an adrenal origin and marked elevations (higher than tr 700 μg/dl) suggest adrenal carcinoma (62). Normal plasma/serum ranges (RIA) and the normal percentage contribution from adrenals and ovaries in the early follicular phase are presented in Table 7.1.

Table 7.1. Normal range of plasma/serum androgens by RIA in adult women and prepubertal children and percentage contribution from adrenals and ovaries to normal circulating levels.

Androgen	Adult women (early follicular phase)	Children (prepubertal)	Adrenal (% total)	Ovary	Peripheral conversion
Testosterone (ng/dl)	20–80	<10	10–25	10–25	50–70
DHT (ng/dl)	10–40	<5	–	–	100
Androstenedione (ng/dl)	50–220	20–80	30–45	45–60	10–20
DHEA (ng/dl)	120–1,000	50–300	80	20	–
DHEA-S (μg/dl)	40–260	10–100	>95	<5	–

DHT, dihydrotestosterone; DHEA, dehydroepiandrosterone; DHEA-S, dehydroepiandrosterone sulfate.

Dexamethasone Suppression Test for Plasma Androgens.

The prolonged DST, proposed by Abraham and Maroulis (60), is based on the suppression of pituitary ACTH and, consequently, the ACTH-dependent adrenocortical zona reticularis androgen production. Oral dexamethasone is administered for 15 (or even more) days at a dose of 0.5 mg every 6 hours (for patients weighing up to 70 kg) or 0.75 mg every 6 hours (for patients 70 kg and up). Two baseline blood samples should be drawn in the early follicular phase and again at the end of the suppression period for hormonal determinations. Cortisol and DHEA-S levels are used to monitor suppression, respectively, of the zona fasciculata and zona reticularis. Appropriate suppression of one or more of the elevated plasma androgens (testosterone, DHT, and androstenedione) characterizes ACTH-dependency of the elevated androgens and suggests its origin in the adrenal cortex. Failure of androgen suppression (when cortisol and DHEA-S are adequately suppressed) demonstrate ACTH independency of the androgen production, suggesting its ovarian origin. Partial responses are typical of a combined source for androgen production (60). The prolonged DST for hyperandrogenism is used less frequently nowadays since it is cumbersome, time-consuming, and often associated with significant dexamethasone-related side effects (epigastralgia, appetite increase and weight gain, insomnia, etc.).

In an attempt to abbreviate Abraham's procedure, we analyzed the 15-day DST (0.5 mg PO every 6 hours) in a sequential fashion in 18 hirsute women, collecting blood samples for

Table 7.2. Mean (± SD) androgen levels obtained in the control (basal) period and after 2 and 15 days of dexamethasone suppression in 18 hirsute patients classified (according to Abraham's criteria) in three groups: ACTH-independent (ACTH/I, $n = 10$), ACTH-dependent (ACTH/D, $n = 4$), and of mixed origin (Mixed, $n = 4$) hyperandrogenism.

Androgen Groups	Basal	Dexamethasone suppression	
		2nd day	15th day
Testosterone (ng/dl)			
ACTH/I	129.9 ± 34.3	114.3 ± 41.9	103.4 ± 26.9
ACTH/D	132.5 ± 10.4	67.8 ± 4.4	69.5 ± 12.8
Mixed	148.0 ± 23.4	83.0 ± 27.7	83.3 ± 12.0
Androstenedione (ng/dl)			
ACTH/I	233.0 ± 82.9	208.2 ± 106.7	228.0 ± 93.0
ACTH/D	215.0 ± 62.5	110.5 ± 62.2	132.5 ± 32.0
Mixed	315.0 ± 141.5	122.5 ± 58.5	202.5 ± 56.8
DHEA-S (μg/dl)			
ACTH/I	175.3 ± 70.0	57.0 ± 33.3	32.4 ± 20.8
ACTH/D	349.5 ± 106.3	128.5 ± 51.5	57.3 ± 31.1
Mixed	303.3 ± 163.0	65.0 ± 51.2	32.2 ± 17.7

androgen measurement before and 2, 5, 10, and 15 days later (63). On the 15th day, hyperandrogenism could be classified as ACTH-dependent (ACTH-D), ACTH-independent (ACTH-I) or of a mixed cause, according to the classic criteria. On the 2nd suppression day both the sensitivity and specificity of testosterone and androstenedione suppression were even better than on the 15th day (63). Table 7.2 shows the mean ±SD levels for DHEA-S, testosterone, and androstenedione for the three groups on the 2nd and 15th day of dexamethasone suppression. This becomes a practical approach for those who postulate using the DST for hyperandrogenism.

Congenital Adrenal Hyperplasia

Congenital adrenal hyperplasia (CAH) is a group of inborn errors of the steroid metabolism resulting from enzymatic deficiencies in cortisol biosynthesis. The most prevalent form of CAH is 21-hydroxylase deficiency, responsible for more than 90% of all cases (64). Excess androgen production is responsible for several degrees of hirsutism and virilization in the affected patient, depending on the severity of the enzymatic deficiency and the onset of the clinical manifestations.

Adrenal synthesis of cortisol and aldosterone from cholesterol involves a sequence of biochemical reactions mediated by specific enzymatic complexes. Deficiency of one of these enzymes (genetically determined by recessive autosomic inheritance) (65), will impair adequate production of cortisol and aldosterone. Chronic cortisol (and aldosterone) deficiency results in marked stimulation of ACTH (and renin-angiotensin) production, which in turn induces adrenocortical hyperplasia and continuous stimulation of the nonimpeded biosynthetic pathways, especially the androgen pathway (64).

Thus, the clinical and laboratory picture results from subnormal cortisol (and aldosterone) levels and the excessive production of precursors (17-alpha-hydroxyprogesterone) and androgens. Excessive adrenocortical androgen production results in virilization of the external genitalia in the female newborn (ambiguous genitalia) and several degrees of hirsutism and virilization in the adult female (when a mild or late form of the enzymatic deficiency occurs) (64). In addition, aldosterone deficiency in the "classic" congenital form will result in inappropriate sodium conservation with sodium loss, dehydration, and cardiovascular collapse.

Determination of 17α-Hydroxyprogesterone (17α-OHP). Plasma or serum RIA for 17α-OHP (66) permits the diagnosis of 21-hydroxylase deficiency with high specificity. 17α-OHP, the immediate precursor to 21-hydroxylase in the adrenal zona fasciculata, is secreted in exaggerated amounts under continuous ACTH stimulation. Measurement of 17α-OHP can be made in small plasma/serum volumes; it is highly discriminative provided the analysis is performed in the newborn after the first 48 to 72 hours of life, because within this period values are normally elevated. Even in this situation, however, the difference between normal and pathologic values are sufficiently great to determine the proper diagnosis. Normal 17α-OHP values after the first 48 to 72 hours are below 200 ng/dl. Affected patients with 21-hydroxylase deficiency present basal levels often greater than 3,000 ng/dl (the average of 25 recently diagnosed children in our service was 18,600 ng/dl).

ACTH Stimulation Test for 17α-OHP. The acute ACTH stimulation test (Cortrosyn, 250 μg IV bolus) permits an additional elevation in plasma/serum 17α-OHP levels; thus, although this test is hardly necessary to establish the diagnosis in the classic forms of the disease, it may be indicated in an attempt to detect non-classic forms (mild or late-onset) of the disease among young adult women complaininng of hirsutism, acne, menstrual abnormalities, and/or infertility. Basal levels of 17α-OHP in these patients are only moderately elevated (values between 500 and 2,000 ng/dl) but in response to ACTH stimulation reach levels in the range of 4,000 to 10,000 ng/dl, confirming unequivocally the diagnosis.

Androgen-Producing Adrenal and Ovarian Neoplasias

Adrenocortical carcinoma may produce a host of different steroid products in excess, leading to combined manifestations of Cushing's syndrome, hypermineralocorticism, and hyperandrogenism. The most common single manifestation of any secreting adrenocortical carcinoma, however, is virilization (61,67, 68). The prevalence of androgen-producing adrenocortical neoplasias (APAN) is higher among children and young adults. In addition, due to its characteristic clinical manifestations APAN is more easily suspected in adult women and children, although men are also affected (68).

Although adrenocortical androgen-producing zona reticularis is potentially able to

Table 7.3. Basal androgen and 17α-OHD levels in patients with androgen-producing adrenocortical carcinomas (Nos. 1–7) and androgen-producing ovarian tumors (Nos. 8–10).

Pt. No.	Age/ Sex	Plasma Testosterone (ng/dl)	Androstenedione (ng/dl)	DHEA-S (μg/dl)	17α-OHP (μg/dl)	Urine 17-Ketosteroids (mg/24hours)
1	35/F	84	430	65	30	–
2	51/F	325	410	394	98	29
3	28/F	210	790	540	142	–
4	31/F	497	430	162	–	–
5	42/M	–	–	–	372	94
6	37/M	88	410	450	50	43
7[a]	33/M	1030	1350	847	4178	198
8	50/F	340	200	32	170	–
9	58/F	292	320	122	480	–
10	41/F	183	120	140	73	–
Normal values						
Female		20–80	90–290	50–340	50–200	5–15
Male		300–1,000	90–290	50–340	50–180	10–20

[a]Patient No. 7 had an androgen- and estrogen-producing (plasma estradiol levels: 94 ng/dl) adrenocortical carcinoma (kindly reported by Dr. Bernardo Liberman at Hospital Brigadeiro, Sao Paulo, Brazil).

synthesize any androgen hormone, the main secretory product of an APAN is DHEA-S. Normal values for DHEA-S vary according to sex and age group: in children up to 2 years of age plasma/serum DHEA-S levels are less than 10 μg/dl, whereas they are greater than 200 μg/dl when an APAN is present; values greater than 600 μg/dl are frequently seen in adults. The diagnosis of an APAN should always be considered if plasma/serum testosterone levels are markedly elevated and especially if not suppressible by dexamethasone administration. Signs and symptoms indicating additional production of excess gluco- or mineralocorticoids and/or the presence of an abdominal mass on exam should increased the diagnostic suspicion of an APAN. Table 7.3 presents individual androgen levels in seven patients with an APAN and three with an ovarian tumor.

Virilizing ovarian tumors (VOT) are uncommon and may be present in different age groups. They vary in size but, not infrequently, are smaller than 6 cm in diameter. VOT should be differentiated from polycystic ovarian disease, hyperthecosis, and luteoma. According to a World Health Organization (WHO) proposal, androgen-producing ovarian neoplasias have recently been classified as tumors of the Sertoli-Leydig cells (69,70) (as opposed to the classic denominations of arrhenoblastoma and androblastoma). Hilus cell tumors (71) are small (less than 5 cm) and generally benign tumors arising in the perimenopausal period; testosterone levels in these malignancies are markedly elevated. There is no specific biochemical maneuver capable of differentiating these tumors from other hyperandrogenic syndromes.

Preoperative Localization Procedures

In addition to all the biochemical investigations presented above, adrenal and ovarian hormone-excess syndromes may, not infrequently, need anatomical (imaging evaluation) confirmation of the suspected pathology and lateralization of the lesion. Several imaging procedures are commonly available today [ultrasound scans, computed tomography (72–74), magnetic resonance imaging (75,76), radioisotopic scintigrams (77,78), angiography, and percutaneous venous blood sampling (79–82)] and may be used to confirm the anatomic and etiologic diagnosis. Accuracy with these methods will heavily depend on the clinician's experience with a given technique; the advantage and accuracy of these techniques are discussed elsewhere in this book.

Pituitary Hormones

ACTH/Beta-LPH in Cushing's Disease, and Ectopic ACTH Syndrome

Although the pituitary gland is a multihormone secretory organ, responsible for the synthesis of several polypeptide hormones, such as growth hormone, prolactin, thyrotropin, LH, follicle-stimulating hormone (FSH), ACTH, and others, pathologies involving excess production of these hormones are sufficiently obvious to preclude needing more sophisticated diagnostic techniques such as the inferior petrosal sinus (IPS) catheterization with hormone determinations. One major exception is ACTH and Cushing's syndrome. The differential diagnosis between an ACTH-producing pituitary microadenoma and the "ectopic ACTH syndrome" is sometimes so intricate that IPS (with measurement of ACTH and beta-lipotropin) is mandatory (83). In this situation, determination of other hormonal "markers" such as prolactin may be necessary to ascertain the diagnosis and location of the anatomic lesion.

Determination of Plasma ACTH Levels

Although the RIA for plasma ACTH is not routinely available, determination of its plasma concentrations can be useful in establishing the etiology of Cushing's syndrome. It is particularly relevant for the diagnosis of the ectopic ACTH syndrome where ACTH levels are usually markedly elevated. Subnormal or undetectable levels of ACTH are unique for the autonomous or primary adrenal source of hypercortisolism, provided exogenous glucocorticoid treatment is not the cause (84,85).

Due to instability, blood samples for ACTH determination should be drawn and handled with extreme care: plastic syringes and tubes (glassware are improper as ACTH may adhere to it) should be kept chilled; EDTA should be used as an anticogulant and Trasylol or NEM (N-ethyl-maleimide) as proteinase inhibitors. Plasma is separated in a refrigerated centrifuge within 30 minutes after collection and kept frozen at $-20°C$ (preferably $-70°C$) until assayed. Specific RIAs use antisera generated against the biologically active 1–24 sequence

of human ACTH which does not cross-react with biologically inactive fragments of the proopiomelanocortin (POMC) molecule. Normal values for plasma ACTH (determined with specific RIAs) range from 20 to 80 pg/ml (between 7 and 9 A.M.) and about half these values in the afternoon (4 to 5 P.M.). The reliability of ACTH determinations will increase when a dynamic test is employed.

Determination of Plasma Beta-Lipotropin (β-LPH) Levels

Beta-lipotropin is co-secreted in the corticotroph in equimolar amounts with ACTH. The molecule of β-LPH is more stable and easier than ACTH to measure with RIA. Since β-LPH and ACTH plasma levels are parallel in disease states (86), determination of β-LPH may be superior to ACTH as a "marker" for Cushing's disease (87,88).

The Metyrapone (Metopirone) Test

Metyrapone is an 11β-hydroxylase (and 18-hydroxylase) inhibitor; this enzyme complex is responsible for cortisol synthesis from its immediate precursor 11-deoxycortisol (compound S), and also for the formation of corticosterone from DOC. Thus, administration of metyrapone (750 mg PO every 4 hours for a total of six doses or, alternatively, an overnight single 3.0-g dose) (89,90) reduces circulating cortisol levels, which in turn stimulate pituitary ACTH release through the negative feedback mechanism. Increased ACTH production stimulates biosynthesis in the adrenal cortex up to the level of compound S and DOS (synthesis cannot proceed beyond that, due to the metyrapone-induced 11β-hydroxylase blockade). Plasma ACTH and compound S can be determined before and 24 to 48 hours later (or the next morning in the overnight test) to assess the response to metyrapone (89,90). Plasma/serum cortisol levels are also determined to confirm the effectiveness of the enzymatic blockade. Figure 7.8 displays cortisol and compound S responses to metyrapone in normal subjects and patients with Cushing's disease. Compound S normally increases from < 1 µg/dl to 10 to 20 µg/dl 24 to 48 hours later, whereas ACTH responds normally to values

Figure 7.8. Serum cortisol and 11-deoxycortisol (compound S) levels in response to oral metyrapone (Metopirone, 750 mg PO every 4 hours or 24 hours) in normal control subjects (NCS) and patients with Cushing's disease.

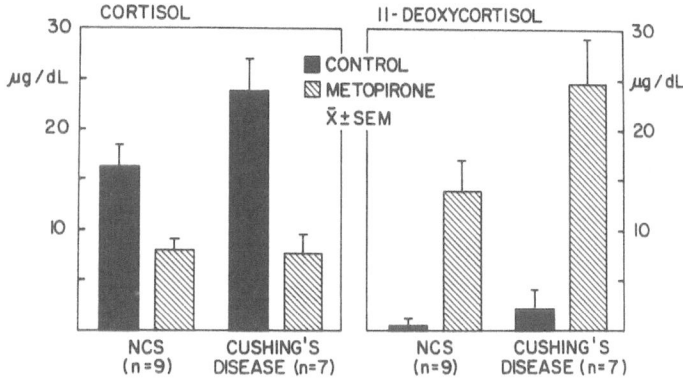

Figure 7.9. Plasma cortisol and ACTH levels in response to synthetic ovine corticotropin-releasing hormone (oCRH) stimulation (1 μg/kg BW IV bolus injection) in normal control subjects (NCS) and patients with Cushing's syndrome (Cushing's disease, $n = 9$; adrenal adenoma, $n = 3$).

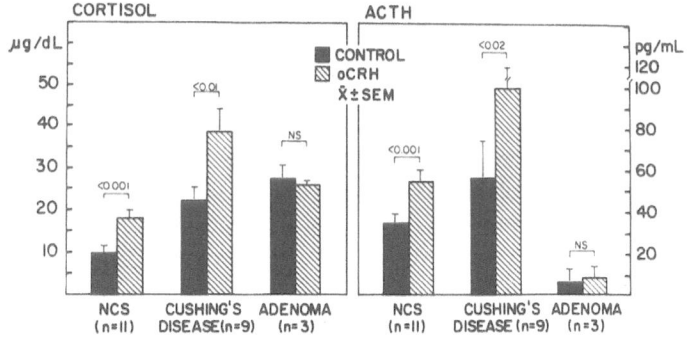

greater than 200 pg/ml. Patients with Cushing's disease often have more exaggerated increases in both compound S and ACTH, whereas responses in patients with adrenal tumors are virtually absent.

Corticotropin Releasing Hormone (CRH) Stimulation Test

CRH has recently been isolated, sequenced, and synthesized (91). Ovine CRH (oCRH) is being used as a pituitary stimulation test to evaluate ACTH reserve and also to tentatively distinguish between ACTH-dependent and primary Cushing's syndrome (92,93). oCRH (1 μg/kg BW or a fixed dose of 100 μg) is administered as an IV bolus injection and blood is collected every 15 to 20 min for 2 hours for determination of plasma ACTH and cortisol.

As with the metyrapone test patients with pituitary-dependent Cushing's disease tend to have a greater than normal response, whereas no response is the rule in primary adrenal disease. Figure 7.9 shows some preliminary cortisol and ACTH results obtained in patients with

Cushing's syndrome and in normal volunteers studied in our service.

Lysine-Vasopressin (8-LVP) Stimulation Test

8-LVP is a synthetic peptide analogue to human antidiuretic hormone (arginine-vasopressin) that has "CRH-like" properties. An intramuscular dose of 10 PU (pressor units) stimulates the release of ACTH and cortisol in normal subjects 30 to 60 minutes later. Since 8-LVP is a more potent CRF (factor) than CRH itself, hormonal responses tend to be more pronounced and distinguishing (94,95). However, side effects such as nausea, vomiting, and significant elevations in blood pressure preclude its use routinely.

Pancreatic Hormones

Insulin and Insulinomas

Insulinomas are rare tumors of the beta cells of Langerhans islets; they present a challenge for diagnosis and treatment. Usually they are single benign tumors of the pancreas (80% of the cases), but can be multiple (11%) or malignant (less than 10%) (96). In approximately 10% of the cases they are part of the so-called multiple endocrine neoplasia type 1 (MEN-1) syndrome, together with primary hyperparathyroidism and pituitary tumors.

Clinical Workup

The clinical presentation of insulinoma is invariably related to signs of severe hypoglycemia: diplopia, blurred vision, sweating, palpitations, weakness. Other signs like confusion, abnormal behavior, unconsciousness or grand mal seizures may also be present. Hypoglycemia is usually detected several hours after meals, most commonly before the evening meal. The laboratory comprobation needs the demonstration of concomitant hypoglycemia and hyperinsulinemia. When a normal fasting sample is not comfirmatory, a prolonged supervised fasting test must be performed, with serial sampling for glucose and insulin measurement. The test can be prolonged for up to 72 hours and the finding of glucose levels lower than 40 mg/dl concomitant with insulin levels greater than 10 IU/l are diagnostic (97). To avoid the risks and discomfort of a prolonged fasting, provocative tests can be employed instead. Tolbutamide is the more often used (98) but is associated with some risks as a consequence of the severe hypoglycemia that can be induced. Calcium infusion can be used as an alternative (99).

Preoperative Localization Methods

Preoperative localization of insulinomas is mandatory, since these tumors are usually small, with an average size of 1.5 cm diameter (97), uniformly distributed throughout the parenchyma of the pancreas, and associated with unacceptable morbidity following blind resection of pancreatic tissue. Of the commonly employed techniques, ultrasound and computed tomography show disappointingly low sensitivity (100). Selective angiography, selective venous sampling, and intraoperative ultrasound show the best results (100,101). Ex-

perience with each methodology varies widely depending on the technical resources, the expertise of different groups, and the choice of methodology.

Hormone Assay

Insulin is the most important secretory product of the beta cells; it can be measured in serum or plasma using standard radioimmunoassay (RIA) techniques. In fact, insulin was the first hormone to have, in 1959, an RIA developed for its measurement (102). Since then, multiple methodological variants have been described but in essence the method is still the same (103). Some points must be considered when analyzing samples collected during venous catheterization of the pancreas:

1. The analysis can be performed either in serum or plasma (104);
2. Samples can stand at room temperature for as long as 4 hours before separation and storage;
3. Hemolysis causes very rapid degradation of insulin (105), and this can be an important problem when blood is collected from small tributary veins;
4. Insulin assay can be performed fast enough so that results may be available in time to repeat sampling if necessary (106);
5. Fasting prior to catheterization (without glucose challenge during the procedure) is of paramount importance to obtain reliable data;
6. 0.5 to 1.0 ml of blood is the minimum sample volume necessary for the assay.

Gastrin and Gastrinoma

Gastrinomas were first described by Zollinger and Ellison in 1955 (107); they are a rare cause of peptic ulcers (0.1 to 1% of the cases), but nevertheless became an obligatory differential diagnosis in this common pathology. The tumors are usually located in the head and tail of the pancreas (108), but other locations, such as the duodenum wall, hilus of the spleen, liver, and the stomach wall, are not uncommon (109). Gastrinomas are reported to be malignant in at least 60% of the cases (110) and are usually metastatic at the time of the diagnosis (108).

Clinical Workup

Patients with the Zollinger-Ellison syndrome usually present with severe and recurrent peptic ulcer disease, associated with persistently elevated basal gastric acid output. The most important diagnostic test is the measurement of fasting serum gastrin, which does not normally exceed 200 ng/ml, whereas in gastrinoma patients it is usually above 1,000 ng/ml. Other causes of hypergastrinemia, such as pernicious anemia and chronic gastritis, have to be ruled out. In cases with borderline basal gastrin levels the secretin stimulation test can be helpful (111).

Preoperative Localization Methods

Gastrinomas can be located by the same techniques employed for insulinomas, but with less satisfactory results. Ultrasound and computed tomography have similar low-sensitivity results. Selective angiography shows a better sensitivity (112), but selective venous sampling (despite good sensitivity) shows low specificity in some statistics (113), and acceptable specificity in others (114). These data stress the need for employing more than one localization method in the study of gastrinomas.

Hormone Assay

The RIA for gastrin, described in 1970 (115), is a widely available method with no special requirements for sampling or storage. Since most of the assays are highly sensitive, sample volumes of serum as small as 0.5 to 1.0 ml are required; after serum or plasma separation, samples can be stored at −20°C, for extended periods without losing immunoreactivity.

Glucagon and Glucagonoma

Glucagonoma is a well-characterized and very rare syndrome produced by tumors of the alpha cells of the Langerhans islets of the pancreas. The syndrome was first described in 1966 (116) and includes skin lesions, weight loss, anemia, depression, and susceptibility to deep vein thrombosis. Tumors are always malignant and usually metastatic at the time of the diagnosis. The primary tumor is found most commonly in the body and tail of the pancreas, where alpha cells are predominant (117).

Hormone Assay

Glucagon is a 29-amino-acid peptide. The first RIA was reported shortly after the introduction of the technique (118), but due to methodological difficulties it is an unusual assay even nowadays. Measurement of glucagon in samples collected during venous catheterization of the pancreas can be useful in locating the tumor; samples must be collected in special conditions such as glass tubes containing 1.2 mg sodium EDTA and 500 U Trasylol (as the protease inhibitor) for each milliliter of blood to be collected. Samples should be kept in an ice bath, immediately centrifuged, and the plasma samples stored at −20°C.

Parathyroid Hormone

Parathyroid Hormone and Primary Hyperparathyroidism

Primary hyperparathyroidism is a common pathology with potentially great health impact on the population (119). The widespead use of serum calcium determinations and the development of sensitive and specific methods for the measurement of parathyroid hormone made primary hyperparathyroidism a common and obvious diagnosis (120). Primary hyperparathyroidism may be due to a solitary parathyroid gland adenoma (in 85% of the cases), to hyperplasia of the four glands, or to carcinoma of the parathyroid gland, a very rare condition. Recent advances in diagnostic procedures unveiled primary hyperparathyroidism as a much more common disease than previously thought (121). In fact, one of the most debated issues in the field today is the treatment of asymptomatic hyperparathyroidism (122,123). In established symptomatic cases surgical intervention is mandatory, and in the hands of an experienced surgeon, success is the general rule.

Clinical Workup

When primary hyperparathyroidism is clinically or biochemically suspected, some diagnostic
procedures are necessary both to confirm the
diagnosis and to evaluate the impact of the disease in the patient. Basic biochemical workup
includes serum calcium and phosphorus and
urinary calcium excretion. Whenever determination of ionized calcium is available should
be made, since its diagnostic sensitivity is higher than that of total serum calcium (124).
Measurement of serum magnesium can be of
interest, in association with urinary calcium, in
cases of asymptomatic patients where the differential diagnosis with familial benign hypercalcemia must be considered (125). Serum
alkaline phosphatase is a good marker for bone
involvement and may be used as a predictor for
the postoperative "hungry bone" syndrome.
Urinary cyclic-AMP measurement can be useful in selected patients, always bearing in mind
that some patients with cancer-associated
hypercalcemia will have high values (126). X-
ray evaluation can be of interest especially of
areas where the typical alterations are usually
more visible, like hands and skull. The measurement of serum parathyroid hormone recently became the obvious conclusive test,
for reasons we will discuss below.

Preoperative Localization Methods

Use of preoperative localization procedures
are highly controversial in cases of first surgery
but considered mandatory in cases that need
reoperation (127). In this condition, the selec-
tion of a localization test depends on the
availability of the specialized equipment and
expertise of the physicians and technicians performing and interpreting these studies. Current
localization techniques can be divided into
noninvasive and invasive methods. Noninvasive methods are always the first choice, since
they have good sensitivity; in a cost-benefit
ranking the first method to be used is high-
resolution, real-time ultrasonography with a
10-MHz transducer. With this technique over
50% of the tumors in patients undergoing reoperation can be identified (128). The second choice would be the technetium-99m/

thallium-201 subtraction scanning, which has
comparable sensitivity. Computed tomography
(CT) scanning and magnetic resonance imaging (MRI), when available, can be used in
sequence with exceptional results. Nonetheless, the incidence of false-positive results
(127) are not neglegible and, in some cases of
persistent hyperparathyroidism, indication for
a localization method with higher sensitivity
and specificity exists. In these cases, invasive
methods such as selective venous catheterization, are evidently indicated. The technique for
performing venous catheterization of the parathyroid glands is described elsewhere in this
book; the important points related to PTH
measurement are discussed in sequence.

Hormone Assay

Parathyroid hormone (PTH) is a linear peptide
comprised of 84 amino acids whose amino-terminal portion, the first 34 amino acids, encompasses the full biological activity (129). PTH is
secreted by the parathyroid cells in its complete form, the 1–84 peptide, as well as in the
form of carboxyl-terminal fragments with no
known biological activity (130). The proportion of molecular forms secreted varies according to several metabolic circumstances, especially serum calcium levels and renal function
(131,132). Unlike the intact PTH molecule,
which is cleared from plasma in minutes, the
carboxyl-terminal fragments have a much
longer half-life that depends on glomerular
filtration (133).

Since its description, by Berson et al. in 1963
(133), PTH radioimmunoassay have been the
subject of much debate, research, development, and controversy. The basis of this debate
was the specificity of the assays; the most
commonly available assay until recently was
carboxyl-terminal specific, with the intrinsic
limitation of measuring PTH fragments with
longer half-lives than the biologically active
molecule (134). The availability of radioimmunoassay methods using antisera specific
for the amino-terminal portion of the PTH
molecule (consequently measuring the biologically active short-lived hormonal forms
[135,136]), and more recently of the immunoradiometric assays for the entire molecule

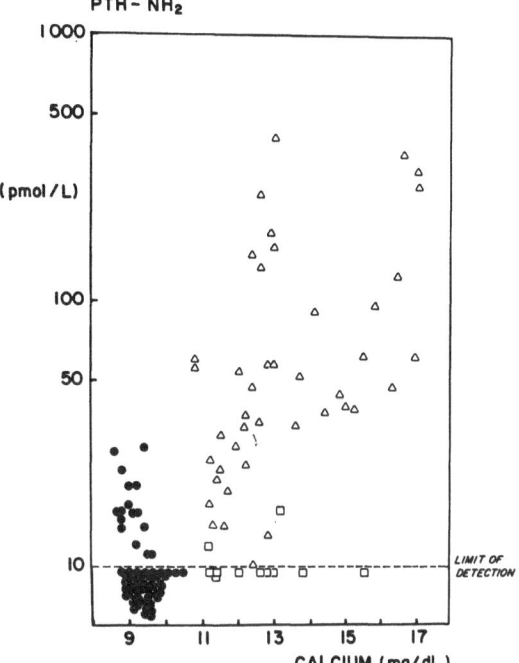

PTH-NH₂

Figure 7.10. Individual levels of serum amino-terminal parathyroid hormone (PTH-NH2) plotted as a function of concurrent serum calcium in normal control subjects (●), surgically confirmed primary hyperparathyroidism (△), and patients with hypercalcemia of different causes (□). Values below the dashed line were all nondetectable (<10 pmol/l).

(137,138), seems to have put an end to all controversy. These are the assays that should be used in any circumstances, especially to measure rapid variations in PTH levels, like those observed in provocative tests, and for the special purpose of detecting hormonal gradients in samples collected from cervical vein catheterization (139).

Figure 7.10 displays individual serum amino-terminal PTH plotted against concurrent serum calcium levels in 74 normal subjects, 42 patients with confirmed primary hyperparathyroidism, and 11 with hypercalcemia of different causes.

PTH assay can be performed in serum or plasma, and due to the high sensitivity of the new assay methods, samples of 0.5 to 1.0 ml of whole blood are sufficient. Serum or plasma should be separated as soon as possible and stored at −20°C.

Renal Hormones

Renin and Renovascular Hypertension/Primary Reninism

Renovascular Hypertension

Renovascular hypertension (RVH) is one of the most common causes of curable hypertension (present in 1 to 3% of the hypertensive population) (140); it results from narrowing of one or both renal arteries due to atherosclerosis, fibromuscular dysplasia, or other unusual causes. RVH may present in a similar way as essential hypertension but its diagnosis may be suspected if any of the following conditions are present: the onset is below ages 20 or after 50 years (especially if the course is severe and of short duration); epigastric or renal artery bruits are present on physical exam; an atherosclerotic process is documented elsewhere; there are variations in the size and/or appearance of the kidneys on X-rays or intravenous pyelogram; during catheterization, there is a gradient of plasma renin activity greater than 1.5 between both renal veins; there is abnormal excretion of radioactive material on renal scintigrams; atherosclerosis or fibromuscular dysplasia can be demonstrated by renal arteriography (140).

The best diagnostic procedure is renal angiography; it is always indicated if anatomic stenosis is suggested by history, physical exam, abnormal intravenous pyelogram, or by the severity of the hypertensive disease (especially sudden deterioration of renal function after administration of angiotensin-converting enzyme inhibitors). Bilateral renal vein catheterization with measurement of plasma renin activity may be attempted to identify and lateralize physiologically significant renal artery stenosis, but the elevated percentage of both false-positive and false-negative results precludes its use routinely.

Primary Reninism (Renin Secreting Tumors)

Excess renin can be produced by a juxtaglomerular apparatus tumor of the kidney, leading to hypertension and secondary hyperaldosteronism in young adults (141). Renin-producing tumors, also referred to as hemangiopericytomas and hamartomas, are small size tumors (1 to 5 cm in diameter) commonly of benign origin; a few reported cases of ectopic renin production originated, however, from extrarenal carcinomas. Hypertension is often severe (diastolic blood pressure usually above 120 mm Hg) and marked hypokalemia is systematically observed.

Levels of plasma renin activity vary from moderate to extremely elevated (5 to 80 ng AI/ml/h) (141) and may result in significant clinical manifestations, such as left ventricular hypertrophy and impairment of renal function, usually reversible following surgical removal of the tumor. Administration of converting enzyme inhibitors (captopril, enalapril) reduces blood pressure significantly. Computed tomography is the most valuable technique for tumor location, whereas selective renal vein catheterization for renin determination is not invariably positive, since topical renin-secreting tumors are usually located at the kidney surface where most of the venous blood is collected by pericapsular veins and not necessarily drained into the main renal effluents. The differential diagnoses include renovascular hypertension and renal infarction, whose diagnoses should be ruled out by previous renal arteriography.

Hormone Assay: Plasma Renin Activity

Renin is a proteolytic enzyme synthesized and stored by cells of the juxtaglomerular apparatus (JGA) in the kidney. The JGA is the center of a feedback loop that participates in the regulation of blood pressure by modulating the rate of renin secretion (142). In general, any condition that reduces renal perfusion will increase renin production. Once in the circulation, renin acts upon a substrate, angiotensinogen, producing angiotensin I, which is converted to angiotensin II, a very potent vasoconstrictor. Currently available methods for measurement of plasma renin activity were developed from the indirect method described by Haber et al. (143) in 1969, which is based on the RIA of angiotensin I generated by a plasma

sample in standardized conditions of temperature and time. Methods vary regarding the time of generation of angiotensin I, the type of enzymatic inhibitor used to block the conversion to angiotensin II, and the pH of the buffers (144,145).

Results obtained with different methodologies (expressed in mass/volume/time) are difficult to compare, and standardization procedures have been advocated (146). Blood must be collected using EDTA as anticoagulant and placed immediately on ice. A minimum of 2 ml of whole blood is advisable. After plasma separation in a refrigerated centrifuge, samples must be stored at $-20°C$, and assayed within 4 weeks (147). A variety of factors can interfere in the final results and must be taken in consideration: the sodium content of the diet; use of drugs as diuretics and beta blockers; and the patient position, since the upright posture increases renin secretion.

Acknowledgments. The authors wish to thank Dr. Edward G. Biglieri (the Clinical Study Center, San Francisco General Hospital, University of California at San Francisco) for granting permission to use data and figures on some of his patients with primary aldosteronism and to Ms. Sonia Kater for skillful elaboration of most of the figures.

Dr. Claudio E. Kater is an established investigator of CNP_q-Conselho Nacional de Desenvolvimento Cientifico e Tecnologico, Brazil, under contract 30.0449/81-CL07.

References

1. Biglieri EG, Kater CE. Disorders of the adrenal cortex. In: Stein JH, ed. *Internal Medicine*, 3rd ed. Boston; Little, Brown; 1990: 2188–2207.
2. Plotz CM, Knowlton AT, Ragan C. The natural history of Cushing's syndrome. *Am J Med* 1952;13:597–614.
3. David DS, Grieco MH, Cushman Jr P. Adrenal glucocorticoids after twenty years. A review of their clinical consequences. *J Chron Dis* 1970;22:637–711.
4. Richardson RL, Greco FA, Oldham RK, Liddle GW. Tumor products and potential markers in small cell lung cancer. *Semin Oncol* 1978;5:253–262.

5. Mason AMS, Ratcliff JB, Buckle RM, Mason AS. ACTH secretion by bronchial carcinoid tumors. *Clin Endocrinol (Oxf)* 1972;1:3–25.
6. Pimstone BL, Uys CJ, Vogelpoel L. Studies in a case of Cushing's syndrome due to an ACTH-producing thymic tumor. *Am J Med* 1972;53:521–528.
7. Cushing H. The basophil adenomas of the pituitary body and their clinical manifestations (pituitary basophilism). *Bull Johns Hopkins Hosp* 1932;50:137–195.
8. Krieger DT. Physiopathology of Cushing's disease. *Endocr Rev* 1983;4:22–43.
9. Schteingart DE, Lloyd RV, Akil H, et al. Cushing's syndrome secondary to ectopic corticotropin-releasing hormone-adrenocorticotropin secretion. *J Clin Endocrinol Metab* 1986;63:770–775.
10. Young Jr WF, Carney JA, Musa BU, Wulffraat NM, Lens JW, Drexhage HA. Familial Cushing's syndrome due to pigmented nodular adrenocortical disease. *N Engl J Med* 1989;321:1659–1664.
11. Streeten DHP, Anderson GH, Dalakos TG, et al. Normal and abnormal function of the hypothalamic-pituitary-adrenocortical system in man. *Endocr Rev* 1984;5:371–394.
12. Crapo L. Cushing's syndrome: a review of diagnostic tests. *Metabolism* 1979;28:955–977.
13. Vieira JGH, Russo EMK, Germek OA, Antunes LAN. A radioimmunoassay method for measurement of serum cortisol (Portuguese). *Rev Bras Patol Clin* 1979;15:125–130.
14. Pavlatos FC, Smilo RP, Forsham PH. A rapid screening test for Cushing's syndrome. *JAMA* 1965;193:720–723.
15. Nugent CA, Nichols T, Tyler FH. Diagnosis of Cushing's syndrome: single dose dexamethasone suppression test. *Arch Intern Med* 1965;116:172–176.
16. Vieira JGH, Accursio WJ, Russo EMK, Maciel RMB, Kater CE, Chacra AR. Usefulness of the rapid dexamethasone suppression in screening suspected patients with Cushing's syndrome (Portuguese). *Rev Assoc Med Brasil* 1985;31:129–132.
17. Aron DC, Tyrrell JB, Fitzgerald PA, Findling JW, Forsham PH. Cushing's syndrome: problems in diagnosis. *Medicine* 1981;60:25–35.
18. Liddle GW. Tests of pituitary-adrenal suppressibility in the diagnosis of Cushing's syndrome. *J Clin Endocrinol Metab* 1960;20:1539–1560.
19. Tyrrell JB, Findling JW, Aron DC, Fitzgerald PA, Forsham PH. An overnight high-dose dexamethasone suppression test for rapid differential diagnosis of Cushing's syndrome. *Ann Intern Med* 1986;104:180–186.
20. Conn JW. Presidential address: Part I. Painting background. Part II. Primary aldosteronism, a new clinical syndrome. *J Lab Clin Med* 1955;45:3–17.
21. Biglieri EG, Irony I, Kater CE. Adrenocortical forms of human hypertension. In: Laragh JH, Brenner BM, eds. *Hypertension: Pathophysiology, Diagnosis and Management.* New York: Raven Press; 1990:1609–1623.
22. Noth RH, Biglieri EG. Primary aldosteronism. *Med Clin North Am* 1988;72:1117–1131.
23. Young Jr WF, Klee GG. Primary aldosteronism: diagnostic evaluation. *Endocrinol Metab Clin North Am* 1988;17:367–395.
24. Arteaga E, Biglieri EG, Kater CE, Lopez JM, Schambelan M. Aldosterone-producing adrenocortical carcinoma: pre-operative recognition and course in three cases. *Ann Intern Med* 1984;101:316–321.
25. Farge D, Chatellier G, Pagny JY, Jeunemaitre X, Plouin PF, Corvol P. Isolated clinical syndrome of primary aldosteronism in four patients with adrenocortical carcinoma. *Am J Med* 1987;83:635–640.
26. Banks WA, Kastin AJ, Ruiz AE, Biglieri EG. Primary adrenal hyperplasia: a new subset of primary hyperaldosteronism. *J Clin Endocrinol Metab* 1984;58:783–785.
27. Biglieri EG, Kater CE, Arteaga E. Primary aldosteronism is comprised of primary adrenal hyperplasia and adenoma. *J Hypertens* 1984;2[suppl 3]:259–261.
28. Biglieri EG, Irony I, Kater CE. Identification and implications of new types of mineralocorticoid hypertension. *J Steroid Biochem* 1989;32(1B):199–204.
29. Gordon RD, Gomez-Sanchez CE, Hamlet SM, Tunny TJ, Klemm SA. Angiotensin-responsive aldosterone producing adenoma masquerades as idiopathic hyperaldosteronism or low renin essential hypertension. *J Hypertens* 1987;5(suppl 5):S103–S106.
30. Irony I, Kater CE, Biglieri EG, Shackleton CHL. Correctable subsets of primary aldosteronism: primary adrenal hyperplasia and renin responsive adenoma. *Am J Hypertens* 1990;3:576–582.
31. Jackson B, Valentine R, Wagner G. Primary aldosteronism due to a malignant ovarian tumor. *Aust NZ J Med* 1986;16:69–71.
32. Todesco S, Terribile V, Borsatti A, Mantero

F. Primary aldosteronism due to a malignant ovarian tumor. *J Clin Endocrinol Metab* 1975;41:809–819.

33. Kater CE, Biglieri EG. Adrenocortical disease and hypertension. In: Sleight P, Freis ED, eds. *Cardiology I. Hypertension.* London: Butterworth; 1982:135–152.

34. Kater CE, Biglieri EG. Diagnosing Cushing's syndrome and primary aldosteronism. An overview on the mechanisms involved in the pathogenesis of steroid-mediated hypertension. *Rev Hosp S Paulo-Esc Paul Med* 1989; 1:77–86.

35. Wenting GH, Man in't Veld AJ, Verhoecen RP, Derkx RP, Schalekamp MADH. Volume pressure relationships during development of mineralocorticoid hypertension in man. *Circ Res* 1977;40(suppl I):I163–I170.

36. Krakoff LR. Measurement of plasma renin substrate by radioimmunoassay of angiotensin. I: Concentration in syndromes associated with steroid excess. *J Clin Endocrinol Metab* 1973; 37:110–117.

37. Ferris JB, Beevers DG, Brown JJ, et al. Clinical, biochemical and pathological features of low-renin ("primary") hyperaldosteronism. *Am Heart J* 1978;95:375–388.

38. Biglieri EG, Kater CE. Mineralocorticoids. In: Greenspan FS, ed. *Basic and Clinical Endocrinology*, 3rd ed. Norwalk: Appleton & Lange; 1991:363–379.

39. Davies DL, Beevers DG, Brown JJ, et al. Aldosterone and its stimuli in normal and hypertensive man: are essential hypertension and primary hyperaldosteronism without tumor the same condition? *J Endocrinol* 1979; 81:79p–91p.

40. Biglieri EG, Slaton Jr PE, Schambelan M, Kronfield SJ. Hypermineralocorticoidism. *Am J Med* 1968;45:170–175.

41. Kater CE, Biglieri EG, Brust N, Chang B, Hirai J, Irony I. Stimulation and suppression of the mineralocorticoid hormones in normal subjects and adrenocortical disorders. *Endocr Rev* 1989;10:149–164.

42. Schambelan M, Brust NL, Chang BCF, Slater K, Biglieri EG. Circadian rhythm and effect of posture on plasma aldosterone concentration in primary aldosteronism. *J Clin Endocrinol Metab* 1976;43:115–131.

43. Ganguly A, Dowdy AJ, Luetscher JA, Melada GA. Anomalous postural response of plasma aldosterone concentration in patients with aldosterone-producing adrenal adenoma. *J Clin Endocrinol Metab* 1973;36:401–404.

44. Weinberger MH, Grim CE, Hollifield JW. Primary aldosteronism: diagnosis, localization, and treatment. *Ann Intern Med* 1979;90:386–395.

45. Aguilera G, Menard RH, Catt KJ. Regulatory actions of angiotensin II on receptors and steroidogenic enzymes in adrenal glomerulosa cells. *Endocrinology* 1980;107:55–60.

46. Brown RD, Wisgerhof M, Carpenter PC. Adrenal sensitivity to angiotensin II and undiscovered aldosterone-stimulating factors in hypertension. *J Steroid Biochem* 1979;11: 1043–1048.

47. Carey RM, Sen S, Dolan LM. Idiopathic hyperaldosteronism. *N Engl J Med* 1984; 311:94–100.

48. Wisgerhof M, Brown RD, Hogan MJ, Carpenter PC, Edis AJ. The plasma aldosterone response to angiotensin II infusion in aldosterone-producing adenoma and idiopathic hyperaldosteronism. *J Clin Endocrinol Metab* 1981;52:195–198.

49. Melby JC. Primary aldosteronism [clinical conference]. *Kidney Int* 1984;26:769–778.

50. Rodriguez JA, Lopez JM, Biglieri EG. DOCA test for aldosteronism: its usefulness and implications. *Hypertension* 1981;3(suppl II): II102–II105.

51. Arteaga E, Klein RF, Biglieri EG. Use of saline infusion test to diagnose the cause of primary aldosteronism. *Am J Med* 1985; 79:722–729.

52. Biglieri EG, Kater CE, Brust N, Chang B, Hirai J. The mineralocorticoid hormone pathways in hypertension with hyperaldosteronism. *Clin Exp Hypertens* 1982;A4(9–10):1677–1685.

53. Biglieri EG, Schambelan M. The significance of elevated levels of plasma 18-hydroxycorticosterone in patients with primary aldosteronism. *J Clin Endocrinol Metab* 1979;49: 87–92.

54. Kater CE, Biglieri EG, Rost CR, et al. The constant plasma 18-hydroxycorticosterone to aldosterone ratio: an expression of the efficacy of corticosterone methyloxidase type II activity in disorders with variable aldosterone production. *J Clin Endocrinol Metab* 1985;60:225–228.

55. Kem DC, Tang K, Hanson CS. The prediction of anatomical morphology of primary aldosteronism using serum 18-hydroxycorticosterone levels. *J Clin Endocrinol Metab* 1985;60:67–73.

56. Corvol P, Claire M, Oblin ME, Geering K,

Rossier B. Mechanisms of the antimineralo-corticoid effects of spironolactones. *Kidney Int* 1981;20:1–6.

57. Conn JW, Hinerman DL. Spironolactone-induced inhibition of aldosterone biosynthesis in primary aldosteronism: morphological and functional studies. *Metabolism* 1977;26:1293–1307.

58. Kater CE, Biglieri EG, Schambelan M, Arteaga E. Studies of impaired aldosterone response to spironolactone-induced renin and potassium elevations in adenomatous but not hyperplastic primary aldosteronism. *Hypertension* 1983;5(suppl V):V115–V121.

59. James VHT. Rippon RL, Jacobs HS. Plasma androgens in patients with hirsutism. In: James VHT, Serio M, Giusti G, eds. *The Endocrine Function of the Human Ovary*. London: Academic Press; 1976:457–470.

60. Abraham GE, Maroulis GB. Effect of dexamethasone on serum cortisol and androgen levels in hirsute patients. *Obstet Gynecol* 1976;47:395–402.

61. Freeman DA. Steroid hormone-producing tumors in man. *Endocr Rev* 1986;7:204–219.

62. Richie JP, Gittes RF. Carcinoma of the adrenal cortex. *Cancer* 1980;45:1957–1964.

63. Moraes CRS, Kater CE. Sequential analysis of the prolonged dexamethasone suppression test in hirsute patients (Portuguese). *Rev Assoc Med Brasil* 1988;34:184–189.

64. New M. Clinical and endocrinological aspects of 21-hydroxylase deficiency. *Ann NY Acad Sci* 1985;458:1–27.

65. Chung B-C, Matteson KJ, Morin JE, Mellon SH, Miller WL. An approach to the molecular biology of congenital adrenal hyperplasia. *Ann Ny Acad Sci* 1985;458:238–251.

66. Vieira JGH, Russo EMK, Maciel RMB, Germek OA, Verreschi ITN. Radioimmunoassay of serum 17-alpha-hydroxyprogesterone: methodological considerations (Portuguese). *Arq Bras Endocrinol Metab* 1980;24:24–30.

67. Costin G, Goebelsmann U, Kogut MD. Sexual precocity due to a testosterone-producing tumor. *J Clin Endocrinol Metab* 1977;45:912–919.

68. Kater CE, Czepielewski MA, Biglieri EG. Androgen-and estrogen-producing adrenocortical tumors causing hypertension. In: Biglieri EG, ed. *Endocrine Hypertension*. New York: Raven Press; 1990:195–206.

69. Roth LM, Anderson MC, Govan ADT, Langley FA, Gowing NFC, Woodcock AS. Sertoli-Leydig cell tumors: a clinicopathologic study of 34 cases. *Cancer* 1981;48:187–197.

70. Roth LM, Sternberg WH. Ovarian stromal tumors containing Leydig cells. II. Pure Leydig cell tumor, non-hilar type. *Cancer* 1973;32:952–960.

71. Boivin Y, Richart RM. Hilus cell tumors of the ovary. A review with a report of 3 new cases. *Cancer* 1965;18:231–240.

72. Abucham-Filho JZ, Albertotti C, Kater CE, Vieira JGH, Chacra AR. Computed tomography of the adrenals in the investigation of Cushing's syndrome (Portuguese). *Arq Bras Endocrinol Metab* 1983;27:145–148.

73. White EA, Schambelan M, Rost CR, Biglieri EG, Moss AA, Korobkin M. Use of computed tomography in diagnosing the cause of primary aldosteronism. *N Engl J Med* 1980;303:1503–1507.

74. Dunnick NR, Doppman JL, Gill Jr JR. Localization of functional adrenal tumors by computed tomography and venous sampling. *Radiology* 1982;142:429–433.

75. Reining JW, Doppman JL. Magnetic resonance imaging of the adrenal. *Radiologe* 1986;26:186–190.

76. Falke THM, teStrake L, Shaff MI. MR imaging of the adrenals: correlation with computed tomography. *J Comput Assist Tomogr* 1986;10:246–253.

77. Hogan MJ, McRae J, Schambelan M, Biglieri EG. Location of aldosterone-producing adenomas with I-19-iodocholesterol. *N Engl J Med* 1976;294:410–414.

78. Miles JM, Wahner HW, Carpenter PC. Adrenal scintiscanning with NP-59, a new radioiodinated cholesterol agent. *Mayo Clin Proc* 1979;54:321–327.

79. Geisinger MA, Zelch MG, Bravo EL. Primary hyperaldosteronism: comparison of CT, adrenal venography, and venous sampling. *AJR* 1983;141:299–302.

80. Espiner EA, Jameson JB, Perry EG. Adrenal venography and sampling in the diagnosis and treatment of primary aldosteronism. *N Z Med J* 1976;83:313–318.

81. Melby JC, Spark RF, Dale SL. Diagnosis and localization of aldosterone-producing adenomas by adrenal-vein catheterization. *N Engl J Med* 1967;277:1050–1056.

82. Moltz L, Pickartz H, Sorensen R, Schwartz U, Hammerstein J. Ovarian and adrenal vein steroids in seven patients with androgen-secreting ovarian neoplasms: selective catheterization findings. *Fertil Steril* 1984;42:585–593.

83. Findling JW, Aron DC, Tyrrell JB, et al.

Selective venous sampling for ACTH in Cushing's syndrome: differentiation between Cushing's disease and the ectopic ACTH syndrome. *Ann Intern Med* 1981;94:647–652.

84. West CD, Dolman LI. Plasma ACTH radioimmunoassay in the diagnosis of pituitary-adrenal dysfunction. *Ann NY Acad Sci* 1977; 28:205–210.

85. Raux MC, Binoux M, Luton JP, Gourmelen M, Girard F. Studies of ACTH secretion control in 116 cases of Cushing's syndrome. *J Clin Endocrinol Metab* 1975;40:186–197.

86. Krieger DT, Liotta AS, Li CH. Human plasma immunoreactive Beta-lipotropin: correlation with basal and stimulated plasma ACTH concentrations. *Life Sci* 1977;21:1771–1778.

87. Krieger DT, Liotta AS, Brownstein MJ, Zimmerman EA. ACTH, Beta-lipotropin and related peptides in brain, pituitary and blood. *Recent Prog Horm Res* 1980;36:277–344.

88. Yamaguchi H, Liotta AS, Krieger DT. Simultaneous determination of human plasma immunoreactive Beta-lipotropin, Gamma-lipotropin, and Beta-endorphin using immune-affinity chromatography. *J Clin Endocrinol Metab* 1980;51:1002–1008.

89. Strott CA, West CD, Nakagawa K, Kondo T, Tyler FH. Plasma 11-deoxycortisol and ACTH response to metyrapone (plasma metyrapone test). *J Clin Endocrinol Metab* 1969;29:6–11.

90. Spiger M, Jubitz W, Meikle AW, et al. Single-dose metyrapone test. *Arch Intern Med* 1975;135:698–700.

91. Vale W, Spiess J, Rivier C, Rivier J. Characterization of a 41-residue ovine hypothalamic peptide that stimulates secretion of corticotropin and Beta-endorphin. *Science* 1981; 213:1394–1397.

92. Boscaro M, Rampazzo A, Sonino N, Merola G, Scanarini M, Mantero F. Corticotropin releasing hormone stimulation test: diagnostic aspects in Cushing's syndrome. *J Endocrinol Invest* 1987;10:297–302.

93. Chrousos GP, Schulte HM, Oldfield EH, Gold PW, Cutler Jr GB, Loriaux DL. The corticotropin-releasing factor stimulation test. An aid in the evaluation of patients with Cushing's syndrome. *N Engl J Med* 1984; 310:622–626.

94. Croughs RJM. Use of lysin-vasopressin in the differential diagnosis of Cushing's syndrome. *Acta Endocrinol (Copenh)* 1970;65:595–607.

95. Toft H, Buus O, Nielsen E. Vasopressin in the diagnosic evaluation of pituitary and hypothalamic function. *Acta Endocrinol (Copenh)* 1971;67:393–400.

96. Service FJ, Nelson RL. Insulinoma. *Compr Ther* 1980;6:70–74.

97. Service FJ. Insulinoma. In: Service FJ, ed. *Hypoglycemic Disorders: Pathogenesis, Diagnosis and Treatment.* Boston: GK Hall; 1983: 111–124.

98. Stefanini P, Carboni M, Patrassi N, Basoli A. Beta-islet cell tumors of the pancreas: results of a study on 1,067 cases. *Surgery* 1974;75:597–609.

99. Brunt LM, Veldhuis JD, Dilley WG, et al. Stimulation of insulin secretion by a rapid intravenous calcium infusion in patients with beta-cell neoplasms of the pancreas. *J Clin Endocrinol Metab* 1986;62:210–216.

100. Fraker DL, Norton JA. Localization and resection of insulinomas and gastrinomas. *JAMA* 1988;259:3601–3605.

101. Kalio H, Suoranta H. Localization of occult insulin secreting tumors of the pancreas. *Ann Surg* 1979;189:49–52.

102. Berson SA, Yalow RS. Quantitative aspects of the reaction between insulin and insulin-binding antibody. *J Clin Invest* 1959;38:1996–2003.

103. Vieira JGH, Russo EMK, Germek OA, Chacra AR. Development of an heterologous radioimmunoassay for the measurement of serum human insulin (Portuguese). *Rev Bras Pat Clin* 1980;16:108–114.

104. Feldman JM, Chapman BA. Radioimmunoassay of insulin in serum and plasma. *Clin Chem* 1973;19:1250–1254.

105. Brodal BP. The influence of hemolysis on the radioimmunoassay of insulin. *Scand J Clin Lab Invest* 1971;28:287–290.

106. Turner RC, Lee ECG, Morris PJ, Harris EA. Localization of insulinomas. *Lancet* 1978;1: 515–518.

107. Zollinger RM, Ellison EH. Primary peptic ulcerations of the jejunum associated with islet cell tumors of the pancreas. *Ann Surg* 1955; 142:709–728.

108. Zollinger RM, Moore FT. Zollinger-Ellison syndrome comes to age. *JAMA* 1968;204:361–365.

109. Ellison EH, Wilson SD. The Zollinger-Ellison syndrome: reappraisal and evaluation of 260 registered cases. *Ann Surg* 1964;160:512–530.

110. Zollinger RM, Martin FW, Carey LC, et al. Observations on the postoperative tumor growth behavior of certain islet cell tumors. *Ann Surg* 1976;184:525–530.

111. McGuigan JE, Wolfe MM. The secretin injec-

tion test in the diagnosis of gastrinoma. *Gastroenterology* 1980;79:1324–1331.

112. Vogel SB, Wolfe MM, McGuigan SE, et al. Localization and resection of gastrinomas in Zollinger-Ellison syndrome. *Ann Surg* 1987; 205:550–556.

113. Burcharth F, Stage JF, Stadel F, et al. Localization of gastrinomas by transhepatic portal catheterization and gastrin assay. *Gastroenterology* 1979;77:444–450.

114. Roche A, Raissonier A, Gillon-Savonret M-C. Pancreatic venous sampling and arteriography in localizing insulinomas and gastrinomas: procedures and results in 55 cases. *Radiology* 1982;145:621–627.

115. Yalow RS, Berson SA. Radioimmunoassay of gastrin. *Gastroenterology* 1970;58:1–8.

116. McGravan MH, Unger RH, Recant L, et al. A glucagon-secreting alpha-cell carcinoma of the pancreas. *N Engl J Med* 1966;274:1408–1413.

117. Wood SM, Polak JM, Bloom SR. The glucagon syndrome. In: Lefevre PJ. ed. *Glucagon II.* New York: Springer-Verlag; 1983:411–430.

118. Unger RH, Eisentraut AM, McCall MS, Keller S, Lanz HC, Madison LL. Glucagon antibodies and their use for immunoassay of glucagon. *Proc Soc Exp Biol Med* 1959;102: 621–623.

119. Heath H III, Hodgson SF, Kennedy MA. Primary hyperparathyroidism. Incidence, morbidity, and potential economic impact in a community. *N Engl J Med* 1980;302:189–193.

120. Mundy GR, Cove DH, Fisken R. Primary hyperparathyroidism: changes in the pattern of clinical presentation. *Lancet* 1980;1:1317–1320.

121. Hodgson SF, Heath H III. Asymptomatic primary hyperparathyroidism: treat or follow? (Editorial). *Mayo Clin Proc* 1981;56:521–522.

122. Scholz DA, Purnell DC. Asymptomatic primary hyperparathyroidism. 10-year prospective study. *Mayo Clin Proc* 1981;56:473–478.

123. Bilezikian JP. Surgery or no surgery for hyperparathyroidism (Editorial). *Ann Intern Med* 1985;102:402–403.

124. Bowers GN, Brassard C, Sena SF. Measurement of ionized calcium in serum with ion-selective electrodes: a mature technology that can meet the daily service needs. *Clin Chem* 1986;32:1437–1447.

125. Heath DA. Familial benign hypercalcemia. *Trends Endocrinol Metab* 1989;1:6–9.

126. Steward AF, Horst R, Deftos LJ, Cadman EC, Lang R, Broadus AE. Biochemical evaluation of patients with cancer-associated hypercalce-

mia: evidence for humoral and non-humoral groups. *N Engl J Med* 1980;303:1377–1383.

127. Levin KE, Clark OH. Localization of parathyroid glands. *Annu Rev Med* 1988;39:29–40.

128. Winzelberg GG, Hydovitz JD, O'Hara KR et al. Parathyroid adenomas evaluated by Tl-201/ Tc99m pertechnetate subtraction scintigraphy and high-resolution ultrasonography. *Radiology* 1985;155:231–235.

129. Potts Jr JT, Tregear GW, Keutmann HT, et al. Synthesis of a biological active N-terminal tetratriancontapeptide of parathyroid hormone. *Proc Natl Acad Sci USA* 1971;68:63–67.

130. Mayer GP, Keaton JA, Hurst JG, Habener JF. Effect of plasma calcium concentration on the relative proportion of hormone and carboxyl fragments in parathyroid venous blood. *Endocrinology* 1979;104:1778–1784.

131. Brandao CMA, Kasamatsu TS, Oliveira MAD, Vieira JGH. Circulating molecular forms of parathyroid hormone in primary and secondary hyperparathyroidism. *Braz J Med Biol Res* 1989;22:963–965.

132. Martin KJ, Hruska KA, Lewis J, Anderson C, Slatopolsky E. The renal handling of parathyroid hormone: role of peritubular uptake and glomerular filtration. *J Clin Invest* 1977;60: 808–814.

133. Berson SA, Yalow RS, Aurbach GD, Potts Jr JT. Immunoassay of bovine and human parathyroid hormone. *Proc Natl Acad Sci USA* 1963;49:513–516.

134. Lufkin EG, Kao PC, Heath III H. Parathyroid hormone radioimmunoassay in the differential diagnosis of hypercalcemia due to primary hyperparathyroidism or malignancy. *Ann Intern Med* 1987;106:559–560.

135. Desplan C, Jullienne A, Moukhtar MS, Milhaud G. Sensitive assay for biological active fragment of human parathyroid hormone. *Lancet* 1977;2:198–199.

136. Vieira JGH, Oliveira MAD, Maciel RMB, Mesquita CH, Russo EMK. Development of an homologous radioimmunoassay for the synthetic amino terminal (1–34) fragment of human parathyroid hormone using egg yolk-obtained antibodies. *J Immunoassay* 1986; 7:57–72.

137. Nussbaum SR, Zahradnik RJ, Lavigne JR, et al. Highly sensitive two-site immunoradiometric assay of parathyrin and its clinical utility in evaluating patients with hypercalcemia. *Clin Chem* 1987;33:1364–1367.

138. Blind E, Schmidt-Gaik H, Armbruster FP, Stadler A. Measurement of intact human para-

thyrin by an extracting two-site immunor-adiometric assay. *Clin Chem* 1987;33:1376–1381.

139. Dunlop DAB, Papapoulos SE, Lodge RW, Fulton AJ, Kendall BE, O'Riordan JLH. Parathyroid venous sampling: anatomic considerations and results in 95 patients with primary hyperparathyroidism. *Br J Radiol* 1980;53:183–191.

140. Pickering TC. Renovascular hypertension. Medical evaluation and nonsurgical treatment. In: Laragh JH, Brenner BM, eds. *Hypertension. Pathophysiology, Diagnosis, and Management*. New York: Raven Press; 1990:1539–1559.

141. Corvol P, Pinet F, Galen FX, et al. Primary reninism. In: Laragh JH, Brenner BM, eds. *Hypertension. Pathophysiology, Diagnosis, and Management*. New York: Raven Press; 1990: 1573–1582.

142. Haber E. The renin-angiotensin system and hypertension. *Kidney Int* 1979;15:427–444.

143. Haber E, Koerner T, Page LB, et al. Application of an angiotensin I radioimmunoassay to the physiologic measurements of plasma renin activity in normal human subjects. *J Clin Endocrinol Metab* 1969;29:1349–1352.

144. Oparil S, Koerner TJ, Haber E. Effects of pH and enzyme inhibitors on apparent generation of angiotensin I in human plasma. *J Clin Endocrinol Metab* 1974;39:965–968.

145. Vieira JGH, Noguti KO, Russo EMK, Maciel RMB. Radioimmunoassay for the measurement of plasma renin activity: technical aspects (Portuguese). *Rev Bras Pat Clin* 1981;17:195–200.

146. Bangham DR, Robertson JIS. Standardization for renin assay. *Lancet* 1976;1:1181.

147. Matsunaga M, Suzuki Y, Nakagawa K, et al. Reexamination of the conditions for processing and storing of blood for plasma renin assay. *Clin Chim Acta* 1986;154:213–218.

Index